CHRONIC ILLNESS, SPIRITUALITY, AND HEALING

CHRONIC ILLNESS, SPIRITUALITY, AND HEALING

DIVERSE DISCIPLINARY, RELIGIOUS, AND CULTURAL PERSPECTIVES

Edited by Michael J. Stoltzfus, Rebecca Green, and Darla Schumm

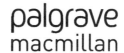

CHRONIC ILLNESS, SPIRITUALITY, AND HEALING
Copyright © Michael J. Stoltzfus, Rebecca Green, and Darla Schumm,
2013.

First published in 2013 by
PALGRAVE MACMILLAN®
in the United States—a division of St. Martin's Press LLC,
175 Fifth Avenue, New York, NY 10010.

Where this book is distributed in the UK, Europe and the rest of the World,
this is by Palgrave Macmillan, a division of Macmillan Publishers Limited,
registered in England, company number 785998, of Houndmills,
Basingstoke, Hampshire RG21 6XS.

Palgrave Macmillan is the global academic imprint of the above
companies and has companies and representatives throughout the world.

Palgrave® and Macmillan® are registered trademarks in the United
States, the United Kingdom, Europe and other countries.

ISBN: 978–1–137–35136–4

Library of Congress Cataloging-in-Publication Data

Chronic illness, spirituality, and healing : diverse disciplinary, religious,
    and cultural perspectives / edited by
    Michael J. Stoltzfus, Rebecca Green and Darla Schumm.
      pages cm
    Includes bibliographical references.
    ISBN 978–1–137–35136–4 (hardcover : alk. paper) 1. Chronically
    ill—Religious life.   2. Chronic diseases—Religious aspects—
    Christianity.   3. Healing—Religious aspects—Christianity.   4. Spiritual
    healing.   I. Stoltzfus, Michael J., 1965– editor of compilation.
    BV4910.C48 2013
    201'.661—dc23   2013011572

A catalogue record of the book is available from the British Library.

Design by Integra Software Services

First edition: September 2013

10 9 8 7 6 5 4 3 2 1

We dedicate this volume to people who live with chronic illness; and to those who are in relationships with people who have chronic illness, whether as friends, partners, spouses, children, parents, or providers of care

CONTENTS

NOTES ON CONTRIBUTORS

Akinmayowa Akin-Otiko is a researcher in the area of African belief systems with particular interest in Yoruba traditional medicine. He teaches African philosophy at the Dominican Institute, Ibadan Nigeria. He has a BA and an MA in Philosophy and is about to defend his PhD thesis in African belief system, at the Institute of African Studies, University of Ibadan, Nigeria.

Paula Arai, author of *Women Living Zen: Japanese Buddhist Nuns* (Oxford University Press, 1999) and *Bringing Zen Home: The Healing Heart of Japanese Buddhist Women's Rituals* (University of Hawaii Press, 2011), received her PhD in Buddhist studies from Harvard University under the mentorship of Masatoshi Nagatomi. She has also published her groundbreaking research on monastic and lay Japanese Buddhist women in numerous journal articles and chapters in edited volumes, and presented widely at national and international venues. Her research has received the generous support of two Fulbright Fellowships. She is currently an associate professor of Buddhist Studies at Louisiana State University and vice-president of Sakyadhita International Association of Buddhist Women.

Kelly Arora, BS, MA, PhD: Dr. Arora lives in the Denver area where she is an adjunct faculty member at the Regis University School of Pharmacy and the Iliff School of Theology. She teaches courses on religion/spirituality and health, intercultural spiritual care, ethics, world religions, and spiritual formation. Kelly also maintains a private practice in spiritual direction and is an active member of the Spiritual Directors International Spirituality and Health Care Initiative.

Delia Birle, PhD, is a licensed psychologist and a lecturer in experimental psychology and psychological statistics at the University of Oradea in Romania. Her research interests that translated into books, numerous articles, and conference presentations include: psychological counseling, gender studies, school psychology, and moral reasoning.

Noel Boyle is an associate professor of Philosophy at Belmont University in Nashville, TN. He holds a PhD in Philosophy from Michigan State University, where he specialized in the philosophy of mind and the philosophy of science. His scholarly work has focused on philosophical issues related to the emerging science of conscious experience. His intellectual passions also include the nature and purpose of liberal education, as well as ancient Greek history, culture, and philosophy.

Nancy J. Burke, PhD, is an associate professor of Medical Anthropology at the University of California, San Francisco. Her research interests include bioethics and clinical trials, technologies of cancer care and therapeutic subjectivity, and social inequalities in cancer treatment and survivorship. She has collaborated on community-based-participatory research in the Filipino community of San Francisco for over six years.

Danielle Rose Costello is a graduate student in Applied Sociology at Valdosta State University. She studies in philosophy and sociology with an emphasis on traditional food-ways, the food industry, agribusiness, and sustainable agriculture. As the vice-president of VSU Blazer Gardens, she has worked to teach her community about contemporary food issues by establishing gardens and teaching sustainable gardening techniques. Most recently she has worked as both a research assistant and indexer for Dr. Lavonna Lovern and Dr. Carol Locust on their book *Native American Communities on Health and Disability*.

Rebecca Green, RN, DNS, is an assistant professor of Nursing at Valdosta State University in Valdosta, Georgia. Her practice specialty is in Community Health Nursing, School Health, and Vulnerable Populations; and her current research focuses on how health-care culture impacts relationships between patients and providers. She has published in the areas of school health, public health, and qualitative inquiry. She has been both a care provider for patients with chronic illness and a receiver of care as a patient with chronic autoimmune dysfunction.

Amy Holte, PhD, MEd, is a research fellow and senior MBSR Teacher at the UCSD Centers for Mindfulness and Integrative Medicine. She teaches meditation, yoga-, and mindfulness-based programs to the general public, patients suffering from a range of conditions, and health-care and education professionals. Her research interests include the spiritual, therapeutic, and healing processes of contemplative traditions; the shifting epistemological grounds of psychology and integrative medicine; conceptual intersections between medicine, neuroscience, and the body; and embodied cognition.

Christine A. James is a professor of Philosophy and Religious Studies at Valdosta State University. She has published a variety of articles and book chapters in scholarly journals such as the *Journal for Philosophical Practice, The Journal for the Study of Religions and Ideologies, The International Journal of Sociology and Social Policy, Essays in Philosophy, The Southwest Philosophy Review, The Journal of Consciousness Studies, Biosemotics, Empedocles: The European Journal for Philosophy of Communication*, and the *Journal for Human Rights*. She has presented her research at conferences throughout the United States, Canada, Austria, Spain, the Netherlands, and the United Kingdom.

Ruth Krall is an Emeritus Professor of Religion, Psychology, and Nursing and Director Emerita of the Peace, Justice, and Conflict Studies Program at Goshen College. She holds degrees in psychiatric-community mental health nursing as well as a doctorate in theology and personality. Dr. Krall is certified as a Guided Imagery facilitator and a Labyrinth facilitator. In 1991 Ruth was diagnosed as having progressive, bi-lateral macular degeneration. In 1995 she was diagnosed with endometrial cancer.

Lavonna L. Lovern is an assistant professor of Philosophy and Religious Studies at Valdosta State University and a founding member in the Native American Studies program at VSU. She has also been appointed to the Florida America Indian Health Advisory Council, where she serves as secretary. Dr. Lovern and Dr. Locust have consulted and conducted seminars on wellness and recently contracted for a book titled *Native American Communities on Health and Disability: A Borderland Dialogue* (2013). Recent publications, involving Indigenous issues in health care and education, include chapters in *Disability and Religious Diversity* (2011) and the *Journal of Qualitative Studies* (2012).

Paul J. Mills, PhD, is a professor of Psychiatry in the Behavioral Medicine Program at the University of California, San Diego (UCSD), Director of the UCSD Clinical Research Biomarker Laboratory, and Co-Director of UCSD Clinical and Translational Research Institute's Translational Research Technologies Division. He is a longstanding NIH-supported clinical investigator with expertise in cardiovascular and sleep physiology, as well as psychoneuroimmune processes in human wellness and disease. His research and teaching efforts include complementary and alternative medicine modalities. He has published over 285 manuscripts and book chapters on these topics. He is an active faculty member in the Behavioral Medicine track of the San Diego State University (SDSU)/UCSD Joint Doctoral Program in Clinical Psychology, and the Health Behavior track of the SDSU/UCSD Joint Doctoral Program in Public Health.

Paul Negrut, PhD (Theology), PhD (Political Science), is a university professor in ethics and counseling at Emanuel University of Oradea, recognized teacher at Queen's University of Belfast, Northern Ireland, PhD program. He is also a licensed clinical psychologist. He has published articles and books in the field of religion, psychology, and the relations between religions and social issues.

Serban Olah, PhD, is an associate professor in sociology at the University of Oradea, Department of Sociology, Social Work and Philosophy, where he teaches Organizational Behavior, Political Sociology, Economic Sociology, and Social Policy. He published articles and books on topics related to: the political and economic elite, the social problems of Roma communities, poverty, quality of life, religious beliefs, and urban transformation.

Salomea Popoviciu, PhD, is a university lecturer in social work, professional ethics, social psychology, and family social work at the Social Work Department at University of Emanuel, Oradea. She has published articles and books on topics related to: family studies, child protection, professional ethics, prejudice and stereotyping, quality of life, spirituality, religious beliefs, and perceptions and experiences of illness.

Ioan Popoviciu, PhD, is a licensed education psychologist and an associate professor in sociology and social research at the Emanuel University of Oradea. He is involved in research related to quality of life, poverty, social entrepreneurship, and educating life-abilities and mental toughness in teens and young adults.

Ruth Stanley, OSB, PharmD, MA, FASHP: Dr. Stanley is a Benedictine sister at St. Benedict's Monastery and director of Holistic Services for the CentraCare Heart and Vascular Center in St. Cloud, MN. She has 30 years of clinical, academic, administrative, and consulting experience in health care and over 25 years of spiritual ministry and holistic practice experience. She holds a doctorate in Pharmacy with postdoctorate clinical residency training and a Masters in Spirituality. Dr. Stanley is certified in formation, spiritual direction, and retreat work as well as numerous holistic healing practices.

Michael J. Stoltzfus is a professor of Religious Studies at Valdosta State University in Valdosta, Georgia. In addition to numerous articles, he is co-editor and contributor to *Disability in Judaism, Christianity, and Islam: Sacred Texts, Historical Traditions, and Social Analysis* and *Disability and Religious Diversity: Cross-Cultural and Interreligious Perspectives* (Palgrave, 2011). He teaches in the areas of religious ethics, religious pluralism and dialogue, religion and culture, world religions, and spirituality and health. His PhD in religion, ethics, and society is from Vanderbilt University.

Ofelia O. Villero is an independent religious studies scholar with a PhD from the Graduate Theological Union. She worked as a community-based participatory researcher at the Helen Diller Family Comprehensive Cancer Center, University of California, San Francisco, for five years. She was also a postdoctoral fellow at the Department of Anthropology, History and Social Medicine, UCSF, for one year.

ACKNOWLEDGMENTS

Most of what we do would not be possible without the love and support of our families, who provide daily inspiration and encouragement and receive our deep gratitude for sustaining us from the beginning to the end of the project.

We would like to thank Editor Burke Gerstenschlager and Assistant Editor Lani Oshimi, who deftly guided us through the process of preparing this manuscript for publication. We are grateful to the editorial board of Palgrave Macmillan for their willingness to bring issues of spirituality and chronic illness to the forefront and publish this book.

We thank Elizabeth Smoak for her help with the editing process. Her attention to detail with initial formatting and editing of submissions was invaluable.

We would most like to acknowledge the support of our institutions, Valdosta State University and Hollins University, in the scholarly efforts necessary to produce work such as this. Creating the time and space for scholarship in a climate that increasingly demands quantifiable indicators of faculty productivity requires a leap of faith for deans and department heads who must justify how faculty time and institutional dollars are being spent. We are happy to be able to offer a tangible, objective measure to justify the hours and dollars spent; but the true justification of this project lies in its potential to transform the lives of those who encounter chronic illness, in immeasurable ways. So we thank our institutions for continuing to make room for scholarly pursuit; and we thank those administrators who continue to advocate for support of scholarship as crucial to maintaining a rich academic milieu in which students and faculty will thrive.

INTRODUCTION

Michael J. Stoltzfus and Rebecca Green

This book presents a unique collection of chapters examining the relationship among chronic illness, spirituality, and healing from interdisciplinary, multicultural, and interreligious perspectives. Contributors to this volume include medical anthropologists, physicians, nurses, psychiatrists, and pharmacologists working in holistic and integrative health care settings, as well as religious studies scholars and spiritual practitioners from diverse religious and cultural contexts. The authors consider how biomedical care might be balanced by spiritual practice that attends to the unique, long-term dimensions associated with chronic illness experiences. The chapters survey the historical and contemporary connections between spirituality and coping with chronic conditions in terms of both mental and physical health through the mind–body–spirit–environment relationship. The chapters explore the direct relationship between spirituality and healing, covering such topics as the role of yoga, meditation, mindfulness, chanting, prayer, music, and a host of distinctive rituals in cultivating well-being in the lives of people living with autoimmune disease, mental illness, addictive illness, cancer, heart disease, diabetes, pain, and other chronic conditions. Religious perspectives integrated into the book include Catholic, Protestant, and Eastern-Orthodox Christian analysis; Buddhism, Hinduism, and Taoism; Filipino, Native American, and African Indigenous traditions; and Goddess-centered practices. The research included in this volume originates from diverse contexts in the United States, Japan, Romania, Australia, Nigeria, and elsewhere.

The three editors represent divergent disciplinary specialties. Two editors are religious studies professors, and the other is a practicing nurse and nursing professor. We made a concerted effort in our call to reach a broad and diverse range of not only scholars and practitioners, but lay people, as well. In addition to the more traditional scholarly call avenues, we made contact via listserv and blogs for chaplains, counselors, addiction recovery specialists, and chronic illness support groups. We asked contributors to focus on the following.

- Augmenting biomedical care with spiritual care from diverse religious and cultural perspectives.

- The role of diverse spiritual insights in understanding and practicing integrated health and well-being.
- The meaning of physical, moral, and spiritual cultivation; healing; renewal; and vitality when an illness is persistent and cure is unlikely.
- Holistic components of well-being and health care that focus upon the relationships among mind, body, spirituality, environment, and making meaning of suffering and loss.
- Exploring the relationship between spiritual practice and the ability to cope with chronic illness.
- Reflections on the theme of invisibility (often associated with chronic illness) in relationship to religious/spiritual understanding and practice.
- Chronic illness as bodily betrayal and the subsequent efforts to find harmony among body, self, and the world.

The contributors employed a wide variety of methodological and practical approaches including ethnography, historical, or cultural analysis; case studies; personal narrative; qualitative and quantitative analysis of clinical and therapeutic encounters; and theological/philosophical reflection and analysis. The authors incorporated into their work literary and theoretical perspectives both from a wide variety of spiritual/religious traditions and from diverse academic and practice disciplines such as sociology, nursing, medicine, disability studies, religious studies, psychology, anthropology, and feminist studies. Scholars from multiple religious traditions and health care professionals working in holistic and integrative clinical settings speak for themselves in their chapter contribution(s); they were not asked to structure their descriptions and analyses into any preordained methodological framework. In addition, two of the editors and multiple contributors approached their thinking and writing from the perspective of lived experience with some form of chronic illness, creating a dynamic of availability to the millions of people living with similar conditions in the United States and around the world.

SPIRITUALITY, CHRONIC ILLNESS, AND HEALING: MAKING THE CONNECTIONS

Spirituality, chronic illness, and healing are all terms that reflect flexibility rather than control, described most often in subjective, experiential ways rather than categorically. No single method or discipline can appropriate these terms, their expressions, or their unique manifestations in particular individual, cultural, or religious voice. Spirituality in the context of chronic illness and healing seeks a broadening of the conversation, expansive enough to incorporate cross-cultural, inter-religious, and trans-disciplinary contexts.

Spirituality can be broadly described as a way of embodied dwelling in a web of changing social and cultural meanings, a lived experience rooted in a holistic availability to learn and grow, to create meaning and purpose, from the dynamic relationship among spirit, body, mind, environment, other people, and multiple sources of transcendence. "Spirit" derives from the

Latin world *spiritus*, which, like its counterparts in Greek (*pneuma*), Hebrew (*ruach*), and *Chinese* (*qi*), means at once breath, wind, spirit, and vital energy (McColman, 1997, pp. 7–10; Kohn, 2007). Breath and breathing are always present with lived experience. Similarly, living with chronic illness, like breathing, is a perpetual part of a person's lived experience, a normal part of the ever-changing rhythm of life. Linking spiritual expression with chronic illness experience requires a multidimensional approach to the art of living in the midst of joy and pain, suffering and healing, disease and health, isolation and unification, religion and culture, hope and dismay, medicine and family.

Chronic illness encompasses a wide variety of conditions including, but not limited to, cancer, rheumatoid arthritis, heart disease, lupus, pain, diabetes, depression, addiction, multiple sclerosis, muscular dystrophy, Crohn's disease, HIV, and others that have physical, mental, emotional, spiritual, relational, vocational, and economic implications. Generally, chronic illness can be described as "a lifelong process of adapting to significant physical, psychological, social, and environmental changes" as a result of illness (Bishop, 2005, p. 219). In 2005, 133 million Americans had a chronic illness; such illnesses are the leading cause of death and disability in the United States (Centers for Disease Control and Prevention, 2009). Due to the unpredictable nature of many chronic illnesses, individuals with chronic conditions, along with their family, friends, and health care professionals are confronted with a challenge to cultivate meaning and healing in the midst of ongoing, long-term illness, pain, suffering, adaptation, and transformation. Faced with all of these uncertainties and complexities, individuals are often forced to question many of their taken-for-granted assumptions and reassess their lives from a new perspective (Bishop, 2005; Charmaz, 1991 & 1995; Garrett, 2002; Gockel, 2009; Kleinman, 1988; Wendell, 2001; Wills, 2007).

For example, most people with chronic illnesses do not fit into, and therefore must question, the dominant acute care model evident in the history of Western medical care and education. The acute care model of illness primarily attends to physical manifestation of the disease in an individual patient and associates health and well-being with eradication of the disease state. Acute care approaches to disease or pain stress a restitution narrative focusing on diagnosis, treatment, and cure (Longmore & Umansky, 2001; Garland-Thompson, 1994). In this model, disease is the enemy to be banished from an individual body by whatever technological or pharmacological means available; self-identity is viewed as existing independently of the experience of illness; and healing is associated with living without the presence of disease. For the chronically ill, disease is an intrinsic element of being alive, a permanent feature of living where people must learn to integrate their illness constructively into their sense of personal, social, medical, and spiritual self-identity. For people living with a chronic illness, the ongoing task is holistic healing rather than curing a specific individual disease state in many cases. This task requires an explicit focus on the human experience of illness in all its multifaceted dynamics and the corresponding flexibility in coping responses, and learning to live well in the presence, rather than the absence, of physical or mental incapacity, recognizing vulnerability as a way of life.

Trans-disciplinary research is making it increasingly clear that many people turn to spiritual and/or religious resources to begin to understand and grapple with illness, suffering, and healing. Surveys suggest that between 70 and 90 percent of people with serious mental or physical health problems in the United States cite religion and spirituality as important means of coping (Koenig et al., 2012; Gockel, 2009; Nichols & Hunt, 2011). Often considered as part of complementary and alternative medicine (CAM), spirituality tends to remain on the fringes of biomedical health care and health scholarship.

The spiritual healing movement, in its many forms, is part of a cultural milieu in which alternative care of myriad types has been proliferating both in terms of quantity and in terms of variety. There is a gradually growing awareness of the inability of biomedicine to cure many chronic diseases, which has contributed to the search for other sorts of healing responses for individuals living with chronic pain, depression, addiction, fatigue, and so on. Holistic healing venues tend to be populated with people living with chronic rather than acute illnesses (Thompson, 2003). People living long term with cancer, AIDS, diabetes, multiple sclerosis, rheumatoid arthritis, or those who serve as the primary caregiver of a family member living with Alzheimer's or mental illness, seek healing and support in the midst of ongoing challenge.

Spirituality and healing are beyond cognitive confinement or categorical definition, and this constitutes their difficulty as a scientific field of inquiry. The experience of spirituality and healing arise through the emergence of novelty and dynamic balance that cannot be captured by objective definitions or abstract models. Nevertheless, researchers in health-care settings increasingly are taking spiritual practices more seriously. In fact, health-care researchers have been investigating spiritual practices like prayer or meditation for efficacy in pain management, recovery time from surgery, and control of chronic conditions for some time and with positive results (Koenig et al., 2012). The area within health-care research that has been most receptive to exploring spiritual practices is the growing field of mind–body medicine. One of the most well documented results of mind–body research is the recognition, long endorsed by diverse spiritual traditions, that how individuals conceptualize and label an illness is predictive of measurable individual health outcomes. However, this type of research is largely based on an acute-model of care in which the efficacy of spiritual practices are measured for quantifiable outcomes in terms of the conventional unit of health-care research, individual bodies, and their physical symptoms.

One of the positions asserted throughout this volume is that spirituality and healing, in the context of chronic illness, always situates the integrated mind/body/spirit in relational contexts that are wider and denser than the individual; that incorporate the interconnections of culture and environment. In experiencing chronic illness, people encounter deep questions of meaning and purpose, medical and religious models that may not fit their experiences, and multiple issues that move beyond measurable and quantifiable physical symptoms. Neither spiritual flourishing nor human healing should be defined exclusively in terms of some ideal standard of individual physical or medical well-being, an ideal that is impossible for many people to attain.

Emerging trends in the tripartite connection between spirituality, healing, and living with chronic illness raise the issue of how to realize a meaningful life as a whole person in a multidimensional personal, medical, social, cultural, and spiritual context. This type of an approach to spirituality and healing, rooted in a willingness to live with flexibility, uncertainty, vulnerability, and without idealistic expectations for cure, can help to transform everybody, from individuals living with chronic illnesses to those with narrow cultural, medical, or religious approaches to health, well-being, and human community. It requires recognition that the concept of "normal" is often a barrier to overcome rather than an outcome to be achieved. This recognition must occur not only for people living with chronic conditions, but also for health-care providers. If spirituality situates people in relational contexts that are wider and denser than the individual, then concepts of spirituality can also be used practically to inform patient care in a variety of ways, and health care can be seen as an avenue for spiritual transformation for both patients and providers.

ORGANIZATIONAL FORMAT AND DIVISIONS

Due to the diversity of disciplinary, spiritual, cultural, methodological, and illness components presented in this book, organizing a coherent and seamless presentation of chapters and topics is challenging. A trans-disciplinary, interreligious, and cross-cultural investigation of the relationship between chronic illness and spiritual practice incorporates paradox, ambiguity, and even inconsistency as a core component of the presentation. Learning to live with and discover balance in the midst of tension, harmony in the midst of difference, is an inevitable component of integrating diverse practical disciplines and academic fields into a single volume. While we have tried to organize the divergent body of work presented here in some orderly fashion, we are left more in hope than certainty that the chapters are both cohesive and fluid.

The book is loosely divided into two parts: (1) Chronic Illness and Healing: Blending Biomedical Care with Spiritual Practice and (2) Chronic Illness: Inter-Religious, Cross-Cultural, and Narrative Perspectives. Contributors include physicians, psychiatrists, pharmacologists, medical anthropologists, and nurses, as well as religious studies scholars and spiritual practitioners from diverse religious and cultural contexts. The first part is authored or co-authored primarily by people from health care disciplines while the second part is authored or co-authored primarily by religious studies scholars and spiritual practitioners, though many are cross-disciplinary practitioners. It is important to note that while each chapter is distinctive and stands on its own as an academic, creative, and literary work, spirituality, chronic illness, and healing are the core themes that navigate broad topics running throughout each chapter and between parts. The collection of chapters as a whole offers a comparative exploration of the intersections between spirituality and chronic illness, gives voice to scholars and practitioners of many of the world's rich and varied religious traditions, actively engages multiple fields of health care, and reflects multicultural and inter-religious attitudes and perspectives.

CHRONIC ILLNESS AND HEALING: BLENDING BIOMEDICAL CARE WITH SPIRITUAL PRACTICE

Mike Stoltzfus and Rebecca Green open Part I by describing some of the unique challenges and opportunities affiliated with integrating the concepts of spirituality, chronic illness, and healing in everyday life, and offer specific implications for a more holistic approach for practical health-care disciplines. Stoltzfus and Green attempt to synthesize some of the diverse disciplinary, religious, and illness components of the book by providing sections that describe and loosely define spirituality, chronic illness, the role of spirituality in coping and healing, and implications for practical disciplines like health care. The basic questions that structure the presentation are the following: What are some of the differences between chronic illness and acute illness and between being diagnosed with a disease and the lived experience of illness? How are religion and spirituality similar and different? How can individuals living with long-term, chronic physical and/or emotional illness respond creatively and meaningfully to a vulnerable and wounded body/mind/spirit? What ideas, attitudes, and values do we find in our culture, society, and spiritual traditions that help or hinder people in this task? How can people address the anger, fear, vulnerability, uncertainty, and longing for a cure that neither biomedicine nor religion can manifest for many forms of chronic illness? How can loved ones and clinical providers who interact with them respond in ways that promote spiritual solace and healing when physical cure is unlikely?

In Chapter 2, Kelly Arora investigates how women with autoimmune diseases often experience psycho-spiritual struggles related to meaning making about their illness experiences and their relationships with the holy or the sacred. Arora demonstrates how psycho-spiritual struggles may result in transformative personal growth, but they can also become chronic struggles that negatively affect health and well-being. Medical, psychotherapeutic, and other spiritual caregiving approaches may not adequately address the unique psycho-spiritual care needs of women with autoimmune diseases. Spiritual direction, grounded in an intercultural approach of not-knowing, offers a long-term relationship in which caregivers and women with autoimmune conditions can co-construct and embody narrative and ritual practices to help women make meaning, lament and acknowledge losses, and enact life-enhancing coping strategies and spiritual practices. Arora uses a poignant case study about a woman who has lupus to illustrate how this care-giving approach might work.

In Chapter 3, Ofelia O. Villero and Nancy J. Burke analyze the findings of a four-year ethnographic inquiry into Filipina transnational workers with experience of breast cancer in the San Francisco Bay area. Hired to work in low-paying, labor-intensive jobs, without health insurance and other safety net, and lacking the language skills necessary to navigate complex cultural and biomedical systems, Filipina transnationals with breast cancer turned to a Filipino spiritual tradition rooted in the indigenous idea of subjectivity (*loób*) and Christian religiosity to frame and manage their illness. Study participants pursued a spiritual track parallel and simultaneous with their biomedical path of cancer treatment. Through spiritual practices that gave them "inner strength," the women were able to overcome fears and anxieties that heightened despair and isolation and served as practical barriers to health-care access and treatment. Villero and Burke demonstrate how spirituality allowed these women to forge a subjectivity separate from their biomedical identity as chronically diseased individuals. From their perspective, they were women who "passed through" (*nalampasan*) tremendous hardships, of which breast cancer was but one, to become whole again.

In Chapter 4, Ruth Stanley connects chronic illness with autonomic nervous system (ANS) dysfunction and demonstrates how ancient spiritual healing practices from diverse traditions share a common pathophysiologic mechanism to modify and restore ANS function, thereby improving quality of life and reducing rates of morbidity and mortality. Four practices have been handed down through the ages as practical and effective means of improving physical, mental, emotional, and spiritual aspects of chronic illness: breathing, simple movements, emotional refocus, and awareness practices. These are remarkably effective means of optimizing the overall well-being in the midst of chronic illness. Stanley explores these four spiritual practices and the basis for their unique effectiveness in chronic illness. The topics include ANS pathophysiology as the gatekeeper of health and well-being; measuring and modifying ANS function using heart rate variability (HRV); and specific improvements in clinical outcomes related to ANS function when using these healing practices in chronic illness.

In Chapter 5, Ruth Stanley investigates how simple ancient chant scales developed by our ancestors to treat chronic illness are remarkably similar to human vocal patterns, suggesting that music and chant trigger a physiological mechanism within the human body. Historically, diverse cultural traditions have believed that the human voice had mystical powers capable of traversing and connecting the temporal and spiritual realms of life. Vocal frequency patterns found in ancient scales function like encoded auditory cues to directly influence ANS control of physical, emotional, spiritual, and psychological states. Stanley explores the origins of ancient scales from vocal intervals and a corresponding ANS pathophysiologic basis for music and healing in chronic illness. The topics discussed are origins of music composition from ancient scales and vocal intervals; physiologic hardwiring for vocal intervals and scales; relationship of vocal intervals and ancient scales to

ANS physiologic states; and finally, practical treatment applications for those who have chronic illness.

In Chapter 6, Amy Holte and Paul J. Mills present a textual analysis of how yoga represents and responds to chronic illness. Drawing from two streams of yoga—Classical Yoga and Modern Yoga Therapy—the authors suggest that yoga depicts chronic illness as a condition of physical disease, but also as a state of suffering that can potentially be healed through yoga's spiritual path. While in its long history yoga has always offered the promise of freedom from suffering, only in modern times has yoga literature directly addressed medically defined chronic illness and elaborated on the specialized applications of yoga for such conditions. Holte and Mills propose that the yogic process shifts the cognitive–motivational framework of chronic illness to a simultaneously embodied and non-dual relational sense of self that can relieve chronic suffering. The analysis concludes with a consideration of the recent emergence of yoga therapeutics within integrative medicine.

Chronic Illness: Inter-Religious, Cross-Cultural, and Narrative Perspectives

In Chapter 7, Paula Arai opens Part II by offering a Zen Buddhist approach to healing rooted in ritual practice. Based on in-depth ethnographic research with Japanese women (some of whom have chronic illnesses) who practice Zen Buddhist teachings, Arai explores how their mode of healing is woven into ritualized activities that imbue their daily lives with power and meaning. In a worldview where the interrelatedness of all things is the primary point of reference, healing means to be in harmony with this impermanent web of relationships that constitutes the dynamic universe. Rituals can be a conduit to an intuitive, bodily based experience of harmony, precisely because rituals can transport people to modes of being that transcend linear and rational thought. Rituals can affect a person more holistically by entering below the radar of cerebral cognition and bypassing dualistic perception. Therefore, rituals that do not explicitly purport to be healing rituals can help someone heal by indirectly facilitating a key dimension of Buddhist healing activity, a non-dualistic experience of reality.

In Chapter 8, Christine James utilizes metabolic syndrome and obesity as a rich test case for those seeking a spiritual response to chronic illness. James offers a comparative study of Christian, Buddhist, and philosophical approaches to metabolic syndrome. The clinical definition and risk factors of metabolic syndrome and obesity are described, including the debate as to whether metabolic syndrome and obesity fit the definition of a chronic illness. The individual and social relationships between weight and the concepts of guilt and shame are examined. The Christian and Buddhist responses and recommendations for overcoming the pathology vary, but they have a common theme in recommending a revision of the individual's approach to control. These various perspectives are summarized and critically evaluated for strengths and weaknesses in terms of their applicability for people living with metabolic syndrome and obesity.

In Chapter 9, Salomea Popoviciu, Ioan Popoviciu, Delia Birle, Serban Olah, and Paul Negrut explore the influence of the relationship among religious beliefs, practices, symbols, and metaphors on the coping strategies of rare disease patients in predominantly Orthodox Romania. The authors structure their presentation into three main sections: (1) an overview of the Romanian Orthodox context; (2) an exploration of the patterns of religious beliefs and practices of rare disease patients or their caregivers and how they correlate with self-reported quality of life; and (3) an analysis of how illness narratives employ religious symbols and metaphors. The results of this study suggest that rare disease patients in Romania are deeply religious. The results also suggest that religious beliefs and practices can be an important coping strategy for people diagnosed with rare diseases. Illness narrative analysis indicates that religious symbols and metaphors serve to reinforce widely shared values of the community regarding health and illness, illustrating the role of religious language on the coping strategies of patients and their power in shaping perceptions of illness.

In Chapter 10, Lavonna Lea Lovern and Danielle Costello describe how and why diabetes is an epidemic among global Indigenous populations. Diabetes and its related issues make it one of the most devastating chronic illnesses in Native American populations. Diabetes-related conditions such as heart disease, stroke, blindness, and amputation continue to be serious challenges in Native American communities. These challenges are exacerbated by poverty and the lack of convenient and affordable health care as well as by environmental degradation and ecosystem contamination. Lovern and Costello focus on the historic and current issues involving colonization and post-colonization tactics that have perpetuated the chronic illness epidemic in Native American populations. The destruction of community and cultural understandings regarding the link between body, mind, and spirit has separated people from traditional practices involving wellness. The final section of this chapter is devoted to an examination of the attempts by Native Americans and communities to re-forge the links between body, mind, and spirit through the reintroduction of traditional ways of being in the world.

In Chapter 11, Akinmayowa Akin-Otiko examines the way chronic illness is understood in the Yoruba traditional healing paradigm in Nigeria and explains how *Ifá* divination is employed to diagnose and treat it. The findings of this ethnographic study demonstrate that chronic illness, for the Yoruba, is *àmódi*, a condition that is difficult to diagnose and treat without the use of *Ifá* divination. *Àmódi* does not follow a predictable pattern of relationship between symptoms and illness causation (as in the Western medical paradigm) because for the Yoruba *Àmódi* is situated in supernatural causation. With *Ifá* divination, patients suffering from chronic illnesses are given hope of recovery and cure, which is different from helping them to cope with chronic illness. This hope is possible because *Ifá* divination is believed to resolve illness conditions, especially when the cause of the illness is supernatural.

In Chapter 12, Ruth Krall offers a riveting narrative centered on a personal encounter with endometrial cancer, the ebbs and flows of her emotional, physical, and spiritual responses to the disease, and how she was able to recover a secure sense of herself as a whole person. In her search for a pathway back to a sense of personal wellness, Krall turned to the mythology of ancient Sumer. In particular, she turned to the myth known as the *Descent of the Goddess* where Sumer's important deity, the Goddess Inanna, journeys into the underworld of death and resurrection, suffering and renewal. The inner balance of destruction and creation; of lost stories and epiphanies; of losing and finding: this is a fragile balance that shifts and moves and dances with illness and recovery. This chapter is a personal narrative centering on how the author gradually learned to reach toward and embrace life in all of its complexities in order to discover a new synthesis, a new set of harmonies.

In Chapter 13, Noel Boyle writes about his son, Ciaran, who suffers from an extreme and destructive seizure disorder, causing him enormous pain, suffering, terror, and isolation. Boyle rejects claims that Ciaran's severe chronic condition was planned by a loving God or that Ciaran's suffering is somehow illusory. According to Boyle, only a false Christian theology would offer comfort by denying the horrors of Ciaran's life. In order to establish a more genuine Christian theological reflection on Ciaran's suffering, Boyle turns to the work of protestant theologian Paul Tillich. Tillich maintained that anxieties regarding such things as death and meaninglessness should not be avoided, but embraced. Such experiences with nonbeing open a window into deeper affirmations of life and meaning. Following Tillich's lead, Boyle does not deny Ciaran's suffering; he asks whether joy exists in spite of suffering. Ciaran's pain serves no divine purpose; his father asks whether meaning emerges in spite of the meaninglessness of his agony.

In Chapter 14, Michael J. Stoltzfus and Rebecca Green offer some brief concluding remarks, highlight some common themes threaded throughout the chapters, and articulate recommendations for future inquiry.

HOPES AND INTENTIONS

It is our hope that this book will appeal to a broad audience including people living with chronic illnesses, scholars and students from many disciplines, health-care professionals, social service professionals, and religious practitioners from diverse traditions and cultural contexts. We believe that this book can function as a useful tool for college and university courses and as resources for more general audiences interested in the intersection of spirituality, chronic illness, and healing. The book might also help people expand what is sometimes a narrow professional and/or personal frame of reference for interpreting and responding to chronic illness, spirituality, and healing. The variety of methodological approaches coupled with differing religious, spiritual, disciplinary, and cultural perspectives represented in the book allows readers to view chronic illness, spirituality, and healing through multiple lenses.

Exploring the spiritual implications of chronic illness and healing from interreligious, cross-cultural, and interdisciplinary perspectives addresses a gap in both academic and popular literature in the more general area of religion/spirituality and health. Much of the available spirituality and health literature focuses on acute rather than chronic health conditions and tends to do so from a single religious perspective. We believe one of the greatest strengths of this edited collection is the interdisciplinary and even "extra-disciplinary" focus that includes both academic and practice disciplines and lay perspectives. Our hope is that this project will make an important contribution to multiple fields including religious studies, psychology, disability studies, anthropology, sociology, and multiple health-related fields such as nursing, medicine, psychology, counseling, social work, and others.

Given the vast and pervasive role that chronic illness and spirituality play in human experience, the chapters included in this volume portray varied and complex perspectives that are by no means exhaustive. Consensus regarding the experience of chronic illness or the understanding of how spiritual traditions and practices should conceptualize and respond to chronic illness is not the objective of this project. Rather, our intention is to foster interreligious, cross-cultural, and trans-disciplinary dialogue about chronic illness, spirituality, and healing and to cultivate creative ways to respond and relate to the fragile yet resilient human condition.

REFERENCES

Bishop, M. (2005). "Quality of life and psychological adaptation to chronic illness and disability: Preliminary analysis of a conceptual and theoretical synthesis." *Rehabilitation Counseling Bulletin, 48,* 219–231.

Centers for Disease Control and Prevention. (2009). "Chronic diseases at a glance: The power to prevent, the call to control". Retrieved from http://www.cdc.gov/nccdphp/publications/AAG/pdf/chronic.pdf.

Charmaz, K. (1991). *Good days, bad days: The self in chronic illness and in time.* NewBrunswick, NJ: Rutgers University Press.

Charmaz, K. (1995). "The body, identity, and self: Adapting to impairment." *The SociologicalQuarterly, 36,* 657–680.

Garland-Thompson, R. (1994). "Redrawing the boundaries of feminist disability studies."*Feminist Studies, 20,* 586.

Garrett, C. (2002). "Spirituality and healing in the sociology of chronic illness." *Health Sociology Review, 11*(1–2), 61–69.

Gockel, A. (2009). "Spirituality and the process of healing: A narrative study." *The International Journal for the Psychology of Religion, 19,* 217–230.

Kleinman, A. (1988). *The illness narratives.* New York: Basic Books.

Koenig, H., King, D. & Carson, V. (eds). (2012). *Handbook of religion and health.* Second edition. New York: Oxford University Press.

Kohn, L. (2007). "Daoyin: Chinese healing exercises." *Asian Medicine, 3,* 103–129.

Longmore, P. & Umansky, L. (eds). (2001). *The new disability history: American perspectives.* New York and London: New York University Press.

McColman, C. (1997). *Where body and soul encounter the sacred.* Georgetown, Massachusetts: North Star Publications.

Nichols, L. & Hunt, B. (2011). "The significance of spirituality for individuals with chronic illness: Implications for mental health counseling." *Journal of Mental Health Counseling, 33*(1), 51–66.

Thompson, C. J. (2003). "Natural health discourse and the therapeutic production of consumer resistance." *The Sociological Quarterly, 44*(1), 81–107.

Wendell, S. (2001). "Unhealthy disabled: Treating chronic illnesses as disabilities." *Hypatia, 16*(4), 17–33.

Wills, M. (2007). "Connection, action and hope: An invitation to reclaim the 'spiritual' in health care." *Journal of Religion and Health, 46*(3), 423–436.

PART I

CHRONIC ILLNESS AND HEALING: BLENDING BIOMEDICAL CARE WITH SPIRITUAL PRACTICE

CHAPTER 1

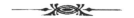

SPIRITUALITY, CHRONIC ILLNESS, AND HEALING: UNIQUE CHALLENGES AND OPPORTUNITIES

Michael J. Stoltzfus and Rebecca Green

Understandings of health, well-being, disease, and illness have changed drastically over the past century, as life expectancy has increased and as treatments for diseases once considered fatal have created an experience we call chronic illness. Prior to the twentieth century, diseases either were resolved or resulted in death, and access to medical treatment was not available to most people. In developed nations today, there has been an epidemiological shift from shorter life expectancy and high death rates from acute, infectious, parasitic diseases to longer life expectancy and ongoing, chronic illness (Lynn & Adamson, 2003). According to Lynn and Adamson (2003), most Americans live their last days in institutional settings rather than at home, and most will spend the final two years of their life coping with chronic illness or disability. Adding to that group younger people with chronic illness, the aging baby-boomer generation which has yet to develop chronic illness, and those who encounter people with chronic illness at work, school, or in social settings, makes the potential range and impact of chronic illness seem overwhelming. In addition, societal changes have occurred that have altered the way people cope with chronic illness and disability. Today's global society and highly transient lifestyle means that many people who live with chronic illness are not in situations in which they can be cared for, assisted by, or supported by nearby family members. These trends have created not only challenges in terms of global health-care delivery, employment, and economics, but they have also raised questions about how society and scholars understand and interpret the material, emotional, psychological, and spiritual meanings and implications of chronic illness.

This chapter describes some of the unique challenges and opportunities associated with integrating the concepts of spirituality, chronic illness, and healing in everyday life, and offers specific implications for a more holistic approach for practical health-care disciplines. How can individuals living with long-term, chronic physical and/or emotional illness respond creatively and meaningfully to a vulnerable and wounded body/mind/spirit? What ideas, attitudes, and values do we find in our culture, society, and spiritual traditions that help or hinder people in this task? How can people address the anger, fear, vulnerability, uncertainty, and longing for a cure that neither biomedicine nor religion can manifest for many forms of chronic illness? How can people discover and live a whole and meaningful life in spite of ongoing illness and pain? How can loved ones and clinical providers who interact with them respond in ways that promote spiritual solace and healing when physical cure is unlikely?

DESCRIBING SPIRITUALITY

As the etymology of the term itself implies, spirituality can be described as the spirit or energy that animates a person's life in each and every moment. "Spirit" derives from the Latin world *spiritus*, which, like its counterparts in Greek (*pneuma*), Hebrew (*ruach*), and *Chinese* (*qi*), means at once breath, wind, spirit, and vital energy (McColman, 1997, pp. 7–10; Kohn, 2007). This association comes most obviously from the observation that if people are alive they are breathing, they are imbued by the spirit of life, and when breathing ceases, the body dies. Breath and breathing are always present in lived experience. With each breath, people exchange carbon dioxide molecules from inside the body for oxygen molecules from the surrounding air in an ongoing transformational process of exchange and renewal. Similarly, living with an incurable chronic illness, like breathing or one's heart-beat, is a perpetual part of a person's lived experience, a normal part of the ever-changing rhythm of life. Perhaps, if people living with chronic illnesses come to see their illness as a natural element of their ever-changing situation, an integral part of life, rather than as a threat or enemy to physical or mental integrity, then they might be in a better position to cope effectively with the pain, stress, and complications that arise. If loved ones and health-care providers can adopt a similar perspective and incorporate it into caring, empathetic interactions, then pain, stress, and complications may be reduced as barriers to spiritual health.

Diverse spiritual traditions have long associated breath and breathing with spirituality and spiritual practice. Multiple forms of Buddhist meditation, Christian contemplative prayer, the Indian practice of *Pranayama*, and the Chinese practice of *Qi Gong*—all seek to cultivate spirituality, healing, and well-being by emphasizing conscious, relaxed, and present-moment breathing. But all of these diverse spiritual traditions also recognize the fact that people live and breathe by paradoxical dispositions rooted in fear and hope, anxiety and compassion, integration and separation. Any such dispositional tendencies, singularly or in combination, can be the spirit that shapes individual and collective lives as people struggle to live creatively and meaningfully moment by moment, day by day, in the presence of the ongoing vulnerability and uncertainty that accompany many forms of chronic illness.

Spirituality, like air or breath, is something that people are filled with, something that connects people with the surrounding atmosphere, something that human bodies depend on for nurture and sustenance, but this link between the spiritual and the material has not always been emphasized in some religious traditions. For example, some forms of Western Christianity have tended to view the spiritual in contrast to the physical, a concern of the soul rather than the body. This viewpoint can lead to a dualistic tendency to see the spirit as sacred and the body as profane. This perspective has found expression in the restriction of Western biomedical care to concern for the body in its disease or pain, sometimes to the neglect of the whole person in his or her spiritual and cultural understanding of suffering and healing. This dualistic approach may associate spirituality as something interior and private, rather than embodied, relational, social, and environmental; and leaves the sufferer to try to integrate a rigid, one-dimensional construct of disease, as explained and treated by the health-care establishment, into a complex, highly dimensional and personal illness experience. For example, health-care providers may be able to easily explain the autoimmune and inflammatory processes associated with a chronic disease like rheumatoid arthritis or Crohn's disease. But all the information in the world about treatment options, possible outcomes, and the expected course of the disease does not prepare patients for the drastic toll the disease will take in every other dimension of life; or equip them to respond in ways that promote spiritual health and well-being. The individual's spiritual response to the literal, embodied rejection of self that occurs in many forms of autoimmune disease is as real and consequential to the whole person as is the physiological response. Spirituality situates people in relational contexts that are much wider and denser than the individual. Spirituality, as it is being broadly described in this chapter, can be understood as a way of embodied dwelling in the world, a lived experience rooted in a holistic availability to learn and grow, to create meaning and purpose, from the dynamic relation among spirit, body, mind, other people, world, and multiple sources of transcendence.

One way that spiritual traditions tend to address this dynamic relationship is through the language of transcendence and immanence, connection and isolation (Garrett, 2001, 49; Cook, 2004; Bouma, 2000; Stoll, 1989). The experience of transcendence is the experience of living in a world that extends infinitely beyond one's immediate, embodied location (Schutz, 1962, pp. 306–356; Schutz & Luckmann, 1983, pp. 106–148). To be human is to be limited by the transcendence of time (past and future); space (here and there); embodiment; and other human beings with their unique perspectives, society, and nature. Yet to be human is to be discontent with these limitations and to seek ways to be more connected to other human beings, to other cultures and societies, and even to other provinces of meaning such as dreams or to a God or Goddess of religious belief. Spirituality is the lived expression of giving meaning and purpose to life in the midst of the ongoing paradoxical relationship of immanence and transcendence, limitation and possibility, isolation and unification, illness and healing, which are always co-presented in embodied encounters with the world. Human beings are perpetually navigating multiple transcendent boundaries and changing dimensions of living while dwelling in a fragile and vulnerable body. The ongoing inner and relational adaptation, coping, or transformation to this perpetual paradox can be described by a variety of spiritual terms such as awakening, enlightenment, grace, wholeness, balance, harmony, mindfulness, or being centered.

The relationship between the terms spirituality and religion has been complicated and controversial (Koenig, 2000; Sawatzsky et al., 2005). The English word religion has as its root the Latin term *relegare*, which means "to tie or bind together" (Fasching & Dechant, 2001). Spirituality, as the term is being described and used in this chapter, is not bound with a specific theological or ideological model. Spirituality neither requires nor negates belief in a god or gods, it does not presume participation in a particular set of rituals, and it is not tied to any specific sacred texts. For many people spirituality is forged and cultivated by participation in a specific religious tradition, while for others it is not affiliated with religious membership. Many people use the religious rituals, values, texts, and beliefs they practice as a framework to understand the purpose and meaning of spirituality in their own lives. Religious traditions tend to be more institutionalized and compartmentalized with standard models for interpreting and responding to ethical questions, the belief in divine beings, or the experience of chronic illness. Looking at spirituality as both integral to, yet distinct from, a particular religious affiliation is important for addressing spirituality with people who might otherwise find it stigmatizing to explore because of its association with organized religious models of interpretation and response. In addition, the concept of spirituality is tempered by humility or an availability to learn from multiple religious traditions and worldviews, rather than an outright rejection of practices and ideas that are not part of a specific religious model or ideological framework. Spiritual humility empowers people to question taken-for-granted assumptions in order to be receptive to new possibilities for creative thought and transformative experience.

Since spirituality is describable but not easily definable, a challenge is to make spirituality more comprehensible while recognizing that for individuals its meaning and experience is largely subjective, unique, flexible, and transforming. The experience of spirituality arises through the emergence of paradox, novelty, and uncertainty that cannot be mastered or categorized by objective meanings or abstract scientific or religious models. Grounded by the perpetual immanence of a vulnerable body, spirituality embraces the full spectrum of human experience including joy and pain, suffering and healing, disease and health, immanence and transcendence, life and death. It is imperative for health-care providers to acknowledge the spectrum that extends beyond the measurable confines of physical disease, and allow a patient's spirituality to inform the provider's response to the patient's multidimensional experience of chronic illness.

Describing Chronic Illness: Personal, Medical, Cultural, and Religious Meanings

Chronic illness encompasses a wide variety of diseases including but not limited to cancer, rheumatoid arthritis, heart disease, lupus, pain, diabetes, depression, addiction, multiple sclerosis, muscular dystrophy, Crohn's Disease, HIV, and many others that have physical, mental, emotional, spiritual, relational, vocational, and economic implications. Generally, chronic illness can be described as "a lifelong process of adapting to significant physical, psychological, social, and environmental changes" as a result of illness (Bishop, 2005, p. 219). In 2005, 133 million Americans had a chronic illness; such illnesses are the leading cause of death and disability in the United States (Centers for Disease Control and Prevention, 2009). Due to the unpredictable nature of many chronic illnesses, individuals with chronic conditions, along with their family, friends, and health-care professionals, are confronted with an ongoing adaptation process and prolonged medical treatment (Kleinman, 1988).

Livneh and Antonak (2005) identified eight life areas affected by chronic illness: (a) frequent and increased stress; (b) psychosocial and physical trauma connected to the onset of the disease process; (c) the experience of grief associated with the loss of abilities, functionalities, roles, or relationships; (d) alterations in body image due to disease and/or side effects of medical treatment for disease; (e) changes in self-understanding associated with present and future vocational and family expectations; (f) coping with uncertainty and unpredictability in terms of disease symptoms like pain and treatment process like side effects of drug therapy; (g) new or increased experiences with prejudicial or biased responses from others; and (h) alterations in quality of life requiring a process of on-going adaptation and adjustment.

Chronic illness can affect all elements of a person's life—physical, social, spiritual, vocational, and psychological. In addition, chronic illnesses and their debilitating symptoms are very real but sometimes undetectable or invisible to the casual observer or even close family members, which may heighten frustration and anxiety (Stone, 1995). Finally, most people can understand and sympathize with episodic illness from which people recover (bone mends, pain subsides, scar heals) or fatal illnesses which end in death. And while health-care providers may understand the long-term physiological implications of chronic disease processes, they encounter patients only episodically when the patient enters the health-care environment. Providers, therefore, may lack insight into the reality of a patient's daily life and needs. Chronic illnesses are neither episodic nor terminal. Therefore, they do not raise the same issues about cure or impending death, but challenge the individual to cultivate meaning and healing in the midst of daily, ongoing, long-term illness, pain, suffering, adaptation, and transformation. Faced with all of these uncertainties and complexities, individuals are often forced to question many of their taken-for-granted assumptions and reassess their lives from a new perspective (Bishop, 2005; Kleinman, 1988; Charmaz, 1991 & 1995; Kaye & Raghavan, 2002; Wills, 2007; Gockel, 2009; Wendell, 2001; Garrett, 2002).

For example, most people with chronic illnesses do not fit, and therefore must question, the dominant acute care model evident in the history of Western medical care and education. The acute care model of illness primarily attends to physical manifestation of the disease in an individual patient and associates health and well-being with eradication of the disease state. Acute care approaches to disease or pain stress a restitution narrative focusing on diagnosis, treatment, and cure (Longmore & Umansky, 2001; Garland-Thompson, 2005). In this model, disease is the enemy to be banished from an individual body by whatever technological or pharmacological means that is available; self-identity is viewed as existing independently of the experience of illness; and healing is associated with living without the presence of disease.

Religious models of interpreting and responding to chronic illness sometimes mimic the restitution narrative associated with the acute care medical model where individual religious diagnosis, treatment, and cure replace individual medical diagnosis, treatment, and cure. There may be an insinuation that chronic illness somehow involves merited suffering (result of or punishment for sin, lesson to learn, test of faith, opportunity for religious repentance) or that suffering itself is somehow meritorious, and well-meaning people from multiple religious traditions may offer religious explanations and solutions to the individual problem (Schumm & Stoltzfus, 2007; Reynolds, 2008; Simundson, 2001). If the restitution narrative is granted a religious legitimacy, then people may feel defective, unworthy, guilty, impure, or even hopeless due to their chronic illness (Arora, 2009). Restitution narratives, whether medical or religious, do not fit well with those who struggle with chronic illnesses and seek balance and healing in the midst of a transforming process, rather than cure.

Chronic illness has the power to alter routine patterns of medical or religious interpretation and response. Cheri Register (1978), writing from her own experience, stated

> Chronic illness does not fit the popular notion of how illness proceeds: You get sick, you go to the doctor and get some medicine, and wait to get better. If there is no remedy for what ails you, you die. An illness that drags on for years, defying diagnosis, treatment, and/or cure is an intolerable anomaly. (p. 3)

Eventually, Register said, people will come to the frightful realization "that illness has become your normal condition" (p. 3). Illness goes from being abnormal to being normal, requiring a shift in perspective, care, interpretation, and response. For the chronically ill, disease is an intrinsic element of being alive, a permanent feature of living where people must learn to integrate their illness constructively into their sense of personal, social, medical, and spiritual self-identity. The nature of such a challenge requires a personal and relational response that is quite different from the restitution narrative associated with the individualistic acute care model.

In his book, *At the Will of the Body*, Arthur Frank (1991) wrote about his own experience with a heart attack and cancer. He drew the helpful distinction between disease talk and illness talk. Disease talk, which is what one hears from many health-care professionals, reduces the body to a physiology that is measured and organized. Illness, by contrast, is the experience of living with the disease.

> Illness begins where medicine leaves off, where I recognize that what is happening to my body is...[happening] to my life....In illness talk there is no such thing as the body, only my body as I experience it. Illness talk is a story about moving from a perfectly comfortable body to one that forces me to ask: What's happening to me? Not it, but me. (p. 13)

A diagnosis of cancer or any chronic illness that may be incurable tends to alienate people from their body because it challenges people to admit their bodily vulnerability, destructibility, and the discomfort present in the unknown. To discover that one's body cannot be fixed, in the context of the acute care mindset of Western medicine, is to experience a sense of powerlessness, helplessness, or loss of control. The fear of the unknown, including the possibility of disability or death, can prompt people to objectify their own bodies.

The sense of alienation from one's body is experienced in illness as the profound loss of possibility. Susan Wendell (2001), writing from her own experience with chronic illness, stated

> When I was disabled by illness, I experienced a much more profound alienation from my body. After a year spent mostly in bed, I could barely identify my body as my own. I felt that "it" was torturing "me," trapping me in exhaustion, pain and inability to do many of the simplest things I did when I was healthy. (p. 12)

Wendell's description helps to articulate how ill people experience their bodies as more than physiological body parts. Bodies are the vehicle through which people interact with others and the means by which people carry out projects in the world. Pain or nausea are not just uncomfortable sensations, they radically complicate giving care and attention to one's spouse, child, or vocation. It may be difficult for health-care providers, who adhere to standard treatment protocols and critical pathways for certain kinds of patients, to step into the individual patient experiences of powerlessness, loss of control, fear, and discomfort that affect the patient's day-to-day functioning and relating.

Discomfort caused by the body in the form of pain, fatigue, nausea, or other symptoms tend to be associated with vulnerability and weakness.

Contemporary cultural dynamics in the United States prefer that these vulnerabilities be kept invisible or shut off in hospitals, retirement homes, hospice facilities, or in silent individual bodies. According to Wendell (2001), "Suffering caused by the body and the inability to control the body are despised, pitied, and above all feared. This fear, experienced individually, is also deeply embedded in our culture" (p. 12). Wendell (1996) argued that contemporary culture idealizes the human body. These cultural ideals are not only about physical appearance, they are also ideals about strength, energy, self-sufficiency, and proper control of the body. "In a culture which loves the idea that the body can be controlled, those who cannot control their bodies are seen (and may see themselves) as failures" (Wendell, 2001, p. 13). Idealizing the body and wanting to control it go hand in hand.

Wendell came to realize how much embracing cultural notions of an idealized body contributed to her own sense of body alienation when she became sick, and how "idealizing the body prevents everyone, able-bodied and disabled, from identifying with and loving her/his real body" (p. 12). Unrealistic cultural ideals of control can cause harm and suffering for everyone, not only for those who struggle with chronic illness. Western biomedicine tends to endorse these ideals to the extent that it focuses on individual cure rather than cultural and personal healing. The incurably chronically ill and the dying can come to symbolize the failure of medicine and science to control nature, to control the body.

If health care or religious care sees its primary focus as the diseased individual body, then the holistic task of addressing the psychological, spiritual, social, relational, cultural, and economic aspects of illness may be considered peripheral or neglected altogether. Yet these aspects are an integral element of the illness experience and a major source of suffering and healing for individuals with chronic illness. The experience of illness, whether acute or chronic, is never simply a bodily disorder that affects only a particular individual. In disrupting a person's life, illness necessarily disrupts family, work, and other social relationships, in addition to causing physical, emotional, and spiritual upheaval.

Kay Toombs (1995), a woman who lived with multiple sclerosis for many years, articulated how an emphasis on the physical pathology of the malfunctioning body contributed to her sense of alienation:

> ... at one time I was under the care of a neurologist, a urologist, a hematologist, a gastroenterologist, a gynecologist, and a vascular surgeon (not to mention the numerous technologists associated with these professionals). Each specialist was focused on a different bodily mechanism, each was "in charge" of that portion of my body, but no one was "in charge" of the whole (in either the mechanistic or holistic sense)—except for me and, at the time, I felt least qualified for the job. (p. 2)

For people living with a chronic illness, the ongoing task is holistic healing rather than curing a specific individual disease state. This task requires an explicit focus on the human experience of illness in all its multifaceted uncertainties and dynamics and corresponding flexibility and adaptability in coping responses; and requires learning to live well in the presence, rather than the absence, of physical or mental incapacity, recognizing vulnerability as a way of life.

An important step in understanding how people might interpret and respond to chronic illness experience is to investigate the cultural metaphors and narratives that invest interpretive meaning and purpose to suffering, pain, illness, and death (Kleinman, 1988; Charmaz, 1991). Personal meaning is uniquely challenged by those boundary situations that take people to the limits of their ability to cope or understand, such as diagnosis of chronic or terminal illness. The dreaded diseases (cancer, AIDS, multiple sclerosis, heart disease, and others) carry with them powerful metaphorical significance. In receiving such a diagnosis, one is forced not only to address the physical symptoms of the illness, as well as the profound uncertainty that accompanies it, but also, as importantly, to confront the personal and cultural meanings associated with the disease. A problem is that the metaphors, the prevailing cultural and religious representations of chronic illness, are sometimes more degrading than elevating, more discouraging than uplifting.

One way to highlight how religious and cultural narratives function to shape personal and social representations of illness is to consider the example of HIV/AIDS. AIDS in the United States emerged in the early 1980s with an unmistakable link to the world of homosexuality. AIDS was linked, however inappropriately, with a group that was for many years openly oppressed; a group whose sexual practices many religious leaders and politicians reviled as unnatural, ungodly, and unspeakable. The popular media first described AIDS as a "gay plague" and some churches labeled AIDS as the "Wrath of God Syndrome" (Hawkins, 1993). People with AIDS often found themselves portrayed by prevailing cultural and religious narratives in the role of self-created victims who deserved whatever pain and suffering they experienced. In such a context, people with AIDS suffered much more than the physical symptoms of the disease. They were shunned, silenced, and shamed in addition to being sick.

In short, the social, cultural, and religious responses to disease can create a "second illness" (Scheper-Hughes & Lock, 1986, p. 137): the layers of stigma, rejection, fear, and exclusion that sometimes attach to particular diseases. Health-care providers must begin to address the "second illnesses" that accompany physical disease. Illness, particularly chronic illness, does not result so much in a deficit of meaning or sense of meaninglessness, but in an excess of meanings, many of them stigmatizing and humbling. Illness experience as disease alone is a form of alienation, a dehumanization of suffering that may perpetuate isolation and self-blame. If healing is to be embraced moment to moment and day to day, it is vital to recognize the extent to which cultural and religious metaphors and narratives may contribute to a weakening of the resolve to live well in spite of ongoing illness. On the other hand, people with chronic illness may be in a better position to question cultural metaphors about controlling the body or medical metaphors about cure because, quite literally, the metaphors are not usual or meaningful to their experiences. However, health-care providers must also be aware of how cultural metaphors influence their relationships with patients; and allow patients' metaphors to guide treatment.

While some people with chronic illness resist being reduced to the prevailing cultural or religious metaphorical meanings that accompany a specific diagnosis, others may feel disempowered by the absence of an official medical diagnosis that legitimates the presence of symptoms as a recognizable medical condition. It is not uncommon for people with chronic illness to go undiagnosed or be misdiagnosed for lengthy periods of time. Some may be told that there is nothing wrong with them or that it is all psychosomatic. There are problems that come with a specific diagnosis and problems that come without one; they may produce unique relations of power, unique tactics of resistance, and unique approaches to healing and renewal (Moss & Dyck, 1999).

Because of the power and legitimacy many modern societies attribute to biomedical models, a diagnosis is invested with broad and powerful social, cultural, economic, religious, and personal meanings. The diagnostic inscription can produce different meanings for different groups. It can act as a script for treating illness. It can affect insurance claims, including health insurance and insurance for lost wages. It can legitimate or de-legitimate a person's claim that their body was ill. In can instigate cultural and religious interpretational responses ranging from alienation, fear, and blame to compassion, care, and nurture. Without diagnosis, symptoms may be attributed to stress, instability, or laziness. With a diagnosis, people may view the illness as their own fault and get caught up in medical or religious restitution narratives. Here again paradox and uncertainty is inherent to the lived experience of chronic illness on many different levels. The diagnosis itself is a complex cultural metaphor that ascribes meaning to a certain set of physical symptoms and measurable characteristics, and even places a monetary value on illness.

In addition, the same chronic illness diagnosis can have very different physical, psychological, emotional, and spiritual effects on different people. For example, two people living with multiple sclerosis may have markedly different symptoms, functional limitations, psychosocial responses, and experiences with health-care diagnosis and therapy. Living with chronic illness is indescribable in the sense that there are no limits to the factors or combinations that make every individual's experience unique. Throughout the literature there is a discussion of the unique meaning chronic illness has for each person, the inability of biomedical, cultural, or religious models to capture this unique meaning, and the need for individuals to integrate shifting horizons of meaning into self-management and perspectives of healing (Schumm & Stoltzfus, 2011; McNulty et al., 2004; Garrett, 2001; Arora, 2009; Gockel, 2009; Krok, 2008; Bishop, 2005; Kleinman, 1988). Facilitation of self-management will be discussed later as a primary means by which health-care providers can promote spiritual healing among their patients with chronic illness; but there is also a need for health-care providers, themselves, to integrate shifting horizons of meaning into their own perspectives of care, and into the greater disciplinary perspective of caring for the chronically ill.

At the same time, individuals with chronic illnesses have a unique opportunity to confront the multidimensional challenges of their illnesses while gaining insight and awareness due to their shifting responses to changing circumstances. For example, individuals with chronic illness have first-hand exposure to the limitations and sometimes narrow views of conventional medicine, conventional religion, and conventional cultural responses to disease; many are looking for alternative ways to gain understanding about their illness and incorporate spiritual insight, meaning, practice, and self-understanding to help achieve healing (Toombs, 1995; Frank 1991 & 1995; Nichols & Hunt, 2011; Gockel, 2009; Stanley, 2009; Garrett, 2001 & 2002). Health-care providers must begin to allow the unique perspectives and understandings of these individual patients to inform their practice.

CHRONIC ILLNESS, SPIRITUALITY, AND HEALING

As a framework for our discussion of chronic illness, spirituality, and healing, we will be using a classification of illness narratives developed by Arthur Frank in *The Wounded Story Teller* (1995). Frank described three types of narrative that people might use when communicating their experience with illness. The chaos narrative emphasizes the disruptions, uncertainty, and unpredictability that illness brings. The restitution narrative tends to focus on diagnosis, treatment, and cure; a story about restoration of the self as it was before illness, though perhaps stronger and wiser. In contrast, Frank advocated for a quest narrative that views illness as part of a person's life journey and as an opportunity for creating new insight, interpretation, and response. A central question in the quest narrative is this: What does physical, mental, and spiritual healing mean when cure is unlikely? A chronic condition requires perpetual healing actively constructed by the person moment to moment, day to day (Charmaz, 1991). This kind of healing involves a transformation of the whole person in all of their social, cultural, spiritual, personal, economic, and medical contexts. Healing cannot be reduced to or associated exclusively with only one of these contexts. Rather, healing is created in the midst of the multidimensional complexity of personal and social dilemmas. Shocked out of ordinary reality by ongoing illness, people turn to those unique sources of meaning that empower transformation in the context of the paradoxical tensions of suffering and healing, pain and joy, alienation and integration. Adopting a quest approach in interactions with and treatment of patients with chronic illness may both transform the practice of the provider and facilitate spiritual healing of individual patients.

Spirituality, chronic illness, and healing are all messy terms, none of which can be contained within stable categories or neat models, and all of them are rooted in flexibility, adaptability, and change. The complexity and multidimensionality of the term healing was captured by Linda Barnes and Susan Sered (2005).

> It can mean the direct, unequivocal, and scientifically measurable cure of physical illness. It can mean the alleviation of pain or other symptoms. It also can mean coping, coming to terms with, or learning to live with that which one cannot change (including physical illness and emotional trauma). Healing can mean integration and connection among all the elements of one's being, reestablishment of self-worth, connection with one's tradition, or personal empowerment. Healing can be about repairing one's relationship with friends, relations, ancestors, the community, the world, the Earth, and/or God. It can refer to developing a sense of well-being or wholeness, whether emotional, social, spiritual, physical, or in relation to others aspects of being that are valued by a particular group. (p. 10)

The experience of healing, like the experience of spirituality and chronic illness described in the previous sections, is distinctive for each person as they face their particular life circumstances and cope with them as best they can. Healing, then, is a dynamic process, not a fixed state that you achieve and hang onto.

Like Frank's quest narrative, the literature associated with spirituality and healing tends to equate spirituality with ongoing seeking and striving (Kaye & Raghavan, 2002; Wills, 2007). Spirituality is not a static event associated with objective meaning, but rather an active process associated with emergent meaning. As such, spirituality engenders an emphasis on transformation and healing rather than cure or an event by which disease is eliminated. For example, addiction programs based on the Alcoholics Anonymous (AA) model of coping with alcohol abuse is understood not as a curative event, but as an active, ongoing process of healing found in the spiritual practices of 12-step support groups, a spiritual approach not based exclusively on the conventions of any specific religious tradition (Eastland et al., 1999). In this approach, spirituality is clearly an active process in that individuals are empowered, purposeful beings capable of seeking healing in the midst of ongoing vulnerability and need for community support. Health-care providers can incorporate a similar perspective and practices into the interventions they design with patients, a perspective in which health is processual, and not a static state of absence of disease that is dependent on cure.

Cross-disciplinary research is making it increasingly clear that many people turn to spiritual and/or religious resources to begin to understand and grapple with illness, suffering, and healing. Surveys suggest that between 70 and 90 percent of people in the United States with serious mental or physical health problems cite religion and spirituality as important means of coping (Koenig et al., 2012; Gockel, 2009; Nichols & Hunt, 2011). Often considered as part of complementary and alternative medicine (CAM), spirituality tends to remain on the fringes of biomedical health-care and health scholarship. Concerning CAM, Sharts-Hopko (2003) noted "more than one third of American adults are seeking alternative solutions to health and illness problems from various non-mainstream sources including spiritual practices" (p. 359). This trend is the case for many reasons including the high cost of health care, large numbers of people without health insurance or access to quality health care, and a growing awareness of the limits associated with conventional biomedicine. Despite a century of progress in surgical procedures, organ transplants, immunization programs, drug therapy for fighting infections and other physical symptoms, and the cracking of the human genome, biomedical successes continue to be limited, as stated by Harold Koenig (2005).

> The focus of biomedicine on the physical alone and the neglect of other parts of the person have left many improving physically but finding themselves wounded emotionally, relationally, and spiritually. The resurgence of interest in many forms of religious healing testifies to this failure of allopathic medicine to heal, despite its increasing capacity to cure. (p. 505)

The spiritual healing movement, in its many forms, is part of a cultural milieu in which alternative care of myriad types has been proliferating both in terms of quantity and in terms of variety. There is a gradual and growing awareness of the inability of biomedicine to cure, let alone heal, many chronic diseases; which has contributed to the search for other sorts of responses for individuals living with chronic pain, depression, addiction, fatigue, limited physical mobility, and so on. Holistic healing venues tend to be populated with people living with chronic rather than acute illnesses (Thompson, 2003). People living long term with cancer, AIDS, diabetes, multiple sclerosis, rheumatoid arthritis, or who serve as the primary caregiver of a family member living with Alzheimer's or mental illness, seek healing and support. At the same time, the emerging recognition of the significance of palliative end-of-life care, especially in the hospice movement, has opened the door to notions of health care and healing that go beyond the emphasis on measurable physical outcomes that has characterized much of the twentieth-century American medicine and research. This emerging trend offers as much, if not more, potential and hope for alleviation of suffering related to chronic illness as does research in genomics, pharmacokinetics, and immunology.

Spirituality and healing are beyond cognitive confinement or categorical definition and this constitutes their difficulty as a scientific field of inquiry. Nevertheless, researchers in health-care settings increasingly are taking spiritual practices more seriously. In fact, health-care researchers have been investigating spiritual practices like prayer or meditation for efficacy in pain management, recovery time from surgery, and control of chronic conditions for some time and with positive results (Koenig et al., 2012). However, this type of research is largely based on an acute model of care in which the efficacy of spiritual practices are measured for quantifiable outcomes in terms of the conventional unit of health-care research, individual bodies and their physical symptoms.

The area within health-care research that has been most receptive to exploring spiritual practices is the growing field of mind–body medicine. The National Institutes of Health (NIH) has committed significant funding to research on "mind–body" medicine, including the connection between faith and health (Wills, 2007). The *Handbook of Religion and Health* (2012), the most complete reference work to survey this field of study, demonstrates the range, depth, and efficacy of interest in such topics. One of the most well documented results of mind–body research is the recognition, long endorsed by diverse spiritual traditions, that how individuals conceptualize and label an illness is predictive of measurable individual health outcomes. With chronic illnesses in particular, people who maintain negative labeling and/or fearful, angry, and anxious emotional responses to illness experience higher rates of morbidity and mortality, greater levels of pain, and poorer quality of life. By contrast, individuals whose subjective response to illness is marked by acceptance of illness and who actively devise strategies for coping, including spiritual practices like meditation or prayer, experience lower rates of morbidity and mortality and greater quality of life (Koenig et al., 2012). However, rarely does this research extend beyond the physical health of the individual or sometimes the immediate family unit. These findings should be used not only to inform providers, in terms of measurable relationships that may exist between dependent and independent variables, but also to transform providers, in terms of their responses to patients. In other words, providers must apply these finding as much to themselves as to their patients.

Yet, from the perspective of the study of spirituality and healing, the mind–body model still tends to restrict itself to the individual, albeit in a more holistic way than the traditional biomedical model. Our argument is that spirituality and healing, in the context of chronic illness, always situates the integrated mind/body/spirit/ in relational contexts that are wider and denser than the individual; that incorporate the interconnections of culture and environment. In experiencing disease and illness, especially chronic or terminal illness, people encounter deep questions of meaning and purpose, medical and religious models that may not fit their experiences, and multiple issues that move beyond measurable and quantifiable physical symptoms. Neither spiritual flourishing nor human healing should be defined exclusively in terms of some ideal standard of individual physical or medical well-being, an ideal that is impossible for many people to attain. Just like women, people of color, and sexual minorities, many people with chronic illnesses have come to equate breaking free of narrow cultural and medical categories as a form of healing and a way to challenge historically contingent ideals of normality. No two human beings experience the same ability levels in terms of speed, strength, eyesight, pain thresholds, or resiliency levels—as such the abnormal is the normal and the normal can be problematic. Emerging trends in the tripartite connection between spirituality, healing, and living with chronic illness raise the issue of how to realize a meaningful life as a whole person in a multidimensional personal, medical, social, cultural, and spiritual context. This type of an approach to spirituality and healing, rooted in a willingness to live with flexibility, uncertainty, vulnerability and without ideal-istic expectations for cure, can help to transform everybody, from individuals living with chronic illnesses to those with narrow cultural, medical, or reli-gious approaches to health, well-being, and human community. It requires the recognition that the concept "normal" is often a barrier to overcome rather than an outcome to be achieved. This recognition must occur not only for patients, but for providers, as well.

FOSTERING SPIRITUAL CULTIVATION AND HEALING BY EMBRACING UNCERTAINTY AND VULNERABILITY

Adapting to uncertainty and vulnerability takes people with serious chronic illness on an odyssey of cultural, medical, religious, and personal meanings (Charmaz, 1991, 1995; Gockel, 2009; Wills, 2007). Their altered lives may transport them into unfamiliar worlds where they may feel alienated. Further-more, the familiar becomes strange when altered bodies or minds pose new constraints, requiring careful scrutiny, and force attending to time, space, culture, movement, and other people in new ways. Facing an ongoing illness that highlights the fragility of the human experience can provide a connection to the exploration of spirituality and healing. Indeed, spirituality and healing are about how people face the paradox of illness and wellness, tragedy and triumph, despair and hope, pain and joy that are always shifting and changing.

Chronically ill people may begin to define their experience as newly authentic and become open to new perspectives and experiences when they stop assuming that fixing their diseased body is necessary to making it acceptable or whole. Arthur Frank (1991) argued that relinquishing cul-tural, medical, religious, or personal notions of cure opens the door to new experiences of healing (pp. 60–62). Kathy Charmaz (1995), discussed relin-quishing the quest to control the body in terms of "surrendering to the sick body," a process where people learn to live with vulnerability and uncer-tainty as an active and intentional process viewing "illness as integral to subjective experience and as integrated with self" (p. 72). Jon Kabat-Zinn (2009) argued that the process of healing, in the context of chronic illness, involves the process of individuals coming to terms with their minds and bodies as they are, not with how people might wish things would be. Encoun-ters with ongoing illness evoke the deepest and most complex of emotions including fear, anxiety, humiliation, and alienation, but also open the door to new awareness, recognition, and healing. As people move from experi-encing themselves as passive victims of disease to experiencing themselves as active creators of meaning and purpose, they may entertain new thoughts, feelings, and relational dynamics. These same concepts—accepting vulnera-bility and uncertainty, acknowledging fear, and creating alternative meanings and purposes—could be incorporated into a provider's understanding and interpretation of the process of healing.

To engage in the full range of human experience, including the regular confrontation with pain, nausea, or fatigue is not a failure but an inevitability of living with many forms of chronic illness. Frank's quest narratives reconstruct illness as an opportunity for discovery, transformation, and awakening; constituting an important element in an emergent subjectivity and spirituality. The process of spiritual discovery and its implications for the adaptation of individuals living with chronic illness can be an affirming approach to exploring the multiple meanings of fragile bodies and their quest for healing.

For example, a woman named Gully (Thompson, 2003), who lives with a compromised immune system that has not responded well to conventional biomedical treatment, actively engaged her quest for healing through her willingness to explore multiple "vehicles of transcendence" (p. 95). Gully interpreted her life as an ongoing narrative of transcending her impoverished childhood by working hard, transcending her physical limitations by combining conventional biomedical care with a willingness to explore alternative avenues of treatment, and transcending the limitations of her orthodox religious experiences by a willingness to engage in spiritual exploration. Gully stated,

> It's mind boggling to me that I have such interests, you know a girl who was poor, seventh of nine children born in the city of Milwaukee. But being sick, honestly, I think now, was a blessing because it exposed me to another world that I would probably have never—I wouldn't have probably dwelled on my spirituality ....You know, I had pain and suffering but it made me a better human being, a better person than before. It's strange but I'm really grateful. I wouldn't have explored acupuncture, Ayurvedic, or met some of the people who enrich my life so much. (pp. 95–96)

In making the commitment to use her compromised immune system as an opportunity for spiritual discovery rather than to shower blame on herself for being sick, she was setting the stage for healing, for the dissolving of medical, cultural, and religious boundaries, for coming to terms with her evolving circumstances.

Through active struggle and active surrender, chronically ill people might paradoxically grow more resolute as they live with uncertainty and adapt to change. Their odyssey of changing experiences might lead them to a deeper level of awareness; of self, of situation, of their place with others. Individuals like Gully endured in their quest for meaningful spiritual insight and healing even as they experienced bodily pain and fragility. In the process, they may grow immune to traditional medical meanings of incurability and social meanings of being less than ideal.

The experience of physical and/or psychological uncertainty and paradox is at the center of the experience of chronic illness. This experience is captured by Adele McCollum (1994), a college professor who lives with an autoimmune deficiency:

> I ... think of my body as the great betrayer. Today it jogs or at least walks briskly. Tomorrow it may gasp for air. Today I pace before the class; tomorrow I teach

from a wheel chair. Today my fingers type flawlessly. Tomorrow they are red, swollen, painful, and can't even open the medicine that brings relief. I can no longer depend on health and energy on a continuum. (p. 128)

McCollum must struggle to embrace healing and wholeness when breathing is easy and when breathing is difficult. Because of the unpredictability of her physical symptoms, she must be flexible in the way she attributes meaning and purpose to her experiences. She stated:

> Notions of fixed reality, permanent ideas or identities, unchanging gods, predictable archetypes or patterns find no match in my present experience. While I hardly think of physical challenges as postmodern, they provide concrete experience of living without certainty, with nothing given or absolute, with no trail more defined than another. (p. 128)

In this context, healing cannot primarily be related to cure for disease, for magically transformed cultural sensitivity, religious miracle, or a new life to come in the future. Nonetheless, to be incurably ill, to live with perpetual physical vulnerability, is not to be without healing. Rather, healing relates to the ability to face forthrightly and with courage whatever comes one's way. Healing is tempered with uncertainty, with flexibility, with a willingness to remain open to the possibilities of different ways of seeing, experiencing, and being in the world. To speak of healing in the context of chronic illness is often to speak of vulnerable healing or wounded healing. Amidst uncertainty and ongoing illness, healing is what makes the human condition livable even when painful, tragic, or difficult. Incorporating this perspective of healing into the personal and collective worldview of health-care providers offers great potential to transform practice, and to transform the experience of chronic illness for both providers and patients.

Historically, some spiritual traditions have distinguished the experience of pain from the experience of suffering. Jon Kabat-Zinn (2009), influenced by a Buddhist worldview, wrote:

> Pain is a natural part of the experience of life. Suffering is one of many possible responses to pain. Suffering can come out of either physical or emotional pain. It involves our thoughts and emotions and how they frame the meaning of our experiences. (p. 285)

Spiritual traditions as a whole tend to embrace pain, disease, and vulnerability as inevitable elements of the human condition while viewing suffering and healing as arising, in part, from the conditioned ideas or emotions that individuals attach to particular experiences of pain or disease. For example, when the chronically ill become attached to the idea of individual cure, these individuals may find that such attachment increases their sense of suffering while doing little to increase their sense of healing. For people thus attached, the biomedical focus on cure that they encounter in clinical settings further alienates them from potential spiritual healing. There is a practical necessity for health-care professionals to habitually consider what is "normal" and to think of illness as deviation of normal. Health-care providers utilize a body of expert knowledge to know exactly what clinical signs and symptoms are significant heralds of disease, and what lab values indicate an aberrant response in what they perceive should be a normal body. Interventions are aimed at returning the body as close to the norm as possible. Success is determined by how close to normal the patient comes. This way of viewing patients and illness is a prime example of how expert knowledge creates a clinical cage in which professionals exist. We (providers) cannot even conceptualize ways in which "not normal" might even be acceptable, much less preferable to "normal." Unfortunately, all too often we ensnare patients with chronic illness in this cage with us, and rather than release them from it, we enlarge the boundaries of it so that even in their day-to-day lives outside the clinical environment, patients define the quality of their lives in terms of limitation, rather than potential or freedom. We need to begin to think of ways in which we can not only free patients from disease processes, but also free them and ourselves from our own personal narrow understandings of healing. Spiritual traditions may be able to promote spiritual practices that aid people with chronic illness in undoing or loosening typical cultural, medical, religious, or personal patterns of thinking, acting, and responding to experiences of pain and disease, as a way to cultivate healing and balance rather than normalcy in the midst of ongoing illness.

For example, nonjudgmental self-observation is a hallmark of a variety of spiritual meditation practices and is thought to foster healing and balance by helping the practitioner to accept, see through, and dissolve destructive thoughts and emotions, revealing a whole and acceptable human being regardless of physical or psychological pain or disease (Kabat-Zinn, 2009). Spiritual practices like meditation, contemplative prayer, or mantra repetition are also used to help people focus on the present moment, rather than being distracted by the past or future. Kay Toombs (1995), reflecting on her experience living with multiple sclerosis, wrote:

> If healing is to be achieved, people with chronic illness have to learn to live fully in the present moment, neither preoccupied by dread of the future, frozen in the act of trying to recapture the past, nor overwhelmed by the everyday demands of debilitating illness and alienated by the experience of uncertainty. (p. 5)

Dwelling in the present moment and acceptance of things as they are (pain or joy, fear or hope) become important components to healing in multiple spiritual traditions and practices and may be seen as important complements to biomedical treatment. Likewise, reflective practice can facilitate a personal transformation of the provider, so that he or she is able to imagine better ways of responding to patients with chronic illness.

Viewing illness, vulnerability, and lament as normal parts of individual and collective life and as opportunities for spiritual cultivation and healing are vitally important. People with chronic illnesses can teach other people, health-care providers, and entire cultures how to integrate pain and uncertainty into an expanded view of spirituality and healing; an understanding not rooted in isolated control or cure. Walter Kleinman (2006) made a similar point when he stated

> ...after three decades of doing psychiatry and anthropology, I don't see any convincing evidence that facing up to our human condition leads to paralysis and pathology. Quite the opposite: seeing the world as dangerous and uncertain may lead to a quiet liberation, preparing us for new ways of being ourselves, living in the world, and making a difference in the lives of others. Surprisingly, confronting our fears can mean giving them up. (p. 10)

Kleinman is not naïve in his appraisal of the power of chronic illness experience to evoke responses of isolation, alienation, and bitterness; yet he also noted the capacity of subjective resilience that illness can instigate:

> The disabling consequences of the disease pathology and the responsiveness or resistance to treatment are influential here, yet what is most important is the patient's subjective self, the quality of their relationships, and the moral life they imagine can be fashioned out of pain and adversity. (p. 156)

The existential condition of vulnerability, pain, and fear often prompts resignation or alienation, yet it also presents opportunities for resolve and transformation. Health-care providers and systems must create new ways in which they can facilitate such resolve and transformation; rather than resignation or alienation both in themselves and among patients with chronic illness.

Victor Frankl (1984), a Jewish psychiatrist who survived Auschwitz, developed a theory of "tragic optimism" rooted in the human ability to discover meaning in every moment of living, regardless of the physical circumstances. Frankl argued that subjective meaning is only possible as a side effect of self-transcendence because meaning always points to something or someone other than oneself. This means that the relational or inter-human experience of love or kindness can be more meaningful and valuable than achieving an individual goal or objective. Physical pain and psychological anguish are more intense when combined with solitary isolation and impersonal social force and less intense when combined with even small acts of care or recognition. This insight has important implications for people living with chronic illness and their quest for healing. It also has significant implications for providers in their relationships with patients.

A powerful temptation, long recognized by diverse spiritual traditions, is to only find life meaningful when one is pain free, safe, healthy, self-sufficient or "normal." The temptation is fed by the illusion that it is possible to somehow free oneself from disease and pain, and is reinforced by the way our society views health and illness. The perpetual uncertainty associated with chronic illness experience may help people to overcome this temptation by recognizing the limits of measuring healing in terms of self-sufficiency or individual cure and the abundance of discovering healing in terms of relational dependency and care (Charmaz, 1983). A basic teaching at the core of spirituality is the recognition that human beings are never free from vulnerability and a need for support. Learning to welcome comfort or aid is a primary form of healing and renewal in human relationships. By recognizing their own dependency to receive healing and comfort from the kindness of others, the chronically ill might also become aware of the importance of responding to human neediness by opening out toward others in self-giving love. This type of healing is centered on the realization that tomorrow may or may not bring new medical treatment but that healing is available nonetheless through concrete acts of loving-kindness available in the present moment. It also creates a mutuality and equity in the patient–provider relationship; in which providers are not only helping patients but are also being helped by them to become better, more compassionate, and more effective in their practice.

Spiritual traditions tend to be grounded in stories of descending into chaos and transforming into new forms of life; feeling isolated by difficult circumstances and discovering meaning in new forms of awareness and relationship. Oliver Sacks (1991) articulated such an experience while he attended synagogue while recovering from an accident in which he lost all sensation in one of his limbs:

> Now, within the religious ceremonies and stories, I found a true parable for my own experience and condition—the experience of affliction and redemption, darkness and light, death and rebirth—the 'pilgrimage' which fortune, or my injury, had forced upon me. Now, as never before, I found relevance in the scriptural symbols and stories. I felt that my own story had the shape of such a universal existential experience, the journey of a soul into the underworld and back, a spiritual drama.... (pp. 146–147)

Spiritual awareness and practice seek to discover a means of maintaining grace, balance, or mindfulness in the midst of joy and pain, suffering and healing, as human life is sure to involve the full gamut of these experiences. In this context, the human community as a whole might be viewed as a chronically ill community where spirituality and healing are present in the midst of vulnerability, dependency, and the relational comfort and care that may result. In this context, providers and the health-care establishment are as much in need of ongoing healing as are sick people and populations.

Arthur Frank (1995) argued that the new self discovered or uncovered by the experience of chronic illness and the quest for healing is not isolated but connected, not autonomous but communicative, not centered on self but centered on self-with-others. Perhaps this is part of the wisdom, inherent in all spiritual traditions, stated positively as treating others as you would want to be treated and negatively as not treating others as you would not want to be treated. From this perspective, whatever blocks this fundamental relational reciprocity blocks healing and spiritual cultivation. Consequently, clinical relationships that are characterized by power imbalance and absence of mutuality may be blocking or even inhibiting the spiritual healing process, even when physical symptoms of the patient's chronic illness seem to be responding to a treatment regimen.

As an example of how the experience of chronic illness can move from a sense of alienation and isolation to a sense of wholeness and transformation, Walter Kleinman (2006) shares the story of Sally Williams. After a series of vocational and personal losses, Sally contracted AIDS while living as a homeless drug addict. Sally articulated that as long as she was preoccupied by her own selfish pain, her own isolated anguish and fear, and her unwillingness to experience anything beyond herself and her cravings, that she remained utterly lost and alone. Only when Sally was able to view herself as a whole person regardless of her circumstances, as someone who was not only larger than her illness but also a part of something larger than herself, was she able to begin a process of healing and renewal. Kleinman wrote,

> [Sally] insists that AIDS and drug abuse, and also poverty and violence and stigma, must be seen as part of all of our worlds. Only this way can we deal effectively with human misery and its sources. In her view, there is no place to hide. There can be no completely secure domain, safe from the dangers that beset most people. (p. 157)

Sally began to view existential vulnerability as an unavoidable element of the human condition, not as an isolated experience. All people are vulnerable to disease and pain in ways that are beyond self-control and all people are on a quest to create healing and renewal in their lives. When Sally began to see and act with the eyes of interconnection and relational reciprocity, she became open to new ways of experiencing, relating to, and being in the world. But why do so many patients have to seek this kind of healing path without support from the environments in which their physical disease is treated? Kleinman went on to say that Sally's spiritual healing is unusual—that many more people who live with chronic illness do not experience liberation but "loss, desperation, and failure cascading into bitterness, isolation, and withdrawal" (p. 156). Perhaps when health-care providers begin to openly acknowledge, as Kleinman did, that no technical terms or professional theories can equip them to deal with the messy human condition, they may be able to seek other means to facilitate spiritual healing.

Implications for the Practical Disciplines

Throughout this chapter references have been made to health care and health-care professionals, and the reader may ask why so much emphasis has been placed on systems and providers when the topic of inquiry is how spiritual practices and traditions can and do inform responses to chronic illness and individuals who have chronic illness. We respond to this potential query in two ways. First, we believe that our culture so values science and health care that faith in these often usurps spiritual faith, often to the detriment of patients' holistic well-being. Therefore, providers of health care have a responsibility to promote and attend to spiritual healing as part of holistic treatment of individuals with chronic illness. Second, we, in both scholarly and practice circles, have too long resided in rigid disciplinary silos and towers in which we blindly promote our own approach to the world and the people we encounter in it. But most people do not live in towers; and even scholars, scientists, and health-care providers leave their silos at the end of the day. It is imperative that we all begin to share and use what we know in ways that will transform the way we all understand our work (and our lives); and will transform the way we work together and live together. This entire volume represents an effort to move in this direction. Too often, references to domains of knowledge outside our own are usually negative or accusatory rather than constructive. Therefore, we hope the reader, whether she/he is a philosopher (as one of us is); a health-care provider (as is the other of us); or someone who lives with or loves someone with chronic illness (as we both do), will consider our reflections about how spirituality can inform society in matters of health care; and the practice of health-care systems and health-care providers, as well.

Concepts of spirituality may be used to inform societal and disciplinary worldviews to spark systemic and institutional change. Attention to spirituality requires attention to the inherent worth of each individual. This approach is not inconsistent with codes of ethics in many practice disciplines that cite values of beneficence, nonmaleficence, social justice, human dignity, and holism as ethical mandates. But the health-care system in the United States has evolved into a system in which profit, rather than patient well-being, has been the primary driver of care. This is not to say that individual providers are more interested in profit than they are in patient well-being; it simply acknowledges that a system rooted in profit has resulted in greater financial incentive to treating complications of disease rather than in preventing the disease. Wielawski (2006) observed, "Doctors and hospitals make more money amputating the limbs of poorly controlled diabetics, performing bypass surgery on patients with advanced heart disease and hospitalizing asthmatics than they do helping these patient avoid such acute exacerbations of underlying illness" (p. 3). Indeed, this perspective continues to be evidenced in how the current argument about health-care reform is framed. Health promotion and disease prevention are being touted primarily as ways to control cost, to save money, and to increase the economic security of the nation and the world. But this argument is inherently flawed, from a spiritual perspective, in that the primary motivator for change continues to be financial. Application of a spiritual framework requires attention to quality of life, human relationship, and human uniqueness over and beyond financial consideration. Otherwise, discussions about issues like health-care reform would quickly degrade into accusations about death panels, euthanasia, and denial of lifesaving treatment and care. Wielawski (2006) described efforts to transform health-care systems in terms "more like the rhetoric of the Prussian military strategist Carl von Clausewitz than modern health reform theory" (p. 3). Systems and providers that prioritize holistic well-being and healing place a priority on what patients with chronic illness face in their daily lives; and facilitate adjustment not only by prescribing medication and treatments, but also by considering how the same patients may need help with negotiating insurance and health-care bureaucracy, transportation, employment, daily chores, and feelings of social isolation and spiritual despair. Realistically, in our society prioritizing these things will probably require a systemic change in financial reimbursement strategies so that there is financial incentive for institutions and providers to spend more time with patients and to better coordinate care and resources outside the acute care setting. As it stands, as stated by a health-care executive, "We only get paid for illness . . . we pray for good flu seasons, we pray for big allergy seasons, because then our office visits go up and we get reimbursed" (Wielawski, 2006, p. 14). This reference to prayer offers a poignant glimpse into how our society deifies both money and health care.

If, as stated earlier, spirituality situates people in relational contexts that are wider and denser than the individual, then concepts of spirituality can also be used practically to inform patient care in a variety of ways, and health care can be seen as an avenue for spiritual transformation for both patients and providers. We see several main categories in which there is rich potential for influence and transformation: (1) Communication; (2) patient self-management; (3) systemic and institutional processes; and (4) personal perspectives of providers in practice. Addressing these broad areas can help providers be part of an environment that supports people with chronic illness in creating lives filled with meaning, purpose, and joy.

Communication is an ongoing and notorious challenge in patient–provider relationships. Widely disparate levels of education, social class, language use, and understandings of health and disease create relational gaps between patients and providers, as well. This gap may not seem like a barrier at all to providers, who in fact see a certain clinical distance as a personal protective factor in avoiding burnout and as essential to maintaining professional boundaries. But numerous studies have shown how essential communication is in improving outcomes in patients with chronic illness (Thorne, 2006). Thorne defined health-care communication as "the focal point at which information, attitudes, and agendas are communicated" (p. 4S). Thorne further discussed the wealth of research available to providers that can provide insight into what people with specific chronic illness struggle with on a day-to-day basis, and cites relevant communication as "a pivotal moment within which damage can be done or benefit can be gained" (p. 5S). Shaw (2007) stated that "patients believe that respectful interactions, where they feel they are listened to and believed by health-care professionals, are more important than having their symptoms alleviated" (p. 36).

So what kind of communication should characterize the interactions between patients and providers, and how does this kind of communication promote spiritual healing? Thorne (2006) recommended an attitudinal shift among providers in which they accept that no matter how compelling population-based evidence may be, that every patient is "confronted with the *n* of 1" (p. 7S), and should be honored as an individual, rather than as one more case of a disease in which the provider is expert. Patients reported that they have more relief from symptoms when listening to their own bodies than they do from following prescribed treatment (Price, 1993; Wellard, 1998). Therefore, when providers thoughtfully incorporate subjective individualized experiences of others into their explanations of standard protocols and treatments, patients will be given an additional set of tools with which to manage their responses to chronic illness. For example, Kralik et al. (2004) interviewed a patient who, because of pain and fatigue related to rheumatoid arthritis, could not pick up her grandchildren. It was not so much the pain and fatigue that troubled her, but the inability to put out her arms and pick up her grandchildren. This patient found new ways of relating to her grandchildren on a physical level, by sitting close to them and reading. Incorporating these kinds of life-based recommendations into their communications with patients will help providers promote less negative perceptions of the illness. Likewise, positive perspectives may be promoted when providers communicate about illness using positive metaphors (i.e. healing as gardening, or a journey) rather than negative ones (i.e. healing as war).

In addition, providers must recognize that chronic illness necessitates a long-term, ongoing clinical relationship. In such cases, closing the relational gap between them and their patients is critical. Closing the relational gap can be achieved relatively easily with just a few changes in the way communication is conducted during clinical encounters. Some of these include increasing the amount of time spent with these patients in clinical encounters; sitting down and engaging in open listening; identifying and referring to commonalities providers share with patients (such as a love of cooking or gardening, or a favored sports team); noting and remembering personal things about the patient (such as employment, children's names, a planned trip, a beloved pet, or favorite hobby) and asking about them during encounters; relevant and appropriate self-disclosure; open acknowledgement of the limits of science and the expertise of the patient in his or her own illness experience; and hearing, prioritizing, and responding to patients' descriptions of how their daily lives are affected by the illness, beyond clinical signs and symptoms (Green, 2012). Prioritizing the patient's experience may mean making recommendations and suggestions that fall outside the realm of clinical treatment to include addressing family relationships, accessing alternative therapies, and seeking spiritual solace. These recommendations may require providers to move beyond the conventional knowledge that has been used in the past and seek other sources of information, and resources beyond the usual clinical referral. When a patient must live with an illness on a day-to-day basis, to that patient, the provider becomes much more than an expert to be consulted episodically; he or she becomes a confidant, a friend, a family member. Like other close relationships, these relationships may include tension, unpleasantness, and struggles for control (Thorne, 2006, p. 9S), but they are more equitable, more meaningful, and more empowering to the patient. Hagerty and Patusky (2003) recommended a framework of relating in clinical interactions that includes more attention to the quality of "here-and-now" interactions and to the potential mutuality that exists in which the provider can be positively impacted by the patient. A sense of mutuality is positive for both the patient, who feels valued by the system and by the provider as more than just a source of income, and for the provider, who may realize that including patient perspectives in holistic care has the potential to reach far beyond the interaction that occurs in the clinical setting. The interaction gains meaning not just as a vehicle for treatment or cure, but as an opportunity for human relationship and spiritual healing.

New ways of communicating with patients require a different perspective on control. Though a great deal of lip-service is given to "patient-centered care" today, providers and systems are still decades behind in terms of relinquishing the control that true patient-centered care requires. Health-care professionals may even label assertive, knowledgeable patients as "demanding" (Shaw, 2007). Simply put, promoting spiritual healing of patients requires providers to relinquish control and allow patients to self-manage their chronic illness. What does self-management look like and how does it promote spiritual healing? Wagner et al (2001) quoted a colleague who described living with rheumatoid arthritis as similar to flying a small plane:

> If it is flown well, one gets where one wants to go with the exhilaration of mastering a complicated set of challenges. If it is flown badly, one either crashes or lands shakily at the wrong airport, reluctant to ever leave the ground again. The patient must be the pilot, because the other possible pilot, the health-care professional, is only in the plane a few hours every year, and this plane rarely touches the ground. (p. 66)

Helping the patient become a successful pilot requires the health-care professional to offer support and expertise "from the ground," so that patients have the confidence, knowledge, and skill to navigate the thrills and hazards they encounter "in the air." One recommendation by these authors was for providers to actively solicit patient perspectives and to provide clinical data and information to patients so that patients can set their own goals and solve their own problems. For example, rather than prescribing either an insulin pump or several daily injections of insulin because the provider feels that one or the other will better control blood glucose in a certain patient with diabetes, the provider can simply provide an explanation of the risks and benefits associated with each, and allow the patient to decide which will better fit his or her lifestyle. This kind of management requires frequent follow-up and more time and personal availability of providers, as patients try a variety of options to see which works best and as clinicians provide realistic information about potential sequelae. In the end, it also requires that the measurement of success may not be an A1C (hemoglobin measurement reflective of average blood glucose over a two to three month period) of less than 7 percent; but a patient's satisfaction that the treatment he or she has chosen is better accommodated into day-to-day life. Wagner made intriguing distinctions between interventions that are designed to improve outcomes among patients with chronic illness: "decision support" interventions, those aimed at improving the knowledge and skills of providers; and "self-management support," those aimed at improving the knowledge and skills of patients so they can successfully manage their own illness. Changing practice to promote self-management requires interventions directed at both provider and patient.

Self-management may facilitate a personal transformation in which "the burden of illness is replaced by the perception that it has enhanced the quality and meaning of life, by enabling people to experience life in a way that was previously inaccessible" (Kralik et al., 2004, p. 260). Kralik et al. mentioned specific ways in which patients could be encouraged to self-manage: (1) by recognizing and monitoring boundaries created by the illness; (2) by mobilizing psychological, physical, and material resources; (3) by managing the shift in identity; and (4) by balancing, pacing, planning, and prioritizing activities and events. These authors recommended that providers embrace processes in practice "that will facilitate interactions with clients without obstructing the diversity of perspectives, create an environment conducive to learning and engage individuals in identifying self-management strategies that have meaning in their lives" (p. 265). The interdisciplinary perspectives that are possible in healing chronic illness are manifest in this quote, in that the concept it represents seamlessly joins with our position that spirituality can be understood as an embodied dwelling in the world, a lived experience rooted in a holistic availability to learn and grow, to create meaning and purpose, from the dynamic relation among spirit, body, mind, other people, world, and multiple sources of transcendence.

Wagner et al. (2001) also identified categories of organizational and system-wide interventions that will improve patient outcomes. These new ways of identifying and labeling interventions is a first step to addressing ways in which poor outcomes result from inadequate, ineffective, or even harmful system behavior, not individual patient behavior. Though at first it may seem as though systemic barriers are not related to spiritual healing, we argue that from a holistic perspective, creating an integrated, holistic approach that allows chronic illness to be treated by providers and managed by patients must necessarily address the entire patient environment. We posit that an integrated, multidimensional approach to chronic illness will promote an environment for optimal healing: this approach must include institutions and systems that deliver care. If care is fragmented and one-dimensional, how can people with chronic illness thrive physically, emotionally, and spiritually in their everyday lives, incorporating illness as just one aspect of a rich and multifaceted life? Wagner et al. (2001) identified inherent systemic and institutional problems and policies that create for patients "obstacles in coping with their condition, not least of which is medical care that often does not meet their needs for effective clinical management, psychological support, and information" (p. 64). These authors identified one of the primary barriers to people with chronic illness as fragmentation of care; and made several recommendations for systemic and institutional change. These recommendations included more systemic emphasis on both communication and self-management; but also redesign of systems that reduces bureaucracy, emphasizes a model of chronic care rather than acute care, better networking among community agencies to assure access to resources, improved access to follow-up and decision-making support outside clinical settings, better interagency communication through use of technology, and more cohesive case management. Making some of these concrete systemic changes can create an environment that supports holistic healing, rather than contributing to suffering. But changing the institutions or systems in which health care is delivered is largely dependent on the perspectives of the individuals practicing within them.

All of the implications we have identified for health-care providers require some measure of personal transformation. Research has shown that health-care providers often approach people with chronic illness with negative attitudes about patients and illness. Shaw (2007) stated that providers may stereotype patients; and make value judgments about whether or not they are worthy of care or whether they have participated appropriately in the prescribed treatment regimen. Providers may blame patients for their illness or failure to recover, and may treat patient reports of their experience or symptoms with suspicion or disbelief, or discount them as malingering. They may shame patients who are deemed noncompliant. Shaw (2007) used the example of reality television shows in which obese "participants are confronted with their problems, put through a challenging regimen to be reformed, monitored throughout and then confess that they realize how aberrant they were and how they have been converted to a healthy way of life" (p. 38). In this medium, health professionals are "presented as experts, monitors and judges of success or failure" (p. 38). Too often, this is how health-care professionals perform and are perceived in real-life clinical settings.

How can concepts of spirituality inform and transform individuals who practice within health-care systems and who treat people with chronic illness? Engaging in personal reflection and reflective practice are at the heart of transforming providers' approaches to the care they deliver and the patients they care for. What is reflective practice? Taylor (2010) defined reflection as "cognitive acts such as thinking, contemplation, meditation and any other forms of attentive consideration, in order to make sense of them, and to make contextually appropriate changes if they are required" (p. 6). Reflective processes can be used by health-care professionals, Taylor went on to say, "to identify the 'truth' of what they do, so they can recognize the traps they fall into routinely, in resorting to unexamined habits to get them through their work" (p. 7). One such unexamined habit is the way health-care providers use concepts of normal, as discussed early in this chapter, but there are countless other routines, habits, and concepts that are ripe for reflection. Reflective practice is what prompts both providers and patients to begin a process of spiritual liberation from ideals, concepts, understandings, and habits that ensnare us.

What specific activities can help health-care providers be more reflective, and begin to change the way they approach the care of patients with chronic illness? Taylor (2010) recommended that providers first identify work constraints (things that they perceive as inhibiting) to the caring relationship with patients: economic, historical, political, social, and personal constraints. Part of this process includes attention to personal tendencies that health-care providers often struggle with, such as self-blame, desire for perfection, and difficulty being assertive. In addition, it is important to acknowledge differences in ideal and real practice expectations, barriers to patient advocacy, and challenges with collegial relationships. Taking the time to think about these things also allows opportunity to imagine how things could be better. Taylor recommended a number of creative activities that promote creative reflection such as journaling, listening to music, drawing, writing poetry, singing, or making pottery. Reflection also requires reflective disposition in which one is purposefully prepared, thoughtful, open, accepting of insight and changing awareness, and tenacious in maintaining the reflective process. Reflection is a deeply spiritual process that can help providers reimagine habitual approaches to patients and traditional understandings about illness, health, and cure.

CONCLUSIONS

The quest for isolated individual cure, so central to the acute care medical restitution narrative and some religious narratives, makes little sense in the context of relational reciprocity and ill prepares all people for the task of living with vulnerability, sickness, pain, and dependency. People tend to think that no amount of pain or disease is acceptable. Consequently, many people spend a great deal of time and energy fighting pain, fighting illness, rather than attempting to learn from them and live with them in a meaningful way. The effort to avoid pain and deny vulnerability contributes to widespread social problems like drug and alcohol abuse, eating disorders, violence, sedentary lives, and a futile quest for isolated independence. In this context, individuals with chronic illness have a lot to teach others about how to experience healing in the midst of pain, vulnerability, or uncertainty; how to embrace connection and relational reciprocity; how to view themselves and their pain as part of a broader communal dynamic that is wider and denser than the individual. Health-care systems and providers have an obligation to hear their stories and incorporate new meanings and new understandings of healing into a more holistic plan of care that promotes well-being in patients' daily lives.

As people with chronic illnesses encounter boundary situations that take them to the limits of their medical, cultural, religious, or personal coping responses, they may shift existing strategies for addressing their issues and become open to making significant changes. Learning to live well with ongoing illness, whether conceptualized as quality of life, coping skills, holistic health and well-being, or some other concepts described in conjunction with chronic illness, often results in a person questioning their existence and purpose in life and working toward acquiring a new sense of meaning and understanding. Health-care systems and providers should seek ways to ease these boundary crossings, rather than creating an additional set of hurdles to cross.

References

Arora, K. (2009). "Models of understanding chronic illness: Implications for pastoral theology and care." *The Journal of Pastoral Theology, 19*(1), 22–37.

Barnes, L. & Sered, S. (2005). *Religion and healing in America.* Oxford: Oxford University Press.

Bishop, M. (2005). "Quality of life and psychological adaptation to chronic illness and disability: Preliminary analysis of a conceptual and theoretical synthesis." *Rehabilitation Counseling Bulletin, 48,* 219–231.

Bouma, G. (2000). "Spirituality and religion," in M. Poole & R. Jureidini (eds). *Sociology: Australian connections.* Sydney: Allen and Unwin.Centers for Disease Control and Prevention. (2009). Chronic diseases at a glance: The power to prevent, the call to control. Retrieved from http://www.cdc.gov/nccdphp/publications/ AAG/pdf/chronic.pdf.Charmaz, K. (1983). Loss of self: A fundamental form of suffering in the chronically ill. *Sociology of Health and Illness* 5(2), 168–195.

Charmaz, K. (1991). *Good days, bad days: The self in chronic illness and in time.* NewBrunswick, NJ: Rutgers University Press.

Charmaz, K. (1995). "The body, identity, and self: Adapting to impairment." *The Sociological Quarterly, 36,* 657–680.

Cook, C. C. H. (2004). "Addiction and spirituality." *Addiction, 99,* 539–551.

Eastland, L. S., Herndon, S. L. & Barr, J. (eds). (1999). *Communication in recovery: Perspectives on twelve-step groups.* Cresskill, NJ: Hampton Press, Inc.

Fasching, D. & Dechant, D. (eds). (2001). *Comparative religious ethics: A narrative approach.* Malden, MA: Blackwell Publishing.

Frank. A. (1991). *At the will of the body: Reflections on illness.* Boston: Houghton Mifflin.

Frank. A. (1995). *The wounded story teller: Body, illness and ethics.* Chicago: University of Chicago Press.

Frankl, V. (1984). *Man's search for meaning.* New York: NY: Simon & Schuster.

Garland-Thompson, R. (1994). "Redrawing the boundaries of feminist disability studies." *Feminist Studies, 20,* 586.

Garrett, C. (2001). "Sources of hope in chronic illness." *Health Sociology Review, 10*(2): 99–108.

Garrett, C. (2002). "Spirituality and healing in the sociology of chronic illness." *Health Sociology Review, 11*(1–2), 61–69.

Gockel, A. (2009). "Spirituality and the process of healing: A narrative study." *The International Journal for the Psychology of Religion, 19,* 217–230.

Green, R. (2012). *African American parents' experiences in their children's health care encounters* (Doctoral dissertation). Retrieved from Kennesaw State University DigitalCommons: http://digitalcommons.kennesaw.edu/etd/498.

Hagerty, B. & Patusky, K. (2003). "Reconceptualizing the nurse-patient relationship." *Journal of Nursing Scholarship, 35*(2), 145–150.

Hawkins, H. (1993). *Reconstructing illness: Studies in pathography.* West Lafayette, Indiana: Purdue University Press.

Kabat-Zinn, J. (2009). *Full catastrophe living: Using the wisdom of the body and mind to facestress, pain and illness.* New York: NY: Bantam Dell.

Kaye, J. & Raghavan, S. K. (2002). "Spirituality in disability and illness." *Journal of Religion and Health*, 41(3): 231–242.Kleinman, A. (2006). *What really matters: Living a moral life amidst uncertainty and danger.* Oxford: Oxford University Press.

Kleinman, A. (1988). *The illness narratives.* New York: Basic Books.

Koenig, H., King, D. & Carson, V. (eds). (2012). *Handbook of religion and health: Second edition.* New York: Oxford University Press.

Koenig, H. (2005). Afterword: A physician's reflections. In L. Barnes & S. Sered (Eds). *Religion and Healing in American.* Oxford: Oxford University Press, 505–507.Koenig, H. G. (2000). "Religion, spirituality and medicine: Application to clinical practice." *Journal of the American Medical Association*, 284, 1708–1731.

Kohn, L. (2007). "Daoyin: Chinese healing exercises." *Asian Medicine*, 3, 103–129.

Kralik, D., Koch, T., Price, K. & Howard, N. (2004). "Chronic illness self-management: Taking action to create order." *Journal of Clinical Nursing*, 13, 259–267.

Krok, D. (2008). "The role of spirituality in coping: Examining the relationships between spiritualdimensions and coping styles." *Mental Health, Religion & Culture*, 11(7), 643–653.

Livneh, H. & Antonak, R. F. (2005). "Psychosocial adaptation to chronic illness disability: Aprimer for counselors." *Journal of Counseling & Development*, 83, 12–20.

Longmore, P. & Umansky, L. (eds). (2001). *The new disability history: Americanperspectives.* New York and London: New York University Press.

Lynn, J. & Adamson, D. (2003). *Living well at the end of life: adapting health care to seriouschronic illness in old age* [White Paper]. Retrieved from The Washington Home Centerfor Palliative Care Studies: http://www.rand.org/pubs/white_papers/WP137.htmlMcCollum, A. (1994). Roundtable discussion women with disabilities: A Challenge to feminist theology." *Journal of Feminist Studies in Religion*, 10(2), 122–129.

McColman, C. (1997). *Where body and soul encounter the sacred.* Georgetown, Massachusetts: North Star Publications.

McNulty, K., Livneh, H. & Wilson, L. M. (2004). "Perceived uncertainty, spiritual well-being, and psychosocial adaptation in individuals with multiple sclerosis." *Rehabilitation Psychology*, 49, 91–99.

Moss, P. & Dyck, I. (1999). "Body, corporeal space, and legitimating chronic illness: Women diagnosed with M.E." *Antipode*, 31(4), 372–397.

Nichols, L. & Hunt, B. (2011). "The significance of spirituality for individuals with chronic illness: Implications for mental health counseling." *Journal of Mental Health Counseling*, 33(1), 51–66.

Price, M. (1993). "Exploration of body listening: Health and physical awareness in chronic illness." *Advances in Nursing Science*, 15(4), 37–52.

Register, C. (1978). *Living with chronic illness: Days of patience and passion.* New York: The Free Press.

Reynolds, T. (2008). *Vulnerable communion: A theology of disability and hospitality.* Grand Rapids, MI: Brazos Press.

Sacks, O. (1991). *A leg to stand on.* London: Picador. Scheper-Hughes N. & Lock, M. (1986). "Speaking 'truth' to illness: Metaphors, reification, and a pedagogy for patients." *Medical Anthropology Quarterly*, 17(5), 137–140.

Schumm, D. & Stoltzfus, M. (2011). "Beyond models: Some tentative Daoist contributions to disability studies," in D. Schumm & M. Stoltzfus (eds). *Disability and religious diversity: Cross-cultural and interreligious perspectives*. New York, NY: Palgrave Macmillan, 103–122.

Schumm, D. & Stoltzfus, M. (2011). "Chronic illness and disability: Narratives of suffering and healing," in D. Schumm & M. Stoltzfus (eds), *Disability and religious diversity: Cross-cultural and interreligious perspectives*. New York, NY: Palgrave Macmillan, 159–175.

Schutz, A. (1962). "Symbol, reality, and society," in M. Natanson (ed.). *The problem of social reality: Collected papers I*. The Hague: Martinus Nijhoff, 287–339.

Schutz, A. & Luckman, T. (1983). *The structures of the lifeworld: Volume II*. Trans. R. Zaner & D. Parent. Evanston, IL: Northwestern University Press.

Sharts-Hopko, N. C. (2003). "Spirituality and health care," in J.T. Catalano (ed.). *Nursing now: Today's issues, tomorrows trends* (2nd ed). Philadelphia: F.A. Davis, 347–371.

Shaw, S. (2007). "Responding appropriately to patients with chronic illness." *Nursing Standard, 21*(24), 35–39.

Simundson, D. J. (2001). *Faith under fire: How the bible speaks to us in times of suffering*. Lima, Ohio: Academic Renewal Press.

Stanley, R. (2009). "Neurobiology of chakras and prayer." *Zygon, 4*(44), 825–846.

Stoll, R. I. (1989). "The essence of spirituality," in V. B. Carson (ed.). *Spiritual dimensions of nursing practice*. Philadelphia: Saunders, 4–23.

Stone, S. D. (1995). "The myth of bodily perfection." *Disability and Society, 10*, 413–424.

Sawatzky, R., Ratner, P. A. & Chiu, L. (2005). "A meta-analysis of the relationship between spirituality and quality of life." *Social Indicators Research, 72*, 153–188.

Taylor, B. (2010). *Reflective practice for healthcare professionals*. Berkshire: UK: Open University Press.

Thorne, S. (2006). "Patient-provider communication in chronic illness: a health promotion window of opportunity." *Family & Community Health, 29*(1S), 4S–11S.

Toombs, K. (1995). "Chronic illness and the goals of medicine." *Second Opinion, 21*(1), 11–22.1

Thompson, C. J. (2003). "Natural health discourse and the therapeutic production of consumer resistance." *The Sociological Quarterly, 44*(1), 81–107.

Wagner, E., Austin, B., Davis, C., Hindmarsh, M., Schaefer, J. & Bonomi, A. (2001). "Improving chronic illness care: Translating evidence into action." *Health Affairs, 20*(6), 64–78.

Wellard, S. (1998). "Constructions of chronic illness." *International Journal of Nursing Studies, 35*, 49–55.

Wendell, S. (1996). *The rejected body: Feminist philosophical reflections on disability*. New York: Routledge.

Wendell, S. (2001). "Unhealthy disabled: Treating chronic illnesses as disabilities." *Hypatia, 16*(4), 17–33.

Wielawski, I. (2006). "Improving chronic illness care," in S. Isaacs & J. Rickman (eds). *To improve health and health care*. Princeton, NJ: The Robert Wood Johnson Foundation, vol. X, 1–17.

Wills, M. (2007). "Connection, action and hope: An invitation to reclaim the 'spiritual' in health care." *Journal of Religion and Health, 46*(3), 423–436.

CHAPTER 2

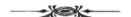

SPIRITUAL DIRECTION AS PSYCHOSPIRITUAL CARE FOR WOMEN WITH AUTOIMMUNE DISEASES

Kelly Arora

By the time I was in my mid 40's, I had established a career in Clinical Social Work; was comfortable with God and my faith of Quakerism; was married to my college sweetheart—with two healthy wonderful children, the home of our dreams, a Golden Retriever, and even two cars! I was set.

Then, in one dramatic 24-hour period, it all began to unravel. Within a short span of time, I was diagnosed first with Lupus SLE then with Parkinson's: two life threatening, chronic diseases. At first, I tried to manage the chaos that the Lupus brought to our lives, all on my own. Within a short time, however, I was driven to the use of drugs and psychiatry for depression when, two years into the diagnosis, the Lupus inflamed my kidneys and my very life was suddenly on the line. It was after stabilizing on an experimental chemotherapy, that I stumbled across "Spiritual Direction" and knew instinctively and immediately that that was my door to sanity, even as I had no idea what spiritual direction really was. In that critical moment, I knew only that I was exhausted, and that therapy could not touch the pain I was in—it was spiritual. I was spinning helplessly—in increasingly tight circles—desperate for relief from relentless questions:

WHERE WAS GOD?

WHAT HAD I DONE TO DESERVE THIS?!

HOW COULD I LIVE WITH THIS MEDICAL NIGHTMARE?

*MY FAMILY SHOULD NOT HAVE TO LIVE WITH THIS LEVEL
OF CHAOS AND LOSS—IT IS NOT FAIR!! WHY ME?!*

GOD HAS BETRAYED ME!!

*Spiritual direction has done nothing short of quieting me down, helping
me to grow up and into my new reality, creating a container for my fears
and extreme panic, and bringing me home to myself and my God. Spiritual direction has transformed my life to one of possibilities out of my now
deepened and renewed relationship with the God-of-my-understanding.*

(Karp, 2010)[1]

This true account illustrates how one woman (I call her Cindy) discovered
the power of spiritual direction to help her cope with her illness experiences.[2] Like the millions of other Americans who live with chronic diseases,
Cindy faces numerous challenges coping with her health conditions on a day-to-day basis, including management of their physical, psychological, social,
and spiritual dimensions. Women who have chronic diseases typically receive
medical care for their physical needs, but psychospiritual struggles associated with their illness experiences are frequently neglected. This chapter
introduces spiritual direction as a long-term strategy to meet the unique
psychospiritual needs of women who have chronic diseases—particularly
autoimmune conditions.

An estimated 14–22 million Americans—75 percent of whom are
women—have autoimmune disorders, incurable conditions in which the
body attacks itself (for example, rheumatoid arthritis attacks connective tissues, primarily at the joints) (Grytten et al., 2006; "Increasing incidence
of rheumatoid arthritis in women," 2008; Uramoto, 1999). Because there
are more than 80 kinds of autoimmune disorders, I focus on three prevalent diseases with similar characteristics: rheumatoid arthritis (RA), multiple
sclerosis (MS), and systemic lupus erythematosus (lupus). With these conditions, symptoms such as pain and fatigue are common and may remain
relatively constant, or they may appear in force during flares or exacerbations that are buffered by periods of remission. As Cindy's story illustrates,
another common experience associated with autoimmune disease is depression, which affects 27–47 percent of women with MS (Pakenham & Cox,
2009, p. 374) and 13–42 percent of people who have RA (Margaretten
et al., 2009, p. 1586). Over 50 percent of people with lupus have psychological struggles and depressive symptoms as a result of that disease (Giffords,
2003, p. 64).

A review of the literature reveals a number of reasons for the high incidence
of depression and other mental health issues associated with autoimmune
diseases. The contributing factors include the unpredictability of the diseases,
side effects of medications (particularly steroids, which are often used to help
patients cope with flares), changes in a woman's appearance, chronic pain,
and losses (see, for example, Giffords, 2003; Keefe et al., 2002). The effects

of autoimmune disease are so emotionally wearing that one study found that "cancer patients were less demoralized by their illness and reported more benefits from it than did patients with lupus. Cancer patients were also less emotionally distressed and reported less pain" (Katz et al., 2001, p. 570).

Experiences of chronic pain, chronic fatigue, and depression can create isolating barriers between the affected person and the outside world. Not only do these experiences make it more difficult to physically engage with others or participate in meaningful activities—including spiritual practices—but these experiences further burden a person psychologically (for example, fatigue heightens experiences of stress) and spiritually (for example, prompting the quintessential question of meaning: Why me?).

Psychospiritual Struggles

Not all women would describe themselves or their experiences as *spiritual*, which is a notoriously "fuzzy" term often confused with *religious* (Zinnbauer et al., 1997). In this chapter, I broadly define spirituality as the lived beliefs, values, and practices that help people make meaning of the world and their purpose in it, including their search for and connection with that which is sacred. For the purposes of this chapter, the sacred encompasses concepts of God, Allah, Brahmin, and other names for theistic understandings of a divine force, as well as nontheistic understandings of that which is transcendent or greater than the self, as might be described in Buddhist or secular spiritualties (for example, ultimate Truth or the highest good). In spite of the idiosyncratic and organic ways that women with chronic illnesses necessarily approach self-management of their conditions over time, living with an incurable condition raises questions of meaning (Schulman-Green et al., 2012, p. 141) and/or affects a woman's sense of connection to that which she calls sacred. The psychospiritual care provided in spiritual direction addresses these dimensions of the illness experience, and therefore, may benefit any woman, irrespective of her self-identification as a spiritual or religious person.

Because symptoms of pain, fatigue, and depression are often invisible, women with autoimmune diseases may appear to others as healthy individuals. On days when disease activity is low, they may also feel and identify as healthy. When the illness reasserts itself, they may re-inhabit the sick role. This ongoing experience of being neither fully healthy nor fully sick—and at the same time, both healthy and sick—has been described by Paterson (2001) as "shifting perspectives": vacillation between times of *illness-in-the-foreground* (IITF) and *wellness-in-the-foreground* (WITF). Illness-in-the-foreground is "characterized by a focus on the sickness, suffering, loss, and burden associated with living with a chronic illness" (p. 23). The focus on day-to-day needs leaves few resources for psychospiritual adaptation. Wellness-in-the-foreground describes times when a woman is not consumed by coping with disease. During times of WITF, she is better able to consider questions of meaning and evaluate coping strategies for the future (Paterson, 2001, p. 23). Awareness of how these experiential shifts affect a woman's ability to cope can help women and their caregivers more effectively address the ongoing psychospiritual concerns associated with chronic health conditions.

In addition to navigating the liminal experience of shifting perspectives, women with RA, MS, and lupus also face many disease-related losses over time. Psychospiritual losses may be associated with a woman's identity, relationships, self-agency, and spiritual beliefs and practices (for example, see Irvine et al., 2009; Philip et al., 2009; Russell et al., 2006; Tang & Anderson, 1999). After her diagnoses, Cindy often felt her new role as patient engulfed her identities as a mother, wife, and professional caregiver. She also noticed the increasing absences of friends whose empathic reserves were depleted from coping with her health crises, and she lost her ability to make sense of the world as she felt abandoned by the just, benevolent, and all-powerful God she had known since childhood.

Like many other women with chronic health conditions, Cindy did not grieve her losses. Suppressed or disenfranchised grief happens when "there is no socially acceptable way of expressing [the loss] and having the physical and psychological experience acknowledged" (Wendell, 1996, p. 40). In general, chronic illness lacks cultural guidelines for what is and is not an "appropriate" loss or an "appropriate" expression of grief[3]—guidelines that extend beyond the differences in mourning identified with cultural groups, gender, and social class (Doka & Martin, 2002, pp. 339–340).

When women who have autoimmune conditions; their families, friends, and social networks; and the cultural milieu in which they live explicitly and/or implicitly suppress expression of loss, the losses become disenfranchised. Spiritual losses in particular are frequently disenfranchised because spiritual dimensions of illness are marginalized within the predominant biomedical context of health care in the United States. The burden of disenfranchised losses can lead to or exacerbate other psychospiritual struggles. In order to limit the potential for disenfranchised losses, women with autoimmune diseases need to share experiences of new and ongoing losses. The ability to lament losses and have losses be supportively acknowledged (not ignored, diminished, or judged), particularly during times when the illness asserts itself, can help a woman sustain her connection with that which is sacred and restore her sense of overall well-being.

Shifting perspectives and disenfranchised losses are two catalysts for psychospiritual struggles. In addition, meaning making about the illness may present as a spiritual struggle or "spiritual crisis" (Agrimson & Taft, 2008, p. 454; Doka, 2009; Fitchett et al., 2004; Fitchett & Risk, 2009). Illness-related meaning making may include reflections on suffering, good and evil, culpability, justice, and personal understandings of and relationship to the sacred (for example, Becker, 1999, p. 65; Reynolds & Prior, 2003, p. 1238; Rowe & Allen, 2004, p. 62; Russell et al., 2006, p. 66). Spiritual struggles are not necessarily problematic. In fact, some faith traditions see such spiritual struggles as an essential component of personal growth,[4] and contemporary psychological studies affirm a positive relationship between loss and posttraumatic growth (Calhoun & Tedeschi, 2001; McConnell & Pargament, 2006, p. 1471). However, longitudinal studies now show that "getting stuck" in spiritual struggles can negatively affect a person's health and sense of well-being (Pargament et al., 2004, p. 727; Trevino et al., 2010, p. 386).

Cindy's story illustrates how "relentless" questions can become problematic. Like many women with RA, MS, and lupus, Cindy found it difficult to cope with the full lived reality of her chronic illness experiences. She was "exhausted . . . [in] pain . . . desperate," and unable to resolve fractured understandings of God. Cindy did not find relief for her struggles within the traditional health care system; she needed a unique approach to cope with the psychospiritual dimension of her illnesses.

Psychospiritual Care for Women with Autoimmune Diseases

Women who have acute physiological conditions can usually find adequate care for their concerns within the dominant biomedical system because short-lived health problems generally do not precipitate ongoing losses or chronic psychospiritual struggles. However, the strength of the biomedical model's short-term, problem-centered focus on curing, a focus that works so well within the acute care context, does little to address needed relief of ongoing psychospiritual suffering associated with chronic diseases. Furthermore, even though many patients want to talk about spiritual concerns, biomedical health care providers usually are not equipped, available, or eager to discuss spiritual issues with their patients (Badaracco, 2007, pp. 120–121; MacLean et al., 2003).

As a clinical social worker, Cindy was aware of a variety of resources to help her cope with her health concerns. She saw a psychiatrist for treatment of depression, but this caregiving relationship did not address the spiritual dimensions of her life with chronic illnesses. Indeed, psychotherapeutic professionals typically do not explicitly talk about spirituality with their clients.[5] Even though spiritually integrated psychotherapy groups engage spiritual concerns, their typical short-term format (6–10 weeks) does not provide ongoing opportunities for women to focus on their evolving relationships with the sacred (Pargament, 2007, p. 325). Pastoral care, pastoral counseling, and chaplaincy explicitly deal with spiritual concerns, but they are also short-term care strategies (often one conversation and rarely more than eight sessions) that do not provide ongoing attention to a person's relationship with the sacred in times of both IITF and WITF (for example, Townsend, 2009; Vander Zee, 2002).

Contemporary spiritual direction,[6] however, is a long-term practice in which at least two people meet regularly—normally once per month for an hour, often over the course of years—to focus on a person's relationship with the sacred. The long-term nature of the relationship and the primary focus on the sacred set the spiritual direction apart from other caregiving relationships. Cindy testified that spiritual direction met her psychospiritual needs in ways other caregiving approaches did not. She discovered that her spiritual director was able to help her lament and acknowledge losses and make meaning of her illness experiences while monitoring the risks posed by getting stuck in chronic struggles.

Over the centuries, spiritual direction has been characterized by silence, contemplation, prayer, and discernment (for example, Cassian, trans. 1997). Today the practice has been enriched by modern psychological understandings of human behavior. In a typical one-on-one spiritual direction session, director and directee collaborate with each other and the sacred in contextual, constructive meaning making. They seek to articulate how the directee understands her experiences, how she understands the sacred, and how she will respond as a result of these understandings. In a group spiritual direction model, each member of the group (typically 3–5 individuals) may function as director when the focus of contemplative discernment within the group moves from one directee to another.

Spiritual directors companion a diverse population of directees, not all of whom share their beliefs or spiritual background. Directors are able to offer a type of intercultural spiritual care[7] through the practice of *not-knowing*: setting aside their own beliefs, values, and biases in order to privilege the directee's experiences and beliefs (Arora, 2011). Not-knowing also helps directors attend to the distinctive ways each woman lives with her illness. To illustrate, Cindy's spiritual director (I call her Jane) recognizes that Cindy's illness experiences take precedence over Jane's knowledge about lupus and Parkinson's disease and their treatments, Jane's expectations of people with chronic health conditions, and Jane's personal experiences of illness. During their sessions together, Jane intentionally and continually notices and sets aside her beliefs, focusing on Cindy's experiences and understandings. Jane is also careful not to impose on Cindy her understandings of the sacred or suffering. At the same time, Jane remains aware that Cindy may hold beliefs that disrupt her relationship with God,[8] beliefs Jane can help Cindy examine and reconstruct if needed.

NARRATIVE PRACTICES

Women with autoimmune diseases may find that simply telling their stories has a healing effect, especially when they share their narratives with someone who listens mindfully, is present to suffering and lament, and acknowledges experiences of loss. The emerging field of narrative medicine recognizes that

> medicine practiced with narrative competence will more ably recognize patients and diseases, convey knowledge and regard, join humbly with colleagues, and accompany patients and their families through the ordeals of illness. These capacities will lead to more human, more ethical, and perhaps more effective care.
>
> (Charon, 2006, p. vii)

Narrative healing is at the heart of spiritual direction, where stories— "spiritual direction is *always* storytelling" (Guenther, 1992, p. 32)—can be told, reinforced, and/or reconstructed safely and confidentially.

Particularly during times of illness-in-the-foreground, a pressing concern for women with autoimmune diseases is lamenting their losses. As noted, it is critical for women with chronic illnesses to have losses heard and acknowledged in order to prevent disenfranchisement and chronic spiritual struggles. "Venting" is helpful, but there is more to be gained in sharing one's illness narrative: studies show that people who derive the greatest healing benefits from sharing their stories are those people who also make meaning of their experiences (for example, Affleck et al., 1987, p. 927).

During times of crisis (such as times when illness is in the foreground), people cope within the context of their embedded meaning-making systems—the beliefs, values, and practices they have carried with them from childhood and young adulthood, often without the benefit of critical reflection. When their embedded beliefs and practices cannot address the depth and/or breadth of their suffering, people experience spiritual struggles until they are able to reconstruct their meaning systems in ways that accommodate their lived experiences, or they disengage from that which is sacred and meaningful in their lives (Pargament, 2007, p. 62). Generally speaking, people are more receptive to, and able to engage in, meaning reconstruction when the time of crisis (IITF) has passed (shifted to WITF), even though times of crisis may highlight the need for such challenging inner work (Klitzman, 2012, p. 136).

Women with chronic health conditions may be most able to reflect on and reconstruct their understandings and practices related to the sacred during times of wellness-in-the-foreground. In typical medical, psychotherapeutic, or short-term spiritual care relationships that focus on crisis resolution, a woman would not typically see a caregiver during times of WITF, diminishing her chances of engaging in valuable meaning making. Spiritual direction, however, is a particularly supportive context for this healing work because director and directee meet during times of IITF *and* WITF.

Spiritual directors facilitate meaning making in the context of stories shared, reinforced, and/or reconstructed safely and confidentially (Bidwell, 2004). Director and directee seek to recognize and interpret connections to the sacred within the directee's narrative. They also seek to understand the meaning of the directee's story in relationship to the sacred, and they determine appropriate responses to these understandings. Narrative reconstruction results in a tentative, yet hope-filled, script for the next chapter in the directee's life story.[9]

In Cindy's case, her narrative was one of confusion and desperation as she tried to understand how a just God (Cindy's embedded image of the sacred) could punish her with two incurable diseases (Cindy's life-limiting interpretation of why she has these health conditions). Because Cindy's experiences of suffering and loss were the focus of her narrative when she met with Jane for the first time, Jane realized that Cindy was in a time of IITF. In response, Jane intentionally provided a safe space for Cindy to describe and mourn her losses and struggles. As Cindy's laments were heard and acknowledged in supportive ways, Cindy was able to reflect on her embedded understandings of God.

Through complex, co-constructive meaning making with Jane over time, Cindy was eventually able to transform life-limiting feelings of personal blame for her illnesses into life-enhancing understandings of illness as an opportunity to learn from and grow stronger in her relationship with a God who was with her in her suffering.[10] It should be noted that if Cindy and Jane's work together stopped at an intellectual level with narrative reconstruction, Cindy might not have experienced the full benefits of new life-enhancing understandings of the sacred. Her coping strategies and spiritual practices also needed to be transformed so that she did not unconsciously reinforce life-limiting beliefs still embedded in existing strategies and practices.

RITUAL PRACTICES

The illness-in-the-foreground and wellness-in-the-foreground perspectives of chronic illness play important roles in helping a woman live well with autoimmune disease. An IITF perspective can prompt a woman to actively attend to her physical needs, such as protecting her body from further irreparable damage by adjusting her activity level, taking appropriate medications, or seeing her doctor for evaluation. During times of WITF, a woman can focus on and develop a strong, holistic self-identity that is not subsumed by illness, but does not deny her health condition either.

Illness-in-the-foreground and wellness-in-the-foreground can also be disadvantageous to a woman's long-term overall well-being. The potential exists for women in WITF experiences to engage in behavior that actually exacerbates health problems in the long run. For example, she might overexert herself, skip medications, put off doctor visits, take on more responsibility than she will later be able to manage, or deny losses. Functioning within an IITF perspective can also threaten her well-being. It might reinforce identification with the sick role and attendant abdication of self-agency, making it difficult for her to engage in spiritual disciplines, or emphasizing the lack of control she feels she has over her body (Mehl-Madrona, 2003, p. 219; Paterson, 2001, pp. 23–24). In order to "liv[e] with illness without living solely for it" (Charmaz, 1991, p. 661), a woman needs a strong self-identity that asserts itself during both IITF and WITF perspectives. Spiritual direction can help women negotiate these shifting perspectives to maintain realistic, holistic, and healthy ways of living with illness and to sustain her relationship with the sacred in all of her illness experiences.

People often use metaphors to describe illness (for example, battle, war, invasion, bomb, or storm) and even personify illness (calling it an enemy, intruder, bug, wolf, bully, or terrorist). Such imagery suggests that during times when illness is in the foreground, illness not only dominates the woman's attention, but it also affects her identity. In other words, IITF perspectives may trigger shifts in her identity from woman, mother, wife, friend, and/or professional to warrior, protector, or exterminator—identities that reinforce the chosen metaphor and focus on illness and the body. In some health situations, such as preparing for surgery or undergoing chemotherapy, imagery that suggests a woman is defending her body from threat may help marshal energies in ways that promote healing or effective coping (Achterberg et al., 1994, pp. 37–55). Although taking on disease as an enemy in a particular battle may be helpful, engaging in an ongoing war against an incurable disease—an enemy that cannot be vanquished—is not a life-enhancing strategy for the long term.

Women with autoimmune disease need a strong, consistent sense of self that does not acquiesce to illness and that supports their connection to the sacred. Spiritual direction can facilitate the transformation of life-diminishing illness metaphors to metaphors that work with the body and strengthen an integrated self-identity. Helping women optimize their awareness of IITF and WITF perspectives through ritually facilitated transitions in the spiritual direction encounter is one way to work toward the construction and conservation of a strong self-identity. Incorporating ritual into spiritual direction to intentionally manage shifts in wellness/illness perspectives may also help alleviate concerns that illness will dominate the spiritual direction session or a woman's life between sessions.

Traditionally, ritual is understood as practices that facilitate shifts from ordinary time and space to sacred time and space in order to affect personal and communal transformation in relationship with the sacred (Kinsley, 1996, p. 121; Smith, 1980, pp. 124–125). Ritual also helps people realize ideals, hopes, values, and beliefs through the embodied integration of thought and action (Bell, 1987, pp. 97–98). Rituals need not be complex. In fact, the simplest rituals are often the most effective (Hogue, 2003, p. 139; Mitchell & Anderson, 1983, p. 142).

Like narratives, rituals tell a story with a definitive beginning, middle, and end (Hogue, 2003, p. 144). Ritual activity within the context of spiritual direction provides another opportunity for constructive meaning making through *poesis*, storytelling that relies on metaphor, symbols, and symbolic action. This type of meaning making may be more accessible than narrative practices as a way for some women to acknowledge and respond to suffering (Graham et al., 2005, pp. 70–73). In addition, nonverbal ritual practices may provide effective means for some women to connect difficult-to-articulate bodily experiences with narrative meaning making (Fischer, 1988, p. 165; Plach et al., 2004, p. 151).

Women's contemporary ritual-making activities tend to be more process-oriented than goal-oriented as they reflect "ongoing struggle and journeying rather than decisive change" (Berry, 2009, p. 93). This feminist understanding of ritual is particularly useful in the context of spiritual direction with women who have autoimmune disease because these conditions are characterized by ongoing struggles (not to be confused with particular struggles that may become chronic) and a perpetual liminal experience that thwarts efforts to "achieve" a particular end state. So, although spiritual direction cannot help women transition out of the liminal reality of chronic illness, ritual may be able to help women negotiate illness-in-the-foreground and wellness-in-the-foreground perspectives within that liminal space.

I return to Cindy's story to illustrate an opening/closing ritual that facilitates IITF and WITF shifts. Jane proposes that the women construct an opening and closing ritual to help establish boundaries for illness experiences within and around their spiritual direction sessions. As the women reflect on the form the ritual might take, their thoughts coalesce on metaphorically containing Cindy's illness experiences in a box that can be opened and closed at will. Before their next session, Cindy selects a small cardboard box that she can easily bring it to spiritual direction sessions in her purse. The box's size also reinforces the notion that Cindy and God are bigger than the illness experiences.

At the beginning of their spiritual direction sessions, Cindy ceremoniously opens the box and places it between herself and Jane, symbolically indicating that the contents of the box are now available for reflection and discernment during their time together. The women hold no expectation about what the box might or might not reveal in a particular session, but in this simple ritual they have explicitly created a safe and sacred space for exploration of Cindy's illness experiences. At the end of each session, Cindy replaces the lid on the box while Jane audibly affirms that illness experiences are but one dimension of Cindy's life and can be appropriately contained. Jane also reminds Cindy that God safely holds both Cindy and her illness experiences. For now, Cindy has chosen a plain box, reinforcing the idea that her illness experiences are neutral entities. Later she might adorn this box or select a new decorative box to reinforce newly constructed, life-enhancing beliefs about positive aspects of her illness experiences.

The illustration of Cindy and Jane's ritual is not prescriptive; every woman and her spiritual director should construct rituals (or choose not to do so) that are meaningful and helpful for a particular directee at a particular time. The salient points embedded within the illustration are that IITF and WITF perspective shifts will occur during a woman's experience of autoimmune disease, but she and her spiritual director can recognize and help the woman cope more effectively with life-limiting aspects of IITF periods by using ritual. The opening and closing moments of spiritual direction sessions are already frequently ritualized, incorporating elements such as silence, prayer, or candle-lighting. This makes them particularly conducive to rituals related to shifting perspectives. Inducing a controlled IITF experience at the beginning of the spiritual direction session can make illness experiences available for reflection without allowing illness to dominate. A temporary shift to IITF at the beginning of the session is accompanied by restoration of a WITF perspective at the end of the spiritual direction encounter. If restoration of WITF is not possible for the woman (there may be times when she is in a prolonged period of IITF), the ritual could serve as a symbolic shift to this hoped-for reality.

Another use of ritual to help women with autoimmune disease cope with their illness experiences is ritual acknowledgment of loss. Public lament of losses, heard and clearly acknowledged by attentive and compassionate spiritual directors (and other directees in the case of group spiritual direction), can help women grieve (potentially) disenfranchised losses asso-ciated with autoimmune diseases. Lament does not necessarily need to take place within the context of a ritual practice; however, pastoral theologians and psychologists agree that ritual can be a powerful means of acknowledging disenfranchised losses (for example, Anderson & Foley, 1998; Doka, 1989; Hogue, 2003). Some women also benefit from more formalized permission to express anger or deep sorrow (Berry, 2009, p. 76)—emotive responses that also may be disenfranchised.

Outside of ritual activity, an informed spiritual director might simply ask a directee to reflect on her losses. In this situation, it is important that the spiritual director listen attentively to the woman's lament and acknowledge the loss in a way that clearly communicates to the directee that her suffering has been recognized and validated. This acknowledgement can consist of a few words, but should not be neglected (Mitchell & Anderson, 1983, p. 118; Montgomery, 2003). That said, spiritual directors should not underestimate the potential for ritual to empower women in ways that transcend narrative means of being heard.

Recall that the definition of ritual I am using includes practices that inte-grate thought and action in order to help realize the ideals, hopes, values, and beliefs of a group. The group with which a woman identifies may sim-ply encompass the partnership she has with her spiritual director, extend to other people she knows, or represent a more abstract identification, such as "women who live full lives in spite of their chronic health conditions." In any of these scenarios, ritual provides a means for women to perform (within the ritual ceremony) and live out (beyond the spiritual direction session) the changes they would like to see in the world, such as the acknowledgment of losses by members of their family or restoration of self-agency over their bod-ies (Berry, 2009, p. 94). Ritual practices to acknowledge losses may be most effective within a group model of spiritual direction because the benefits of ritual construction and performance are amplified within a group of women who support each other (Hogue, 2003, p. 141).

Group Practices

Studies indicate that people benefit in a number of ways from group care settings. Both the social support found in groups and the opportunity to participate in reciprocal caregiving relationships are associated with enhanced well-being (Koenig et al., 2001, p. 100; Pargament, 1997, p. 212). Group models of care are often particularly attractive to women because of their collaborative relational dynamics (Fischer, 1988, p. 21).

In the case of spiritual direction, the group model—also grounded in the practice of not-knowing—encourages relational development while still rec-ognizing the diverse relationships with and views of the sacred operating within and among the women in the group. In the group spiritual direction context, women learn how to step into each other's spiritual worlds, which are shaped in unique ways by their illness experiences and relationships with the sacred. Women benefit from this exposure to different understandings of illness, understandings of the sacred, spiritual coping resources, and spiritual practices. In addition, women in group direction can learn from and share success stories of adapting to life with chronic illnesses, serving as examples of hope for one another. The opportunity to learn from each other and the support of the community can help women in their efforts to understand and reconstruct life-limiting embedded beliefs, psychospiritual work that is challenging to both initiate and sustain.

Not all women with autoimmune diseases would embrace a group caregiving context, especially if group members came together around the topic of illness. Some people do not want to spend time focusing on symptoms, disabilities, doctor visits, treatment regimens, and other disadvantages of living with an incurable condition. They avoid illness support groups because this focus implicitly threatens their efforts to hold onto wellness perspectives that allow them to experience life in full (Paterson, 2001, p. 24). Other women may avoid groups in order to deny limits related to their illnesses. One-on-one spiritual direction relationships (rather than group direction) may be a better way to engage women who have these concerns.

SUMMARY

Cindy's poignant story illustrates how women with autoimmune diseases may benefit from augmenting traditional biomedical health care with spiritual direction, a caregiving approach that is well-suited to address the unique, long-term psychospiritual dimensions of chronic illness experiences. As a result of their health conditions, women with autoimmune diseases may experience spiritual struggles related to meaning making about their illness experiences and their relationships with the sacred. In addition, psychospiritual struggles may be initiated or exacerbated by ongoing— and often disenfranchised—losses and by the liminal nature of chronic illness, experienced as ongoing shifts between illness-in-the-foreground and wellness-in-the-foreground perspectives.

When the chronic illness experience asserts itself, a woman may be challenged to cope with and make meaning of physical, psychological, and spiritual suffering and loss. When the illness experience shifts to the background, she may be better able to engage in deliberative meaning making and choose coping strategies that prepare her for future assaults on her meaning-making system. While ongoing threats to a woman's spirituality may result in transformative spiritual growth, they may also give rise to chronic spiritual struggles that can negatively affect her already vulnerable health and well-being. For women living with these progressively degenerative autoimmune diseases, the risk of chronic spiritual struggles does not diminish and may even increase over time.

Evaluation of medical, psychological, and spiritual caregiving approaches to address the unique long-term care and psychospiritual concerns of women with autoimmune diseases reveals that the practice of spiritual direction may be an optimal way to complement biomedical care. The focus on the sacred—the core of a person's spirituality—is what sets spiritual direction apart from other psychospiritual caregiving relationships. Spiritual direction grounded in not-knowing, an intercultural approach to care, can provide an ongoing relational context that respects a woman's highly idiosyncratic illness experiences.

Spiritual direction, in either a one-on-one or a group format, is a safe and confidential space where directors and women with autoimmune disease can co-construct and embody narrative and ritual practices that help facilitate meaning making, facilitate shifts between illness-in-the-foreground and wellness-in-the-foreground experiences, lament, and acknowledge disenfranchised (or potentially disenfranchised) losses. Women can also attend to coping strategies and spiritual practices that enact life-enhancing understandings of illness and the sacred. In this long-term caregiving relationship, spiritual directors can help balance a woman's need to engage in transformative spiritual struggles with the risks posed by getting stuck in chronic struggles. As a complementary approach to biomedical care, spiritual direction offers what no other caregiving approach can provide to meet the psychospiritual needs of women with autoimmune conditions.

NOTES

1. The vignettes that follow are based on this illness narrative, but factual details may have been altered for purposes of illustration or confidentiality.
2. *Disease* describes a medically defined condition in which physiological structure and/or function are impaired. *Illness* refers to the subjective, holistic experience of living with disease, including the way disease affects members of a person's family and extended community.
3. Pastoral theologians, such as Anderson and Foley (1998), are working to increase awareness of and develop rituals for grieving many common life experiences. Chronic illness, however, has not been addressed in the current literature.
4. For example, Christianity acknowledges the transformative power inherent within "dark night of the soul" experiences (Cross, trans. 1959), and Buddhism teaches acceptance of suffering in all forms as the means of release from successive rebirths (*Buddhist scriptures*, trans. 1987).
5. Kenneth Pargament, Len Sperry, and Edward Shafranske are among psychotherapists attempting to change this professional norm.
6. Spiritual guidance, spiritual companionship, and spiritual direction are but a few names for the practice of seeking insight into one's relationship with the sacred. Although contemporary practitioners use a variety of terms, the most common referent remains spiritual direction. In this chapter, I refer to the caregiver as the spiritual *director* and the careseeker as the *directee*.
7. In his description of the intercultural care paradigm, Lartey uses the term intercultural to push spiritual caregivers beyond recognition of diverse cultures to a critical awareness and engagement with that which is 'other' in careseekers" (2003, p. 2). Doehring (2010) further describes spiritual care within the context of the intercultural care paradigm as she invites caregivers

to specifically recognize diversity in religious and spiritual beliefs and practices.

8. In privileging Cindy's spiritual belief system, I use Cindy's language for the sacred, God.

9. Hope-filled narratives do not always include finding benefits in the illness experience (Davis, 2001, p. 146). Hope may consist of asserting the possibility that a woman can live with her illness without struggling against it.

10. "Life-limiting" and "life-enhancing" are contextual terms relative to particular experiences and personalized meaning-making systems. What is a life-enhancing practice or belief for one person (for example, believing that God or the universe brought on or allowed a health condition to manifest may be interpreted as an opportunity to experience a valuable life lesson) may be life-limiting to another person (for example, believing that God or the universe brought on or allowed a health condition to manifest may be understood as punishment for wrongdoing).

REFERENCES

Achterberg, J., Dossey, B. & Kolkmeier, L. (1994). *Rituals of healing: Using imagery for health and wellness.* New York, NY: Bantam Books.

Affleck, G., Pfeiffer, C., Tennen, H. & Fifield, J. (1987). "Attributional processes in rheumatoid arthritis patients." *Arthritis and Rheumatism, 30*, 927–931.

Agrimson, L. B. & Taft, L. B. (2008). "Spiritual crisis: A concept analysis." *Journal of Advanced Nursing, 65*(2), 454–461. doi: 10.1111/j.1365-2648.2008.04869.x.

Anderson, H. & Foley, E. (1998). *Mighty stories, dangerous rituals: Weaving together the human and the divine.* San Francisco, CA: Jossey Bass.

Arora, K. R. (2011). "Not-knowing in spiritual direction: Reflections on social identity." *Presence: An International Journal of Spiritual Direction, 17*(2), 19–26.

Badaracco, C. H. (2007). *Prescribing faith: Medicine, media, and religion in American culture.* Waco, TX: Baylor University Press.

Becker, G. (1999). *Disrupted lives: How people create meaning in a chaotic world.* Berkeley, CA: University of California Press.

Bell, C. (1987). "Discourse and dichotomies: The structure of ritual theory." *Religion, 17*, 95–118.

Berry, J. (2009). *Ritual making women: Shaping rites for changing lives.* London, England: Equinox Publishing Ltd.

Bidwell, D. R. (2004). "Real/izing the sacred: Spiritual direction and social constructionism." *Journal of Pastoral Theology, 14*(1), 59–74.

Buddhist scriptures. (trans. 1987). (E. Conze, Trans.). London, England: Penguin Books Ltd.

Calhoun, L. G. & Tedeschi, R. G. (2001). "Posttraumatic growth: The positive lessons of loss." In R. A. Neimeyer (Ed.), *Meaning reconstruction and the experience of loss.* Washington, DC: American Psychological Association, 157–172.

Cassian, J. (trans. 1997). *John Cassian: The conferences* (B. Ramsey, Trans.). New York, NY: Newman Press.

Charmaz, K. (1991). *Good days, bad days: The self in chronic illness and time.* New Brunswick, NJ: Rutgers University Press.

Charon, R. (2006). *Narrative medicine: Honoring the stories of illness.* New York, NY: Oxford University Press.

Cross, J. (trans. 1959). *Dark night of the soul* (E. A. Peers, Trans.). New York, NY: Image Books.

Davis, C. G. (2001). "The tormented and the transformed: Understanding responses to loss and trauma." In R. A. Neimeyer (Ed.), *Meaning reconstruction and the experience of loss* . Washington, DC: American Psychological Association, 137–155.

Doehring, C. (2010). "Pastoral care and counseling in a postmodern context." In G. H. Asquith (Ed.), *The concise dictionary of pastoral care and counseling*. Nashville, TN: Abingdon Press, 70–74.

Doka, K. J. (1989). "Conclusion." In K. J. Doka (Ed.), *Disenfranchised grief: Recognizing hidden sorrow*. Lexington, MA: Lexington Books, 329–333.

Doka, K. J. (2009). *Counseling individuals with life-threatening illness*. New York, NY: Springer Publishing.

Doka, K. J. & Martin, T. L. (2002). "How we grieve: Culture, class, and gender." In K. J. Doka (Ed.), *Disenfranchised grief: New directions, challenges, and strategies for practice* . Champaign, IL: Research Press, 337–347.

Fischer, K. (1988). *Women at the well: Feminist perspectives on spiritual direction*. New York, NY: Paulist.

Fitchett, G., Murphy, P. E., Kim, J., Gibbons, J. L., Cameron, J. R. & Davis, J. A. (2004). "Religious struggle: Prevalence, correlates and mental health risks in diabetic, congestive heart failure, and oncology patients." *International Journal of Psychiatry in Medicine, 34*(2), 179–196.

Fitchett, G. & Risk, J. L. (2009). "Screening for spiritual struggle." *Journal of Pastoral Care and Counseling, 63*(1–2), 1–12.

Giffords, E. D. (2003). "Understanding and managing systemic lupus erythematosus (SLE)." *Journal of Social Work in Health Care, 37*(4), 57–72. doi: 10.1300/J010v37n04_04.

Graham, E., Walton, H. & Ward, F. (2005). *Theological reflection: Methods*. London, England: SCM Press.

Grytten, N., Glad, S. B., Aarseth, J. H., Nyland, H., Midgard, R. & Myhr, K. (2006). "A 50-year follow-up of the incidence of multiple sclerosis in Hordaland County, Norway." *Neurology, 66*(2), 182–186. doi: 10.1212/01.wnl.0000195549.95448.b9.

Guenther, M. (1992). *Holy listening: The art of spiritual direction*. Boston, MA: Cowley Publications.

Hogue, D. A. (2003). *Remembering the future, imagining the past: Story, ritual, and the human brain*. Cleveland, OH: Pilgrim Press.

Increasing incidence of rheumatoid arthritis in women. (2008). *Medical News Today*. Retrieved from http://www.medicalnewstoday.com/articles/126886.php.

Irvine, H., Davidson, C., Hoy, K. & Lowe-Strong, A. (2009). "Psychosocial adjustment to multiple sclerosis: Exploration of identity redefinition." *Disability and Rehabilitation, 31*(8), 599–606. doi: 10.1080/09638280802243286.

Karp, M. (2010). What has spiritual direction opened for you? *SDI Membership Moments*. Retrieved from http://info.sdiworld.org/post/what-has-spiritual-direction-opened-for-you.

Katz, R. C., Flasher, L., Cacciapaglia, H. & Nelson, S. (2001). "The psychosocial impact of cancer and lupus: A cross validation study that extends the generality of 'benefit-finding' in patients with chronic disease." *Journal of Behavioral Medicine, 24*(6), 561–571. doi: 0160–7715/01/1200–0561/0.

Keefe, F. J., Smith, S., Buffington, A. L. H., Gibson, J., Studts, J. L. & Caldwell, D. S. (2002). "Recent advances and future directions in the biopsychosocial assessment and treatment of arthritis." *Journal of Consulting and Clinical Psychology, 70*(3), 640–655. doi: 10.1037//0022–006X.70.3.640.

Kinsley, D. (1996). *Health, healing, and religion: A cross-cultural perspective.* Upper Saddle River, NJ: Prentice Hall.

Klitzman, R. L. (2012). *Am I my genes? Confronting fate and family secrets in the age of genetic testing.* New York, NY: Oxford University Press.

Koenig, H. G., McCullough, M. E. & Larson, D. B. (2001). *Handbook of religion and health.* New York, NY: Oxford University Press.

Lartey, E. Y. (2003). *In living color: An intercultural approach to pastoral care and counseling* (2nd, revised ed.). London, England: Jessica Kingsley.

MacLean, C. D., Susi, B., Phifer, N., Schultz, L., Bynum, D., Franco, M. & Cykert, S. (2003). "Patient preference for physician discussion and practice of spirituality." *Journal of General Internal Medicine, 18,* 38–43.

Margaretten, M., Yelin, E., Imboden, J., Graf, J., Barton, J., Katz, P. & Julian, L. (2009). "Predictors of depression in a multiethnic cohort of patients with rheumatoid arthritis." *Arthritis and Rheumatism, 61*(11), 1586–1591. doi: 10.1002/art.24822.

McConnell, K. M. & Pargament, K. I. (2006). "Examining the links between spiritual struggles and symptoms of psychopathology in a national sample." *Journal of Clinical Psychology, 62*(12), 1469–1484. doi: 10.1002/jclp.20325.

Mehl-Madrona, L. E. (2003). *Coyote healing: Miracles in native medicine.* Rochester, VT: Bear and Company.

Mitchell, K. R. & Anderson, H. (1983). *All our losses, all our griefs: Resources for pastoral care.* Louisville, KY: Westminster John Knox Press.

Montgomery, G. A. (2003). Grief needs a witness: A psychological study of the witness, from the perspective of Jungian psychology and self psychology. Doctoral dissertation, Pacifica Graduate Institute, Carpinteria, CA. ProQuest Dissertations and Theses database. (AAT 3128808).

Pakenham, K. I. & Cox, S. (2009). "The dimensional structure of benefit finding in multiple sclerosis and relations with positive and negative adjustment: A longitudinal study." *Psychology and Health, 24*(4), 373–393. doi: 10.1080/08870440701832592.

Pargament, K. I. (1997). *The psychology of religion and coping: Theory, research, practice.* New York, NY: Guilford Press.

Pargament, K. I. (2007). *Spiritually-integrated psychotherapy: Understanding and addressing the sacred.* New York, NY: Guilford Press.

Pargament, K. I., Koenig, H. G., Tarakeshwar, N. & Hahn, J. (2004). "Religious coping methods as predictors of psychological, physical and spiritual outcomes among medically ill elderly patients: A two-year longitudinal study." *Journal of Health Psychology, 9*(6), 713–730. doi: 10.1177/1359105304045366.

Paterson, B. L. (2001). "The shifting perspectives model of chronic illness." *Journal of Nursing Scholarship, 33*(1), 21–26.

Philip, E. J., Lindner, H. & Lederman, L. (2009). "Relationship of illness perceptions with depression among individuals diagnosed with lupus." *Depression and Anxiety, 26,* 575–582. doi: 10.1002/da.20451.

Plach, S. K., Stevens, P. E. & Moss, V. A. (2004). "Corporeality: Women's experiences of a body with rheumatoid arthritis." *Clinical Nursing Research, 13*(2), 137–155. doi: 10.1177/1054773803262219.

Reynolds, F. & Prior, S. (2003). " 'Sticking jewels in your life' : Exploring women's strategies for negotiating an acceptable quality of life with multiple sclerosis." *Qualitative Health Research, 13*(9), 1225–1251. doi: 10.1177/1049732303257108.

Rowe, M. M. & Allen, R. G. (2004). "Spirituality as a means of coping with chronic illness." *American Journal of Health Studies, 19*(1), 62–67.

Russell, C. S., White, M. B. & White, C. P. (2006). "Why me? Why now? Why multiple sclerosis?: Making meaning and perceived quality of life in a Midwestern sample of patients with multiple sclerosis." *Families, Systems, and Health, 24*(1), 65–81. doi: 10.1037/1091-7527.24.1.65.

Schulman-Green, D., Jaser, S., Martin, F., Alonzo, A., Grey, M., McCorkle, R. & Whittemore, R. (2012). "Processes of self-managment in chronic illness." *Journal of Nursing Scholarship, 44*(2), 136–144. doi: 10.1111/j.1547-5069.2012.01444.x.

Smith, J. Z. (1980). "The bare facts of ritual." *History of Religions, 19*(4), 112–127.

Tang, S. Y. S. & Anderson, J. M. (1999). "Human agency and the process of healing: Lessons learned from women living with a chronic illness—rewriting the expert." *Nursing Inquiry, 6*, 83–93.

Townsend, L. (2009). *Introduction to pastoral counseling.* Nashville, TN: Abingdon.

Trevino, K. M., Pargament, K. I., Cotton, S., Leonard, A. C., Hahn, J., Caprini-Faigin, C. A. & Tsevat, J. (2010). "Religious coping and physiological, psychological, social, and spiritual outcomes in patients with HIV/AIDS: Cross-sectional and longitudinal findings." *AIDS Behavior, 14*, 379–389. doi: 10.1007/s10461-007-9332-6.

Uramoto, K. M. (1999). "Trends in the incidence and mortality of sytemic lupus erythematosus, 1950–1992." *Arthritis and Rheumatism, 42*(1), 46–50. doi: 10.1002/1529-0131(199901).

Vander Zee, J. (2002). "The chronically ill patient." In R. B. Gilbert (Ed.), *Health care and spirituality: Listening, assessing, caring.* Amityville, NY: Baywood Publishing, 179–187.

Wendell, S. (1996). *The rejected body: Feminist philosophical reflections on disability.* New York, NY: Routledge.

Zinnbauer, B. J., Pargament, K. I., Cole, B. S., Rye, M. S., Butter, E. M., Belavich, T. G. & Kadar, J. L. (1997). "Religion and spirituality: Unfuzzying the fuzzy." *Journal for the Scientific Study of Religion, 36*(4), 549–564.

CHAPTER 3

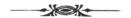

BEYOND COPING: SPIRITUALITY AND FILIPINA TRANSNATIONALS WITH EXPERIENCE OF BREAST CANCER

Ofelia O. Villero and Nancy J. Burke

INTRODUCTION

Like thousands of Filipino transnationals before her, Carina left the Philippines for the United States hoping to build a bright future for her family. She came to California in 1999 to look for work, leaving her husband, 13-year-old daughter and 6-year-old son behind. After a year, she was able to petition for her husband, who needed her care because he was diabetic. Unfortunately, she and her husband did not get along and he became physically abusive. In addition, when she asked him to go back to the Philippines a year later to bring their children to the United States, he did not follow through with a petition for their daughter, only arranging for their son's papers. Six months after she was reunited with her son, her husband abandoned them for good.

As a single mother, Carina rented a room in a house owned by a Filipino family. She worked at a hamburger eatery during the day and went to school at night, still aiming to provide for a better future for her children (she filed a new petition for her daughter) and also financially support her parents in the Philippines. But her hopes were suddenly dashed when she was diagnosed with breast cancer in 2003. Carina told us her story on a sunny afternoon in San Francisco. She said:

> When I was told I was positive for cancer, my first thought was about my children. What will happen to them when I'm gone? One more thing, what about

my son? We don't have relatives here in the US. We're alone. I was scared. I had
a feeling that my life was over.

Carina's fears were understandable. Among the Filipinos, cancer is seen as a
death sentence, or as Carina put it, "Your timer is clicking away." Her job
did not offer health benefits, so she had no idea how she would pay for her
medical care. Without relatives close by, who would care for her son while
she was undergoing cancer treatment? Or for that matter, who would be
her caregiver? If she survived the surgery, how would she pay for further
treatment and medications? How would she be able to pay their rent and buy
food? She was also worried about not being able to send some money to her
parents and siblings in the Philippines.

In spite of overwhelming odds, Carina was able to overcome her fears and
recover from breast cancer. She has passed the five-year survival mark, and
although there is no guarantee that her cancer will not return, she is confident
that she would no longer be as desperate and forlorn as before. She was able
to find an office job with health insurance and has been reunited with her
daughter, whom she sees as her closest friend and would be her caregiver if
and when cancer strikes again. Carina recounted how she prevailed in such
dire circumstances:

> At the time I was crying and crying. I was always sad and didn't know what
> to do. But my friend told me to be strong and pray. I called my mom and my
> brothers and sisters and told them to pray for me. Then I just became strong.
> I really pulled myself together and prepared myself because I knew that I was
> going to be alone with this and I had to do it by myself. By the grace of God,
> I was able to get through it.

Through her prayers and those of others, Carina believed that she found the
courage to talk about her breast cancer diagnosis in spite of her paralyzing
fear of being stigmatized. "At first I didn't want people to know I was sick.
I didn't want them to feel sorry for me. I wanted them to treat me the same as
any normal person." But when she admitted openly that she had breast cancer
and asked for help, she realized that "people did not distance themselves."
Instead, they were supportive and those who helped her initially had become
her friends later on. She also followed their advice and approached social
service agencies, which offered money to pay her rent for a limited period of
time. Then she was referred to a city hospital, which provided free medical
care. Acquaintances from her son's school brought food and looked after
him. But in summing up her experience, Carina underplays her own and other
people's actions and highlights instead the positive impact of spirituality not
only on her struggle against breast cancer but also on her life as a whole.

Carina's narrative is not unique among Filipina transnational workers
whom we interviewed as part of a four-year ethnographic study of Filipinas
with experience of breast cancer. Burdened with family responsibilities, without health care resources and any safety net, missing kin support and lacking

the language skills necessary to navigate complex cultural and biomedical systems, the women turn to Filipino notions of spirituality and practices of religiosity to frame and manage their illness. From their perspective, recovery from breast cancer was not only the result of their persistent efforts to seek medical and social assistance, or the care that they received from charitable hospitals and skilled medical professionals, or even their strict adherence to several courses of cancer treatment. Equally important were prayers, devotions, and other religious practices that gave them inner strength to face the challenges of treatment and recovery.

Several studies have linked religious beliefs and attitudes to health outcomes. Psychologist Kenneth Pargament (1997) developed the theory of *religious coping*, which views religion as a way of coping during stressful situations such as chronic illness. He also classified religious coping as being positive or negative, with corresponding positive or negative effects on those undergoing stress.

Examining the validity of Pargament's claim, a study of 198 women with breast cancer concluded that positive religious coping did not result in any measures of well-being, yet negative coping predicted worse mental health and life satisfaction in women with breast cancer (Herbert et al., 2009). A longitudinal study of the role of spirituality in response to the diagnosis and treatment of breast cancer concluded that there is limited support for Pargament's hypothesis, and that women with cancer who were not religious to begin with but who turned to religious coping after diagnosis may experience long-term adjustment problems (Gall et al., 2009). A study on the use of prayer alone in religious coping, among individuals with various types of cancer, did not negate the practice of praying. However, it cautioned that praying presents underlying complexities and challenges that may lead to difficulties in coping with the disease (Taylor et al., 1999). The authors posited that praying negatively influences coping when patients lack a "secure attachment to God," which could lead to internal tensions about wanting to be in control versus relinquishing that control to God, feelings of unworthiness when the petitioners' prayers were "unanswered" and spiritual pain from perceptions of unfairness or capriciousness of God (p. 391).

However, among women belonging to ethnocultural minorities, research suggests a greater correlation between religion and coping. A synthesis of 15 qualitative research studies focusing on women from various ethnocultural groups—African American, Asian American, Native American, and Hispanic American—revealed that reliance on religious practices such as prayer, meditation, church attendance, and consultation with spiritual leaders increased after diagnosis with breast cancer (Howard et al., 2007). These findings are in line with Pargament's claim that religious coping is greater for people within certain cultural and socioeconomic contexts—members of ethnic minorities, the poor, and women and elderly who face threatening and harmful situations. In a study of ethnocultural influences in cancer, Johnson (1998) states that ethnocultural factors affect patients' responses to cancer diagnosis, treatment compliance, and adjustment, and for persons with metastatic terminal cancer, their emotional/behavioral reactions to death and bereavement are likewise impacted. With an understanding of ethnicity as "shared social and cultural heritage among members of a group" (Sue et al., 1991, p. 535) and culture as a "general design for living and pattern for interpreting reality" (Airhihebuwa, 1985, p. 7), Johnson's research suggests that both ethnicity and culture play a central role in people's conception of health and disease, particularly in the case of cancer where lifestyle and cultural beliefs can influence recognition of early symptoms.

Our own ethnographic study confirms that Filipina transnationals with breast cancer turn to religious coping in order to offset the stressful effects of their illness. It also corroborates the idea that ethnocultural factors play a major role in the management of the disease. Our findings show that religious coping for our participants is an expression of a hybridized Filipino spiritual tradition rooted in the indigenous idea of subjectivity and Christian practices that foster spiritual strength as their physical bodies undergo debilitation and fragmentation. Our findings also differ from previous research on religious coping with regard to the link between religious coping and the outcome of the disease itself. We found that Filipino expressions of spirituality emphasize the non-physical or spiritual aspect of the illness experience, meaning that improvement is expected to take place on the spiritual side first and foremost, which in turn could lead, but not necessarily, to an improvement in the physical aspect of illness elsewhere identified as physical health or disease outcome (Ellison & Levin, 1998; Johnstone et al., 2008; Campbell et al., 2010). As far as our participants were concerned, the impact of Filipino spirituality extended beyond physical manifestations and experiences of the disease to include personal empowerment and identity formation.

This outlook is evident in Carina's assessment of her experience—that prayers made her strong so she was able to begin her fight against breast cancer *before* her treatment. Her courage to surmount her fear of stigmatization and reach out to other people made the difference in her survival. This is not to suggest that our participants did not pay attention to the medical care they were given or ignored their treatment regimen, but they equally focused, and in fact, insisted on practices that took their spiritual well-being into consideration and saw their spiritual state as a measure of the success of their recovery from breast cancer.

We argue that by caring for their spiritual selves, Filipinas in our study developed a subjectivity differentiated from the biomedical standpoint that perceived them as diseased bodies, or after having completed treatment as "breast cancer survivors." At the same time that they conscientiously and rigorously followed the course of treatment prescribed by their oncologists and physicians, they continued to fulfill their roles as useful members of their families and transnational communities, although with great sacrifice on their part. They took their identity from their courage and determination in surmounting seemingly endless challenges, of which breast cancer was but one of many. As we will explain later in this chapter, from their illness experience our study participants constructed a specific identity as Filipino transnational women who have "passed through" (*nalampasan*) and became whole again.

Our findings highlight the ways in which tying Pargament's theory of religious coping to specific health outcomes limits its relevance to understanding the complex nature of spirituality in the context of chronic illness. Filipino transnationals see their spirituality and the practices it engenders as having a wider meaning and effect, encompassing not just the course of a disease but the trajectory and context of their entire lives. In other words, their spirituality in times of chronic illness is not restricted to instrumental purposes like influencing the direct outcome of a disease (although it could certainly be one of the factors). It includes accessing spiritual power for inner transformation, which generates broader and deeper consequences before physical recovery from the disease occurs.

BACKGROUND

Breast cancer is a major health concern among Filipino Americans. It is the number one cause of cancer death in Filipino women (Maxwell et al., 2003), who have nearly twice the incidence of breast cancer than Chinese, Korean, and Vietnamese women, second in incidence only to Japanese women (Keegan et al., 2007). According to Surveillance, Epidemiology and End Results (SEER) data, the incidence of breast cancer in Filipinas is 73.1 per 100,000, which is higher than in Hispanic women but lower than the incidence in African American and White women (Wu & Bancroft, 2006). Unfortunately, the rates of certain breast cancers are also not declining. For the period 1990–2002, incident rates of *in situ* breast cancer have actually increased for Filipino women (Keegan et al., 2007). Additionally, Filipino women have five-year survival probabilities similar to those of African Americans (Lin et al., 2002), a group that fares far worse than Whites in survival probabilities for breast cancer (Baquet et al., 2008). Filipino women also look similar to African American women in the proportion diagnosed with late-stage breast cancer (Gomez et al., 2010). Women with breast cancer who are diagnosed at its earliest, most treatable stage have a 97 percent probability of surviving five years or more (California Cancer Registry, 2012). Unfortunately, foreign-born Filipinas have consistently more advanced breast-cancer-stage diagnosis and, consequently, lower survival rates than US-born Filipino women (Gomez et al., 2010).

Filipinos are the second largest immigrant group in the United States, numbering 1.7 million, next only to Mexican immigrants (Terrazas & Batalova, 2010). In addition, there are 1.4 million native-born US citizens of Filipino ancestry. Half of all Filipino immigrants reside in the state of California, with the largest number (16.5 percent of the total Filipino-born population) concentrated in the metropolitan areas of Los Angeles, Long Beach, and Santa Ana, followed by San Francisco, Oakland, and Fremont

(9.4 percent). Our ethnographic study of Filipinas with breast cancer was conducted in the San Francisco Bay Area.

Unlike the early migration pattern of Filipinos wherein men greatly outnumbered women (Takaki, 1998), three of every five Filipino immigrants living in the United States in 2008 were women (58.8 percent, compared to 41.3 percent men) (Terrazas & Batalova, 2010). For this study, we distinguish between Filipino immigrants and transnationals. Our participants interacted on a regular, patterned basis with the Philippines, not only economically through remittances to kin but also through periodic visits, constant phone calls with families and friends, maintenance of cultural and social ties with fellow Filipinos, and the conscious pursuit of news and information about their country of origin. We see transnationals as "migrants who are fully encapsulated neither in the host society nor in their native land but who nonetheless remain active participants in the social settings of both locations," as defined by Petron (2008, p. 4). In analyzing the behavior patterns of transnationals, Guarnizo (2003) calls attention to the concept of "transnational living," which he defines as "crossing borders characterized by wittingly or unwittingly maintaining and reproducing the social milieu from afar" (p. 666). This could help explain the sociocultural context of religious coping among some ethnic communities.

Religion plays a major role in the lives of both native-born and foreign-born Filipinos. The 1991 and 1998 International Social Survey Program studies on religion declared Filipinos the most religious people in the world (as cited in Gonzalez, 2009, p. 15). Based on the Pew Forum on Religion and Public Life's report on global Christianity (2011), 93.4 percent of the Philippine population is Christian, with Catholics at 81.4 percent, Protestants at 11 percent, and those that belong to local religions that classify themselves as Christians at 1 percent. The religious environment in the Philippines is so vibrant that it is a common occurrence for Catholic masses to be held in public places—in airports, shopping malls, parks, and streets—and for community leaders and ordinary citizens to perform prayers and devotions almost everywhere, with no legal restrictions (Gonzalez, 2009). For instance, while shopping at one of the biggest department store chains in Metro Manila, the first author (Villero) observed that shoppers and sales people alike paused to pray when the Angelus was played over the loudspeaker throughout the store, complete with a recording of church bells and the solemn voice of a prayer leader.

Filipino immigrants bring their religious affiliations, beliefs, and practices to the United States, and second-generation Filipino Americans generally follow the religion of their parents. According to Carnes and Yang (2004), Christianity constitutes the bulk of Filipino American religious identification, with 68 percent identifying as Catholics and 18 percent as evangelical Protestants. They also consider Filipino Americans the most religious among Asian Americans, with 94 percent regularly attending worship services. In assessing the impact of religion on Filipinos living in the Philippines and in the San Francisco Bay Area, Gonzalez (2009) states:

Behaviorally, then, religion greatly influences the way Filipinos respond to the situations they face daily, whether in the Philippines or anywhere else in the world. Because of this influence, Filipino migrant faithful have a strong tendency to exhibit...religion-reinforced Filipino traits, values, and actions. (p. 19)

METHODS

Narratives and observations included here were recorded over the course of four years of ethnographic fieldwork with Filipinas who had experienced breast cancer in the San Francisco Bay Area. We collaborated with community-based organizations serving Filipinos, attended Filipino cultural events, spent time in women's homes and with their families, and followed them to oncology appointments and support groups. Throughout the course of the study, we participated in 63 support groups. These were both Filipina-only ($n = 42$) groups and those open to women of any ethnicity ($n = 21$). We also conducted life history (Goldman et al., 2003) interviews with 63 Filipinas and their families. Interview participants included those who had attended a support group ($n = 27$, 21 women, six male family members), women who had never attended a group ($n = 27$), and women who attended and stopped ($n = 3$). Nine of our participants took part in two small group interviews. Lastly, we interviewed six support group facilitators and staff. We conducted the interviews either in English ($n = 9$) or in Tagalog ($n = 62$), and translated all Tagalog interviews into English for analysis. All interviews took place from 2007 to 2011. We transcribed all interviews and used Atlas.ti ethnographic software to organize our data. Both authors read and coded all transcripts and fieldnotes. All participants provided written informed consent prior to participation.

SPIRITUALITY AND CANCER TREATMENT

As we sat in her dimly lit living room in a housing project in San Francisco, Loreta recounted her life story. At the age of 12, she was sent to Malaysia from the Philippines to work as a nanny and make a life for herself there. As a full-grown woman, she went back to the Philippines to visit her ill mother, who then asked her to leave with her for the United States as her caregiver. Before moving to San Francisco, Loreta was sexually assaulted, resulting in an unintended pregnancy. After her mother's death and with a daughter to raise, Loreta worked as a caregiver until she was diagnosed with breast cancer.

Loreta talked about her reaction when the doctor informed her she had stage-three breast cancer: "Yeah, so, just my tears come out and after that I said, 'Oh, never mind.' I just, uh, what I do, I pray. The doctor come out, I pray." Praying comforted her not just at the beginning but throughout her treatment, including eight cycles of chemotherapy. Although she admitted that her initial despair gave way to optimism with the encouragement of her doctor and the support of family members, she nevertheless pointed out that prayers were the constant in her life from diagnosis to her present stage of remission.

Just like Loreta who immediately turned to prayer upon learning of her disease, Marietta, 65-year old and a caregiver, recalled that she did exactly the same thing.

> Right after the doctor told me that I had breast cancer, I went to church to pray. I did not tell anybody until after I had been to church. There was no mass, but the church door was open and I went in. I was in shock, thinking about what will happen to me, the effect on my children and grandchildren. From the time I had the diagnosis, to the surgery, to chemotherapy and radiation, up to now before my five years [of hormone therapy] is up, I have not stopped praying. My family has not stopped praying for me.

Another participant, Cora, told us that her spiritual practice consisted of attending Sunday masses without fail. "After I found out I had breast cancer, I never missed a Sunday mass. The first Sunday I was in the hospital, but there was a TV mass. The second Sunday I was at home . . . was able to get up and go to church. After that just continued."

Aside from prayers and masses, study participants took part in other religious activities while undergoing treatment. The most popular were novenas to saints, in particular to St. Peregrine, patron of people with cancer, and St. Anthony, patron of miracles. The women also performed devotions to the Sacred Heart of Jesus, the Divine Mercy, and Our Lady of Perpetual Help, which they had begun before their move to the United States. The women usually had more than one novena and devotion to fulfill.

Our analysis of the life-history interviews we conducted revealed that participants pursued a spiritual track parallel and simultaneous with their biomedical path of cancer treatment. Their calendars highlighted not only their doctor's visits and treatment schedule but also times for novena and devotion services. Marivic, a security guard, stated that she had two novenas to perform, one to Our Lady of Perpetual Help and the other to St. Patrick. Her work shifts and treatment timetable did not allow for regular church visits, but she nevertheless kept her promise to her patron saints to attend novenas in their honor. She related:

> I go to St. Patrick's [church] and to Epiphany. If I miss the Wednesday eight a.m. [Perpetual Help] novena in Epiphany, I go to Corpus Christi at seven at night. If I can't make it on Wednesday, I go to St. Patrick's on Tuesday night. It is already Wednesday morning in the Philippines [Perpetual Help novena day]. If I cannot make any of those days, I go to Daly City, the church up the hill, on Saturday.

Pilgrimages supplemented novenas and devotions. After completion of intensive cancer therapies, many of the women visited the Philippines not only to reassure worried family members but also to do pilgrimages. Mely, who used to be a bookkeeper, had devotions to two popular Filipino religious symbols, the Holy Nazarene of Quiapo and Our Lady of Manaoag, in addition to the Holy Infant of Prague and Our Lady of Guadalupe. With her husband who had also recovered from a serious illness, Mely went on pilgrimage:

> You know when we got cured, it's been almost six years since we last went home to the Philippines because of our sickness. We immediately went to Quiapo to visit the Holy Nazarene. I was at the door of the church and I shouted, "Holy Nazarene, we are here now. Manny and I are cured now." It was so wonderful because my voice echoed inside the church. I did the same when we went to Manaoag.

Our Lady of Lourdes in France also attracted many of our study participants. They saved up to take part in church-sponsored pilgrimages to Lourdes, often going together with close friends who were members of the same church.

Micha described the simultaneous and parallel tracks of her religiosity and cancer treatment as having two physicians: "I told Him that the doctor did everything that he could do and that the rest would be up to Him. God is also my physician and He will do everything that He can." As far as she was concerned, both "physicians" worked at the same time to make her whole.

Spiritual practices continued through survivorship, and in many cases intensified post-treatment. In gratitude for their recovery, some sought to fulfill the religious pledges they made by going on pilgrimages, not just once but several times. As an extension of their devotions, others took on annual financial sponsorships of religious events in the United States and in the Philippines, which were dedicated to their patron saints. There were a few who established foundations to help the needy.

Some participants who were also members of a breast cancer support group for Filipinas and had survived much longer than five years still maintained a heavy schedule of novenas and devotions. Prior to the start of support group meetings, participants updated each other on changes and locations of novenas and devotions in the Bay Area. Their membership in the support group, which offered talks on caring for their bodies, was more than a way to increase their biomedical knowledge. It was an extension of their spirituality. As part of the support group's regular activities, they initiated a class on the craft of rosary making, requested members of the clergy as speakers in the group's weekly talks and the inclusion of Catholic mass in their celebrations.

Our participants' tenacity in observing religious practices in spite of the heavy demands of their treatment regimen indicates the high value the women placed on spirituality in times of illness. Clarita concisely summed up the reason: "I agree with a lot of people who are spiritual, that with a lot of prayers you will survive. It's not only physical healing that is important. Your spiritual and emotional healing is the most important." If spiritual well-being is necessary for physical healing, then the road to breast cancer recovery will necessarily traverse a spiritual path. This accounts for statements by our participants like Paulita who concluded:

> Yeah, I was diagnosed with colon cancer when I was 57-years-old, then when I was 58 it was breast cancer. Things happen in your life, and then after that one thing I can say I was blessed. Well, I guess it's all our Divine Lord. Divine Providence. I say prayers. It's the thing that kept me going.

In one indicator of religious coping—consultation with members of the clergy—our findings revealed a noticeable divergence from the Howard et al. (2007) study, which found that ethnocultural women's reliance on consultation with spiritual leaders increased after breast cancer diagnosis. Except for one, our participants did not speak with priests and other clergy on a one-to-one or personal basis outside regular church activities like novenas, devotions, and masses. Our in-depth interviews and participant observations revealed only one incident wherein an informant saw a priest several times; it was not voluntary on her part although she did feel it ultimately aided her recovery. Pacita related that without her knowledge, her sister had requested an Irish priest to visit her at home:

> So yeah, he came over and he says, "You know I'm here. If you don't want to talk I'm here. I can just sit here and read. If you want I can read a passage, something from the bible, or if you want I can leave, too." So it was awkward, in the beginning. It was very, you know, you have respect for the priest, but on the other hand, what are you doing here? And I was still in my nightgown. So it was, uh, awkward, and it was also good that we had that . . . that common ground, that it's the religious side. It helped.

The only other one-on-one contact with clergy that two of our participants mentioned was participation in "healing masses," where the priest "pray over you" by laying their hands over the head of each individual present. Socorro said that she could hear the priest muttering a prayer and could feel his breath as he laid his hand over her head. Yet even though she recommended going to healing masses, she preferred communicating with the divine without any religious mediator. "I do pray a lot by myself and I talk to the Lord. There's so many ways of praying, but the best prayer is when you talk to Him like I am talking to you now." Participants expressed preference for a relationship with the divine that was highly personal, intimate, and direct.

Aside from providing a straight line to the divine, prayers also reinforced the women's social and community relationships. The women requested prayers for their recovery not just from members of their family and close and distant relatives and acquaintances, but also from total strangers, widening their support network and decreasing the disease's stigmatizing effect. Our participants admitted to being energized and responding well to their treatments after receiving prayer pledges and being prayed over. Vesta said:

I found out around Christmas time that I had cancer, but I never became negative about it. My son did have worries and was depressed at the beginning. What helped me and my son was the fact that he told his school. He goes to a Catholic school, and the teacher and his classmates sent me prayer pledges.

Ernan gave a similar story:

In my case, when I learned I had breast cancer I told all my friends. I said that if I was to have an operation, please pray for me. I was lucky to have this group of Born-again Christians. The sister of my sister-in-law took me to her church and this group prayed over me. It was a group of over 300. It was the day before my operation. After my operation I was fine. They took out 14 lymph nodes and not even one had cancer.

From a biomedical perspective, it is disputable that prayers would have a direct impact on the result of surgical procedures. However, participants reported a lift in spirits from prayer offerings. They saw these as gestures of concern, perhaps a symbol of the power of community to safeguard and sustain the individual. In their time of trouble and need, the presence of a group of people pledging prayers and imparting words of encouragement recreated the social body.

Filipino Subjectivity

Carmela was working as a caregiver when she found out she had breast cancer. While visiting relatives, she noticed a small, hard lump in her left breast. Carmela's worst fears were confirmed when the oncologist told her that she had breast cancer, and recommended mastectomy as a first step in a series of treatments. While the oncologist assured her that many women had survived the illness and thrived, Carmela did not hear this. As far as she was concerned, cancer meant imminent death.

While dealing with the shock of her diagnosis and impending surgery, Carmela also had to face the loss of her employment as personal caregiver for older persons. Although her job did not come with any health benefits, it was her only source of income. Without it she was dependent on her relatives' goodwill for survival. It was no wonder she felt scared and depressed.

At her mother's recommendation, Carmela attended a meeting of a support group for Filipinas with breast cancer, consisting of about 20 women in their 60s and 70s. The support group met every Monday in the basement of a rundown building in San Francisco's South of Market district to eat a potluck lunch and listen to talks related to breast cancer. Like Carmela, most of the support group members used to work as caregivers. Some of them were still caregivers, this time unpaid, for their own relatives in exchange for food and lodging. A few of the women held down jobs as security guards and hotel housekeepers.

At the meeting, Carmela requested to hear the women's stories and to ask questions about their experiences. In response, the women stood up one by one to narrate how they handled surgery, chemotherapy, radiation and hormone therapies, and ongoing struggles to remain cancer-free. The survivors prefaced their stories with "By the grace of God, I am alive today" or "Thank God that I made it through," before continuing with details of how they managed and endured the emotional and physical trauma associated with cancer and its various treatments. The women concluded their stories with the advice, "*Magdasal ka*" ("You have to pray"). They all pointed out that prayers were responsible for giving them *lakas ng loob* (inner strength).

After the sharing of stories, the group's facilitator said that it would be a good idea for those present to pray for Carmela. Instead of just agreeing verbally, the group stood up as one and gestured in a laying on of hands over Carmela's head. The facilitator motioned to one of the women, who appeared to be the oldest person present, to lead the prayers. In Tagalog, for a full ten minutes, the prayer leader asked God to bless Carmela and give her *lakas ng loob* to survive her surgery and subsequent medical treatments. Teary-eyed and moved by their concern and prayers, Carmela touched her heart and thanked everyone. Several of the women went up to Carmela and urged her, "*Lakasan mo ang iyong loob*" (lit., "Keep your inside strong").

Before the meeting ended, Carmela shared the name of her oncologist and site of her surgery. She said she knew that the oncologist and hospital were well regarded, but that she was still afraid. "After the prayers here," she said, "I know that everything will be all right. I am no longer scared."

The incident illustrates an important concept of Filipino subjectivity, the *loob* (pronounced lo-ób), literally translated into English as "interiority." In contrast to the palpable physical body, the *loob* is hidden, felt rather than seen. It consists of emotions, sensations, attitudes, and perceptions, which do not stand separate from the body because they are felt by and within the body. Nevertheless, the *loob*, as articulated by our study participants, is distinct from the body. *Katawan* is the Tagalog term for body, similar to *corpus* in Latin, and refers to the physical, structural aspects of the body.

The support group prayed to ask God to strengthen Carmela's *loob*, thus revealing the underlying reason for their religious behavior. Although Carmela was confident of her oncologist's ability and the hospital facilities, it was not enough to reassure her. The prayer ritual and the gathering of women who had undergone cancer treatment and survived to tell the tale with smiles and encouragement gave her strength and peace of mind. For Carmela and the women in the support group, spiritual practices that addressed the needs of the *loob* went hand in hand with medical intervention to set the context for survival and recovery.

The *loob*'s prominence in Philippine culture is evident in its grammatical usage as the root of numerous words that express physical, emotional, psychological, and spiritual states. Examples include *looban* (interior space or area), *sama ng loob* (resentment/hurt feelings), *buo ang loob* (determined/whole), and *kagandahang loob* (generosity). It is also seen as the opposite of *labas* or exteriority, which often figuratively stands in for the body and the physical world.

An anthropologist from the University of the Philippines, Prospero Covar (1998) argues that Filipino culture distinguishes between the biological and the metaphysical processes of becoming human. *Pagigingtao* refers to being born human—a term often used to describe Jesus Christ's birth into the material world—and *pagpapakatao* to becoming a person. Both terms describe the *tao* (human being), but the elements, processes, and end products differ, with the former emphasizing human physical formation, and the latter stressing the ontological. However, with regard to the relationship between the body and the *loob*, a correspondence exists. For example, the visage or face is equivalent to consciousness. The heart stands for love, compassion, or kindness. As the historian Vicente Rafael (1993) puts it, the *loob* is juxtaposed to the body, rather than opposed to it. Although the body and *loob* are distinct, they interact and influence each other, with emotional distress weakening the body and disease affecting the *loob*.

Another anthropologist, Albert Alejo (1990), defines *loob* as the "very principle that gathers and governs the intellectual, emotional, volitional, and ethical dimensions of [Filipino] humanness" (p. 28). He states that in the process of becoming human, the *loob* interacts with the body, and together they bring forth a world of consciousness, feelings, attitudes, possibilities, desires, creations, and intentions.

Yet the *loob* cannot be collapsed into the body and vice versa. *Sakit* (pain/illness) is felt both in the body and in the *loob*. Carmela's despondence was not merely the result of having breast cancer. If it were so, she would have been heartened by her doctor's assertion that she would get better after the surgery. But she requested for the support group's prayer ritual to get rid of her anxiety. Like the physical body, the *loob* can weaken, get sick, and be manipulated. Hence, the need to strengthen, nurture, and purify it constantly through appropriate rituals and relationships. Our study participants associate a strong *loob* with improvement in their health outlook.

Reynaldo Ileto (1997), a historian who popularized the study of the *loob* and named it as a factor in the armed struggle against Spanish colonialism by the Filipino peasantry, links it to the Javanese idea of power, which is derived from Animism. The religion of the indigenes of the Philippine archipelago before Spanish colonization and conversion to Catholicism was Animism, a belief that spirits can be found everywhere in the universe (Vitebsky, 1995). According to Ileto, Javanese see the universe as suffused with a creative energy that can be accessed through such practices as extreme asceticism, meditation, sexual abstinence, and various types of sacrifices. The *loob* can absorb this power or cosmic energy through rites of renewal and purification, including prayers, controlled bodily movements, and other forms of self-discipline. Ascetic practices and sacrifices are closely related to concentration of power, and distractions like the world and the flesh are linked to diffusion or disintegration of power (Anderson, 1990). The more cosmic energy the *loob* can access, the greater its power, which can be used in battle and for healing. Using this framework, the support meeting attended by Carmela, which involves prayers and ritualized sacrifices such as cooking, bringing of food for the potluck, and cleaning up afterwards, is a setting that enables the concentration of cosmic energy, thus cultivating and strengthening the *loob*.

In his research among the Tagalogs in Central Luzon, Philippines, Robert Love (2004) explains that access to power is not automatic, but is dependent on an adept who has the ability to mediate between the individual seeking power and the source of power. What gets passed on to the individual from the power source through the mediator is not the power itself but the *galing*, the capacity or ability to attain excellence or perfection particularly with regards to one's well-being, health, and fortune. A sign of the transference of the *galing* is the strengthening of the *loob*. The adept and the power-seeker perform various rituals for the transfer to occur. Based on Love's paradigm, one could argue that our study participants were following a hybridized Filipino spiritual tradition that calls for spiritual practices aimed at boosting the *loob*.

Although strengthening the *loob* may not have a direct bearing on the outcome of cancer treatments, women in our study reported its positive impact in other ways. Yoly recalled:

> In the beginning I was crying and crying and of course it was the evil spirit coming in. When your body is weak, the more the cancer will spread within you. I asked the Lord and Mama Mary to help me. I was dreaming one time and Mary came down and really touched me. I told her, "Mama Mary, I still have children and they are very young, help me, let me know if I should have this surgery or not." You know, after that I really dreamt about it and She touched me. I woke up and I was crying. She told me, "My child, go ahead I will help you and you will get through this." You really have to have lakas ng loob through prayers. See?

As our participants indicated, while they clearly recognized the differences between spirituality and biomedical approach to cancer treatment, they saw the need for both. The support group visited by Carmela gave ample evidence of this awareness. Its organizer emphasized breast cancer education, and to that end, invited doctors and other medical personnel as speakers for its Monday meetings. In addition, it issued a guideline banning the imposition of one's religious beliefs on another, as well as proselytizing during meetings. Although the women looked forward to the educational lectures, limited their interaction with the speakers to medical matters, and admitted to learning considerably about breast cancer from these sessions, they continued to attribute their recovery from cancer to God, to encourage prayers as part and parcel of cancer treatment, to ask for the inclusion of clergy in the educational series and endorsed Chi Gong classes that included meditations on compassion and forgiveness.

The manifold biomedical and spiritual activities that the women engaged in call into question the observation made by anthropologists Lynch and de Guzman (1964) that Filipinos are fatalistic, based on his study of the cultural value *bahala na* (come what may). Ostensibly, it is an attitude equivalent to habitual resignation to one's fate that permeates Philippine society. However, as psychologist Virgilio Enriquez (1990) explains, *bahala na* is resorted to when Filipinos are faced with "unstructured, indefinite, unpredictable and stressful situations" that must be confronted and overcome, and instead of passivity its utterance is a signal of courage and determination in spite of highly problematic and uncertain conditions (p. 302). Like strengthening the *loob*, *bahala na* is a way of coping whose value lies in fostering resiliency in the midst of demoralizing and debilitating situations such as those faced by Filipina transnationals with breast cancer.

Breast Cancer Survivorship

Several of our participants expressed unease about being referred to as "breast cancer survivors." Panching pointed out: "I am a stroke survivor but not a cancer survivor. May be I got better with my stroke but the cancer is a lifetime illness. It will forever be there, so how can you say that you are a survivor?" Lourdes, a 58-year-old former warehouse worker, reasoned:

> I am about to pass the five-year mark and my doctor said that I will be a survivor. But I just found out I have lupus. I will not be able to return to work. I am worried about what will happen to me. I will be a burden to my daughter. So I told my doctor that I don't feel like a survivor.

Their objection to the label may be discounted as the women's way of articulating the difference between acute and chronic illness, but an analysis of their narratives paint a more complicated picture. These narratives reveal a focus on the survivorship process, which our participants called *nalampasan*. The root of nalampasan is *lampas*, which can be translated as "reaching beyond," "passing ahead," or "passing through." When inflected, as in nalampasan, it pertains to the past. Its root can also be repeated, as in *lampas-lampasan*, to mean "through and through." By using nalampasan, the women likened their experience of breast cancer to a journey. The word connotes passing someone or something as one travels along on the same path. The emphasis is on the process of journeying, rather than the place of departure or destination. The journey's progress is not measured on the basis of distance or time but on circumstances and people encountered while traveling. In other words, our participants did not view their illness as separate from concurrent experiences happening in their lives. Although coping with breast cancer was a priority, the women viewed it as just one of the many hardships that they had to pass through (Burke et al., 2012).

Consider Letty's story. Trained as a certified public accountant, Letty came to the United States to work in various menial jobs to support her three children and an unemployed, philandering husband in the Philippines. She finally found a job as a bookkeeper for a small-business owner who rewarded her hard work by sponsoring her work visa. After five years of self-deprivation to save money, she was able to bring her family to San Francisco. While working on two jobs, without health insurance, she was diagnosed with breast cancer. She asked her sister living in another city to care for her children on Fridays and Saturdays for several months so that she could undergo medical treatments on her own. Letty took the children back on Sundays, as soon as she was able to withstand the side effects of her chemotherapy. Like our other study participants, Letty credited her *lakas ng loob* for her ability to make it through.

Letty regarded herself as a single mother worried about her children's welfare throughout her treatment. Moreover, she had to deal with domestic violence when her husband arrived from the Philippines. Weakened by cancer therapies, Letty nevertheless managed to get a restraining order against her husband and divorce him, while protecting her children. In narrating her struggle with breast cancer, she situated her illness in relation to other events in her life and her role as mother rather than focusing on her medical condition. As she told us, she passed through and moved ahead not just regarding breast cancer, but the other trials that made up her journey. Similarly, Loreta, whose story appeared earlier, placed her experience of breast cancer within the context of the discrimination she had experienced as a child laborer in Malaysia, the violence and assault she experienced in the Philippines as an adult, and the struggles she had faced since coming to San Francisco as she worked to care for her own mother and young daughter.

Because *lampas* or passing happens in relation to others, survivorship involves helping others pass through adversity (Burke et al., 2012). This was mirrored in a statement by Mitring who had accepted the burdens of her illness, but was worried about her daughter's reaction: "My problem was how to make my daughter pass beyond [the pain] when she finds out I have breast cancer." Another participant, Tekla, added a novena to San Ramon, patron saint of pregnant women, for her daughter-in-law who was experiencing a complicated pregnancy. She also became caregiver to her grandchild while her daughter-in-law recovered. Passing ahead of someone implied a successful journey but also called for a sense of responsibility to help those who are having troubles of their own.

Another layer of meaning embedded in *nalampasan* is a sense of complete and thorough penetration. The trauma of breast cancer and its ripple effects not only impacted their physical bodies but also penetrated their *loob*'s deepest recesses, leaving no relationships and circumstances untouched. The experience was transformative because the women were able to put their shattered lives back together again in spite of the pain that they endured. From their perspective, survivorship, therefore, is about a return to wholeness.

Our participants' objection at being called breast cancer survivors rested partly on the understanding that cancer was not an acute disease with a set ending, either of recovery and resumption of prior activities or of death (Lubkin & Larsen, 2006). Remission in cancer does not mean one is cured because of the possibility that it will return and affect other parts of the body as well. The other, more important reason for the women's discomfort with the label was its marginalization of their experience and identity as women who have passed through hardships. Their biomedical path and its marker such as the number of years a patient has survived breast cancer from the time of diagnosis did not capture the totality of their experience as Filipino trasnationals who overcame multiple, and sometimes simultaneous, difficulties of which breast cancer was only one. The label also did not encompass the inner transformations that they had undergone to address those difficulties. Our participants believed that inner transformations were necessary for their recovery.

Conclusion

Our study of Filipino transnationals with experience of breast cancer reveals that spirituality plays a significant role in their management of and recovery from breast cancer. Our findings support to a degree Pargament's theory of religious coping—that religion can be used as a coping mechanism in situations of stress, particularly by certain groups of people such as ethnic minorities with a vigorous religious culture. However, our findings indicate that our participants' turn to spirituality in dealing with breast cancer served more than instrumental purposes. This turn was influenced by the notion of Filipino subjectivity or personhood rooted in the *loob*. Our participants engaged in religious activities like prayers and novenas not merely to ask God to get rid of their disease, but more importantly, to strengthen their *loob* in order to have the capacity to confront difficulties related and unrelated to their breast cancer.

A strengthened *loob* set the context for breast cancer recovery as it enabled the women to conquer fears and anxieties that heightened despair and isolation and served as practical barriers to health-care access and treatment. As they fulfilled their medical appointments and underwent surgery and various therapies, the women also insisted on continuing their spiritual practices. They refused to let their medical schedules interfere with their other goal of nurturing the *loob*, not only to vitalize their spirit for their ongoing breast cancer treatment but also for the struggles that awaited them outside the clinics and hospitals. For Filipino transnationals with breast cancer, the disease was but one of many hurdles that had to be surmounted if they were to improve their lives and those of loved ones.

The women's insistence on paying attention to their *loob* through spirituality allowed them to forge a subjectivity separate from their biomedical identity as chronically diseased individuals. In their attempt to seek courage and determination from within their persons, they experienced the ability to gain control of their situation, giving them a sense of agency to seek outside intervention for their medical as well as other equally pressing needs. While facing mortality and abusive situations, they did not only cope but also become empowered. Thus, participants described themselves as more than survivors of breast cancer, but women who have passed through incredible hardships and deserve a respected place among their families and transnational communities.

Our study shows that the relationship between spirituality and chronic illness is more complex, going beyond standard measures of health outcomes such as psychological stress and illness adjustment. Our findings illustrate the impact of spirituality on issues of health-care access, identity, gender, and empowerment, which can influence health and quality of life, albeit indirectly. Our findings also indicate that spirituality plays a crucial role in the management of chronic illness. It not only decreases the level of stress after a disease diagnosis, but also offers a parallel and balancing perspective to intense and physically debilitating medical treatment regimens.

For the participants in our study, the Filipino spiritual tradition rooted in the *loob* provided a framework from which to view their illness and the challenges it posed. They regarded strengthening the *loob* through spiritual practices as a crucial step in countering their illness, which affected not only the body but also the inner self. Thus, management of chronic illness involved two parallel and simultaneous tracks—inner spiritual transformation and disease treatment. One without the other constituted an incomplete response to chronic illness.

REFERENCES

Airhihebuwa, C. O. (1985). *Health and culture: Beyond the western paradigm.* Thousand Oaks, CA: Sage Publications.

Alejo, A. E. (1990). *Tao po! Tuloy po!* [It's a person! Please come in!]. Quezon City, Metro Manila: Ateneo de Manila University Office of Research and Publications.

Anderson, B. R. (1990). *Language and power: Exploring political cultures in Indonesia.* Ithaca, NY: Cornell University Press.

Baquet, C. R., Mishra, S. I., Commiskey, P., Ellison, G. L., & DeShields, M. (2008). Breast cancer epidemiology in blacks and whites: Disparities in incidence, mortality, survival rates and histology. *Journal of the National Medical Association, 100*(5), 480–488.

Burke, N. J., Villero, O. V., & Guerra, C. (2012). Passing through: Meanings of survivorship and support among Filipinas with breast cancer. *Qualitative Health Research, 22*(2), 189–198.

Carnes, T., & Yang, F. (Eds.). (2004). *Asian American religions: The making and remaking of borders and boundaries.* New York, NY: New York University Press.

California Cancer Registry. (2012). *Geographic variations in advanced stage breast cancer in California, 1999–2003.* Retrieved from http://www.ccrcal.org/Data_and_Statistics/GISBreast/index.shtml.

Campbell, D. J., Yoon, D. P., & Johnstone, B. (2010). Determining relationships between physical health and spiritual experience, religious practices, and congregational support in a heterogenous medical sample. *Journal of Religion and Health, 49*(1), 3–17.

Covar, P. C. (1998). *Larangan: Seminal essays on Philippine culture.* Manila: Sampaguita Press.

Ellison, C. G., & Levin, J. S. (1998). The religion-health connection: Evidence, theory, and future directions. *Health Education and Behavior, 25*(6), 700–720.

Enriquez, V. (1990). Indigenous personality theory. In *Indigenous psychology: A book of readings* . Quezon City, Metro Manila: Akademya ng Sikolohiyang Pilipino, 285–310.

Gall, T. L., Kristjansson, E., Charbonneau, C., & Florack, P. (2009). A longitudinal study on the role of spirituality in response to the diagnosis and treatment of breast cancer. *Journal of Behaviorial Medicine, 32*(2), 174–186.

Goldman, R., Hunt, M. K., Allen, J. D., Hauser, S., Emmons, K., Maeda, M., & Sorensen, G. (2003). The life history interview method: Applications to intervention development. *Health Education and Behavior, 30*(5), 564–581.

Gomez, S. L., Clarke, C. A., Shema, S. J., Chang, E. T., Keegan, T. H. M., & Glaser, S. L. (2010). Disparities in breast cancer survival among Asian women by ethnicity and immigrant status: A population-based study. *American Journal of Public Health, 100*(5), 861–869.

Gonzalez, J. L. (2009). *Filipino American faith in action: Immigration, religion, and civic engagement.* New York, NY: New York University Press.

Guarnizo, L. E. (2003). The economics of transnational living. *International Migration Review, 37*(3), 666–699.

Herbert, R., Zdaniuk, B., Schulz, R., & Scheier, M. (2009). Positive and negative religious coping and well-being in women with breast cancer. *Journal of Palliative Medicine, 12*(6), 537–545.

Howard, A. F., Balneaves, L. G., & Bottorff, J. L. (2007). Ethnocultural women's experiences of breast cancer: A qualitative meta-study. *Cancer Nursing, 30*(4), E27–35.

Ileto, R. C. (1997). *Pasyon and revolution: Popular movements in the Philippines, 1840–1910.* Quezon City, Metro Manila: Ateneo de Manila University Press.

Johnson, K. R. S. (1998). Ethnocultural influences in cancer. *Journal of Clinical Psychology in Medical Settings, 5*(3), 357–364.

Johnstone, B., Franklin, K. L., Yoon, D. P., Burris, J., & Shigaki, C. (2008). Relationships among religiousness, spirituality, and health for individuals with stroke. *Journal of Clinical Psychology in Medical Settings, 15*(4), 308–313.

Keegan, T. H., Gomez, S. L., Clarke, C. A., Chan, J. K., & Glaser, S. L. (2007). Recent trends in breast cancer incidence among six Asian groups in the Greater Bay Area of Northern California. *International Journal of Cancer, 120*(6), 1324–1329.

Lin, S. S., Clarke, C. A., Prehn, A. W., Glaser, S. L., West, D. W., & O'Malley, C. D., (2002). Survival differences among Asian subpopulations in the United States after prostate, colorectal, breast, and cervical cancer. *Cancer, 94*(4), 1175–1182.

Love, R. S. (2004). *The Samahan of papa God: Tradition and conversion in a Tagalog peasant religious movement.* Manila: Anvil Press.

Lubkin, I. M., & Larsen, P. D. (2006). *Chronic illness: Impact and interventions.* Sudbury, MA: Jones & Bartlett Publishers.

Lynch, F., & de Guzman, A. (Eds.). (1964). *Four readings on Philippine values.* Quezon City, Metro Manila: Ateneo de Manila University Press.

Maxwell, A. E., Bastani, R., Vida, P., & Warda, U. S. (2003). Results of a randomized trial to increase breast and cervical cancer screening among Filipino American women. *Preventive Medicine, 37*, 102–109.

Pargament, K. I. (1997). *The psychology of religion and coping: Theory, research, practice.* New York, NY: Guilford Press.

Petron, M. A. (2008). Negotiating borders with "Valores del Rancho". *Latin American Perspectives, 35*(1), 104–119.

Pew Forum on Religion and Public Life (December 19, 2011). *Global Christianity: A report on the size and distribution of the world's Christian population.* Retrieved from http://www.pewforum.org/Christian/Global-Christianity-philippines.aspx.

Rafael, V. L. (1993). *Contracting colonialism: Translation and Christian conversion in Tagalog society under early Spanish rule.* Durham, NC: Duke University Press.

Sue, S., Fujino, D. C., Hu, L. T., Takeuchi, D. T., & Zana, N. W. (1991). Community mental health services for ethnic minority groups: A test of the cultural responsiveness hypothesis. *Journal of Consulting and Clinical Psychology, 59*(4), 533–540.

Takaki, R. (1998). *Strangers from a different shore: A history of Asian Americans.* Boston: Little, Brown.

Taylor, E. J., Outlaw, F. H., Bernardo, T., & Roy, A. (1999). Spiritual conflicts associated with praying about cancer. *Psycho-Oncology, 8,* 386–394.

Terrazas, A., & Batalova, J. (2010). Migration Policy Institute. *Filipino immigrants in the United States.* Retrieved from http://www.migrationinformation.org/usfocus/display.cfm? ID = 777.

Vitebsky, P. (1995). *The Shaman.* London: Little, Brown and Company.

Wu, T., & Bancroft, J. (2006). Filipino American women's perceptions and experiences with breast cancer screening. *Oncology Nursing Forum, 33*(4), 71–78.

CHAPTER 4

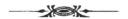

PATHOPHYSIOLOGIC BASIS AND APPLICATION OF SPIRITUAL HEALING PRACTICES IN CHRONIC ILLNESS

Ruth Stanley

Ancient healers from diverse spiritual traditions were remarkably keen to the correlation of illness with our emotional self-regulation, attitudes, and perceptions. From their perspective, spirituality encompassed the deepest desires of being human and the ongoing expression and fulfillment through human thoughts, feelings, and actions. As such, spirituality lay at the core of human mental, physical, and emotional health, forming the bedrock of our perceptions, both positive and negative. In these traditions, spirituality facilitated a sense of well-being and connection to life even in the face of stressors such as debilitating or terminal illness. Thus, physical health was always considered within the framework of spiritual health or enlightenment. To be healthy was something far beyond physical cure or physical health. The emphasis was to become whole in mind, body, and spirit with a deliberate focus on integration and acceptance within the limitations of any given disease or circumstance. There was one common pathway to wholeness, which fostered freedom *from* negative, destructive, or habitual emotional and thought patterns in order to be free *for* positive, compassionate living grounded in trust and love. The designs of many ancient spiritual or healing practices from a variety of traditions emphasized physical calm, promoted perceptual awareness, and cultivated heartfelt safety and trust.

Science is beginning to teach us to better appreciate and trust the wisdom of our ancient healing traditions. We now know there is a high correlation between integrated spirituality and positive clinical outcomes across all demographics in chronic disease states (Koenig et al., 2001). Patients who regularly practice spiritual techniques consistent with their belief system receive the greatest health benefits, including reduced rates of morbidity and mortality. As such, spiritual practices appear critical for maintaining a sense of optimism, peace, joy, and comfort in chronic, debilitating, or terminal disease. Why is this so significant? The answer is quite simple. Chronic illness is often associated with baseline autonomic nervous system (ANS) dysfunction, and effective spiritual healing practices have been demonstrated to improve ANS function.

Our ANS determines overall physical, cognitive, emotional, and spiritual health by serving as our body's well-being gatekeeper, constantly controlling perception, emotional self- regulation and behavioral responses to any given stimuli (Porges, 2011). Because expectations and desires frame our perception of any given disease diagnosis, it follows that our attitudes toward chronic illness directly affect ANS function and thus quality of life and clinical outcomes. Even though perceptions do not cause disease, they significantly influence how effectively our ANS can respond to ongoing disease processes and our felt sense of mental, physical, emotional, and spiritual well-being in the midst of chronic illness. Although not linked as a single specific etiology of any given disease state, severely negative attitudes interfere with innate healing processes. Negativity and poor emotional self-regulation further worsen the ANS dysfunction already seen with any disease process, impede our natural defenses against disease, and lead to poorer clinical outcomes. Compared to patients with neutral or positive attitudes, patients who are excessively negative toward their chronic illness can experience more rapidly debilitating disease processes, unrelieved pain, functional impairment, emotional instability, and emergence of coexisting disease states. From a mental health perspective, overly negative attitudes can result in a two to five times higher prevalence of depression and a greater than 50 percent incidence of coexistent general anxiety, panic, or post-traumatic stress disorder in chronic illness. In contrast, patients who maintain a sense of positivity, hope, or optimism in chronic illness exhibit better overall coping skills, emotional stability, natural defenses against disease, and higher quality of life (Koenig et al., 2001).

Since ANS function can be practically measured and modified with heart rate variability (HRV), techniques improving HRV mirror improved ANS function and overall well-being (McCraty et al., 2006; Kok & Fredrickson, 2010). Effective spiritual techniques measurably improve HRV and result in improved emotional self-regulation, clinical outcomes, and quality of life across all chronic disease states. Therefore, ancient spiritual techniques from diverse traditions can be practical complements to routine medical treatment for enhancing overall clinical outcomes and mental health in chronic illness. It seems our ancestors' understanding of holistic health and healing was far more accurate and integrative than ever previously imagined given the remarkable emphasis on our ANS as the pathway to well-being.

In this chapter, we explore the pathophysiologic basis of spiritual healing practices in chronic illness. We examine first the fascinating pathophysiology of our body's gatekeeper, the ANS, followed by the pivotal role of the ANS in emotional self-regulation. We will then look at practical applications of measuring and modifying ANS function with the use of heart rate variability (HRV) as related to clinical outcomes in chronic illness. Finally, we explore the impact of universal spiritual healing practices on HRV and emotional self-regulation in chronic illness by specifically focusing on breathing, simple movement, emotional refocus, and awareness techniques. First, we begin with nurturing a basic understanding of how our ANS controls overall health and well-being.

PATHOPHYSIOLOGY OF OUR ANS

Although once thought very simple and dualistic, the ANS is now understood as a much more complex family of neural systems, which evolved to support both survival and social engagement. Our ANS has three distinct phylogenetically ordered neural response systems to assess safety and respond effectively to perceived danger (Porges, 2009, 2011). Found in all invertebrates and reptiles, the oldest phylogenetic ANS is a simple unmyelinated or "vegetative" vagus nerve controlling bodily systems below the diaphragm, which of course is vitally important in these creatures since they spend their days primarily seeking, eating, and digesting food (Porges, 2007a, 2009, 2011). In response to danger, stimulation of the vegetative vagus produces severe neurogenic bradycardia and immobile freeze (i.e. feign death) or passive avoidance. Activation of this oldest vegetative vagus in humans is normally inhibited unless the other two newer systems catastrophically fail.

Of significantly more importance is the sympathetic system, a second phylogenetic ANS system which evolved for vertebrates like humans. Opposite of the vegetative vagus, stimulation of the sympathetic system results in mobilization or active avoidance (i.e. fight or flight) in response to perceived danger or environmental changes (Porges, 2009, 2007a, 2011). The ability to mobilize rapidly requires a lot of energy and quick fuel (i.e. glucose), which is provided by immediate release of cortisol (i.e. stress hormone), breakdown of protein and amino acids to sugar, and insulin resistance. Our sympathetic system is routinely reserved for active response to immediate perceived danger, thus the nickname "fight or flight." Chronic stimulation of the sympathetic system weakens our ANS and causes the emergence of cardiovascular, systemic, immunologic, infectious, endocrine, and autoimmune diseases. Fortunately for us, evolution did not stop with two opposing systems (i.e. total immobilization versus mobilization) since uncontrolled stimulation of either can result in great harm, even death. Under normal circumstances, the sympathetic system is selectively inhibited or suppressed by our newest, most integrated phylogenetic system, the "smart" vagus nerve.

The final and clearly dominant phylogenetic ANS is a highly myelinated "smart" vagus neural network, which controls all emotion, motion, and communication. The smart vagus is our ANS gatekeeper: Without its proper function we cannot thrive, much less survive (Porges, 2011; Porges &

Furman, 2011). Unlike reptiles, we are dependent on socialization for optimal health and survival, so the smart vagus is focused above the diaphragm
to control a vastly expanded repertoire of social engagement functions. This
system gives us the critical and sophisticated ability to assess, communicate,
and respond to our environment and each other. Our smart vagal network
controls the other two more primitive ANS phylogenetic systems in order
to regulate homeostasis (i.e. physiologic stability), which normally favors
calm states of energy conservation, restoration, and maintenance. Myelinated
vagal parasympathetic tone, or more simply vagal tone, is normally high
to inhibit or suppress sympathetic response (i.e. fight or flight) during safe
conditions. Our smart vagal myelinated network is also called our social
engagement system because it regulates activities necessary for healthy socialization such as muscles controlling head, neck, and facial gestures, emotional
expression of eyes and face, hearing, talking, swallowing, and breathing.
As a gatekeeper, our social engagement system processes affective experience, emotional expression, facial gesture, vocal communication, sounds, and
social behavior in order to assess safety. Once stimuli are interpreted as safe
or threatening, vagal tone is adjusted much like a volume control dial to
regulate communication and behavior by inhibiting or allowing sympathetic
response (i.e. fight or flight). Flexibility or adaptability in adjusting vagal tone
up or down is necessary to properly manage homeostasis between calm and
threatened states. How does vagal tone affect emotional self-regulation?

EMOTIONAL SELF-REGULATION AND VAGAL TONE

The ability to accurately perceive danger or detect whether another person
is trustworthy is the primary focus of our ANS and absolutely critical to
health and well-being. Clearly stated, basic ANS regulation of physiologic
and emotional states is dependent on one thing: assessment of safety or
threat. ANS response can be easily categorized as either approach (i.e. safety)
or withdrawal (i.e. threat) with corresponding emotional perceptual correlates of positive (i.e. approach, safe) or negative (i.e. withdrawal, threat)
(Porges, 2011, 2011b). Based on perception of safety or threat, our gatekeeper (i.e. social engagement system) adjusts vagal tone to control emotional
self-regulation and conscious choices to inhibit behavioral impulses, make
decisions, or persist in difficult tasks (Kok & Fredrickson, 2010; Appelhans &
Luecken, 2006; Thayer et al., 2009).

When properly functioning, our gatekeeper fosters relationship in safe
environments by maintaining a high vagal tone (dial volume at high) to
inhibit the sympathetic withdrawal response (see Appendix A). We experience high vagal tone or safety as a sense of calm, decreased emotional or
cognitive arousal with negative stimuli, more positivity (i.e. joy, love, peace,
gratitude), socialization, and increased self-regulating capacity to control
destructive emotional, cognitive, and behavioral patterns. If our gatekeeper
perceives threat or negative stimuli, vagal tone is quickly reduced (dial volume lowered) to allow appropriate sympathetic response, including negative

emotions (i.e. fear, anger, anxiety, and aggression) and withdrawal from danger (i.e. fight or flight). Ideally, high vagal tone is quickly restored once an immediate threat is over, and vagal inhibition (dial volume back to high) of the sympathetic response (i.e. fight or flight) is re-engaged. If our vagal tone dial is faulty, impaired, or unable to function, insufficient vagal tone means continued sympathetic response (i.e. fight or flight) domination, erosion of emotional self-regulation, misinterpretation of neutral or positive stimuli as negative, increased negativity and destructive patterns, and increased potential of chronic disease (Porges, 2011). Thus, ANS assessment of safety (i.e. gatekeeping) and response (i.e. vagal tone) are critical to our overall health and physiologic capacity for self-regulating emotions, thoughts, and behaviors. Given the importance to overall health, is there a way to clinically measure ANS function in chronic illness?

MEASURING VAGAL TONE FOR CLINICAL PRACTICE

Both respiratory sinus arrhythmia (RSA) and heart rate variability (HRV) are excellent measures of vagal tone and the overall ANS function. RSA measures vagal tone as reflected in the normal variation of heart rate (i.e. increase with inspiration, decrease with expiration) that accompanies respiration (Porges, 2007a, 2007b; Ysauma & Hayano, 2004). Vagal tone as measured by RSA is optimal at our resonant breathing rate of 4.5–7 breaths per minute. HRV, the other measureable index, correlates well with RSA (i.e. correlation coefficient 0.95) and provides a more practical and useful working measure for ANS and emotional self- regulatory capacity (McCraty et al., 2006; Porges, 2007a; Lehrer et al., 2000; Berntson et al., 1997; Shields, 2009; Segerstrom & Nes, 2007; Kok & Fredrickson, 2010; Thayer et al., 2009; Appelhans & Leucken, 2006). Recorded as distinct frequency patterns or time domain intervals from the electrocardiogram (ECG), HRV is the brief time interval between heartbeats reflecting ANS function, vagal tone, and the interplay between sympathetic and parasympathetic activity (i.e. vagal tone volume dial). HRV essentially measures ANS adaptability. At around 0.1 Hz frequency, the body naturally enters a profound innate healing state of maximal adaptability, resetting gatekeeping and vagal tone dial to restore proper vagal tone and maximal self-regulatory capacity (see Appendix B). As would be expected, 0.1 Hz is the same frequency associated with resonant breathing and optimal RSA. The 0.1 Hz healing frequency reflects one of our body's most powerful restorative states for achieving emotional, physical, cognitive, and spiritual well-being, even in the midst of disease.

HRV, then, is an excellent overall measure of ANS function, emotional self-regulatory capacity, and RSA. Simply stated, chronically low HRV usually denotes faulty gatekeeping or an inflexible vagal tone dial and typically corresponds to more negative emotional valence, low self-regulatory ability, and higher cortisol (i.e. stress hormone) levels. As with ANS dysfunction, chronically low HRV is associated with most chronic disease states and correlates well with significantly decreased quality of life and worsened prognosis, morbidity, and mortality (McCraty et al., 2006) (see Appendix C). Not surprisingly, very low HRV is consistently found in chronic conditions with documented poor self-regulation, such as addictive or compulsive pathologies, personality disorders, anxiety, panic, depression, and bipolar. In contrast, normal or high HRV usually suggests a good gatekeeper and very flexible dial function. Normal or high HRV is associated with increased quality of life, more positive emotions, better cognitive performance, stronger social engagement and connection, and decreased morbidity and mortality in chronic illness. People with higher baseline HRV are better able to self-regulate and overcome destructive emotional and behavioral patterns as would be expected with normal ANS function.

Most importantly, HRV also appears to be a good measure of our ability to overcome genetic predispositions and habitual preferences regarding emotional self-regulation in response to negative stressors. Improving HRV from a chronically low initial baseline restores gatekeeping and vagal tone, thus correcting emotional self-regulatory deficits and restoring optimal adaptability to our ANS. Thus, a faulty gatekeeper or impaired vagal tone dial can be internally modified or reset by increasing HRV to improve physical, emotional, cognitive, and behavioral well-being. This is good news for patients with chronic illness, since the opportunity to improve overall sense of well-being (i.e. emotional, spiritual, cognitive) is possible even in the face of debilitating disease. The magnitude of clinical improvement is related to the degree of overall improvement in HRV, vagal tone, or ability to consistently achieve our innate healing frequency (i.e. 0.1 Hz). How then do we improve HRV? Astute ancient healers knew the answer to this question, so let us now take our understanding of ANS pathophysiology and explore spiritual healing practices.

Pathophysiology and Healing Practices

As stated earlier, core attitudes, expectations, and desires frame our perception of any given person, event, or disease diagnosis. Consciously and unconsciously, every person, event, or circumstance is evaluated, judged, and labeled as positive, negative, or neutral by our ANS as it relates to our deepest needs, desires, and sense of safety. Something or someone perceived as positive or neutral results in approach behaviors, calm, and a sense of safety and well-being. In contrast, anything or anyone labeled as negative is threatening, which results in withdrawal behaviors, fear, and a sense of danger. Stressors in our life are simply something or someone we assess as negative or threatening because it is not the way we want, think, or feel it should be to meet our needs. When we label something or someone as negative, it only becomes detrimental to our health when we are driven to change it to meet our needs. Overwhelming fear fueling our need to change a situation or person signals overt danger to our ANS. Fear, denial, and desire to change any new diagnosis of chronic illness are normal responses. However, consistent fear of the uncontrollable, of not having needs met or of death result in exaggerated physiologic defensive strategies including significantly reduced vagal tone (dial volume lowered) and chronic activation of the sympathetic response (i.e. fight or flight). With chronic illness, people who maintain ongoing negative labeling of their illness through destructive thought and emotional patterns experience a greater sense of hopelessness and helplessness, increased levels of pain, poorer quality of life, higher morbidity and mortality, and significantly more mental and somatic complaints (Koenig et al., 2001; Thayer et al., 2009). From a holistic standpoint, ancient healers understood that the most important factor is not that chronic illness is good or bad, but that we perceive it as significantly negative. It is this negative labeling of disease that results in lowered vagal tone and chronic sympathetic response (i.e. fight or flight), both of which only complicate an already compromised ANS in chronic illness. Thus, a primary purpose of ancient spiritual practices in chronic illness was to transition someone from physiologic "fight or flight," negative labeling and fear toward safety, positive labeling, and neutrality.

Fortunately, humans have the ability to perceptually and emotionally reframe negative stimuli as neutral or even positive through fostering a sense of security and acceptance. We can re-educate and reset our gatekeeper's assessment regarding what is actually safe or threatening, and we can adjust our vagal tone dial. Ancient healing traditions were very effective at this, sharing a common emphasis on transforming negative stimuli into neutral or positive ones in order to restore health. Ancient traditions from both the East and the West accurately recognized that normal fear-related patterns associated with chronic illness are not in and of themselves unhealthy; they are, rather, to be expected. Learning to accept what "is," versus fighting against it, allows us to live within the healthy boundaries of our limitations, maximizing our health as much as possible. Ancient healing remedies emphasized spiritual practices focused on physically calming the body, increasing neutral awareness of destructive patterns, and overcoming the tendency to dwell on negative emotions or thoughts in overly excessive or repressive ways (Cassian, 2000). In doing so, we facilitate our body's ability to fight disease and utilize its innate wisdom for wholeness. Therefore, some ancient spiritual practices may be highly effective at restoring ANS function by resetting our gatekeeper and vagal tone dial using techniques designed to refocus our body, thoughts, feelings, and spirit on calm, safety, security, and trust. As would be expected, effective spiritual healing practices improve HRV, significantly increasing vagal tone and fostering innate healing (i.e. 0.1 Hz frequency). Given the relationship among poor ANS function, low HRV, and chronic illness, it is no surprise that a pathophysiologic basis for spiritual practices is simply restoration of maximal possible ANS adaptability, which results in improved vagal tone and emotional self-regulation regardless of disease process.

Four core spiritual practices are found in some form throughout every ancient healing tradition, regardless of religion, geography, or historical timeframe. These practices are: breathing, simple physical movements, emotional refocus, and awareness practices. Breathing and simple movement are calming physical practices to negate the sympathetic response (i.e. fight or flight). Emotional refocus and awareness are directed more toward specifically altering perceptions to prevent or neutralize sympathetic response (i.e. fight or flight) by overcoming negative, destructive thought and emotional patterns. Let us begin with the simple practice of breathing.

BREATHING PRACTICES

The first universal holistic practice for improving HRV and ANS function is also the most fundamental... breathing. Reflective of the mystery of life, breathing is at the core of most spiritual traditions and has always been correlated to mental, spiritual, emotional, and physical health. For example, the divine association of breath to life is evident in the Jewish name for God, YHWH. When pronounced in the native Hebrew language, the word reproduces only the sound of inhalation and exhalation and expresses the belief that the source of life is mystically the very breath sustaining us each moment. All healing traditions, regardless of belief system, share breathing practices as a core practice to calm the body, and in turn also the mind and spirit. The importance placed on breathing across traditions reflects an intuitive, deep understanding of human breathing patterns as they relate to health, healing, and wholeness. The quality and rate of respiration is the most immediate, reliable holistic method for modifying ANS function. As the only vital ANS function in the body open to both conscious and unconscious awareness and modification, breathing directly impacts psychological, spiritual, physical, and emotional states. Controlled by our ANS gatekeeper, the direct relationship between respiration and vagal tone can be easily observed in our patterns of breathing. For example, low vagal tone (i.e. volume dial set low) results in shallow, rapid breathing patterns consistent with increased sympathetic response (i.e. fight or flight). Slowed, deep breathing calms us by dialing back up vagal tone, reducing sympathetic response (i.e. fight or flight), and allowing an overwhelmed gatekeeper the opportunity to reassess more accurately environmental cues for safety or danger.

The goal of most breathing techniques is to invite the body into the natural rhythm of resonant breathing associated with optimal RSA, 0.1 Hz frequency, and physical calm (Lehrer, 2007; Lehrer et al., 2000). As discussed earlier, RSA is directly correlated with vagal tone and represents the normal variation in heart rate seen with respiration (i.e. increase with inhalation, decrease with exhalation). Respiratory efficiency and highest oxygen exchange occur between 4.5 and 7 breaths a minute, which is a much slower respiratory pace than the 9–24 breaths per minute normally seen in healthy adults. Breathing at a pace of around six breaths per minute (range 4.5–7) usually results in resonant breathing or optimal RSA, producing a rise and fall in heart rate completely in unison with each inhalation and exhalation (Bernardi et al., 2001; Lehrer, 2007; Adams et al., 2009; Wang et al., 2010; Shields, 2009; Oveis et al., 2009). Resonant breathing optimizes high vagal tone and ANS function, resulting in innate healing (i.e. 0.1 Hz frequency) and improved emotional self-regulation. People who practice resonant breathing have a decreased hypoxic ventilatory response, better oxygen saturation when stressed, and better tolerance to exercise or high altitudes. Breathing practices promoting resonant breathing at 0.1 Hz result in clinically significant improvements in overall gatekeeping, vagal tone, exercise tolerance, emotional self-regulation, quality of life, pain, anxiety, fatigue, insomnia, depression, morbidity, mortality, pulmonary function, blood pressure, and psychosocial/emotional burden of disease (Lehrer, 2007; Lehrer et al., 2004; Karavidas et al., 2007; Courtney et al., 2011; Wang et al., 2010; Adams et al., 2009). People with chronic illness often develop dysfunctional breathing patterns consistent with decreased physiologic resilience, loss of ANS adaptability, and worsened self-regulatory capacity. Simply changing the quality and pace of our breathing can result in significant emotional, psychological, spiritual, and physical improvement. Breathing practices are effective free treatment strategies in chronic illness . . . if we are willing to do them. A good philosophy is that since we are breathing anyway, why not breathe in a way that helps us!

There are many breathing techniques that can produce RSA, and breathing is often combined with physical movement, emotional refocus, and awareness practices to maximize benefit. HRV biofeedback is a simple way to learn how to breathe at a resonant frequency (Lehrer, 2007). By counting or synchronizing breathing with sound or object, one can easily be taught resonant breathing as verified with HRV measurement and feedback. To determine patient-specific resonant frequency, different rates of breathing between 4.5 and 7 breaths per minute are tested to determine optimal breathing pace (i.e. RSA) as identified by 0.1 Hz HRV pattern. With deliberate practice of 15 minutes or more two to three times daily, a person can quickly condition himself or herself to breathe easily at this frequency anytime. Commercial, easy-to-use HRV biofeedback software are available, as are simple-to-use hand-held devices. HRV biofeedback is particularly effective in chronic pulmonary disease: Patients achieving optimal RSA have improved pulmonary function test, lower use of rescue and maintenance medications, fewer symptoms, and fewer exacerbations (Lehrer et al., 2004,). Resonant breathing can result in one full level of clinical improvement based on the National Heart Lung and Blood Institute classification of asthma severity. Similarly robust positive clinical outcomes have been noted with HRV biofeedback to facilitate RSA across multiple chronic disease states, including cardiovascular, cancer, diabetes, autoimmune, pain syndromes, anxiety, panic or post-traumatic stress disorder, and major depression (Lehrer, 2007; Wang et al., 2010; Karavidas et al., 2007). Significant increases in vagal tone associated with breathing practices directly correlate with acute and long-term clinical benefit in chronic illness.

Not surprisingly, other methods of eliciting RSA without the benefit of HRV biofeedback training have been shown to positively improve HRV with frequency patterns observed at 0.1 Hz. Deep abdominal breathing improves HRV and clinical outcomes associated with a variety of medical and mental health disorders (van Dixhoorn, 2007; Kulur et al., 2009; Rossi-Caruso et al., 2011). Paced breathing devices that facilitate deep breathing are now approved by the FDA to treat hypertension and are equally as effective as drug therapy in managing mild hypertension. These devices use sound to slow breathing and to pace each inhalation and exhalation. Spiritual masters through the ages have employed rote prayers, poetry, chants, and mantras designed to pace breathing at around six breaths per minute for similar purposes (Cysarz et al., 2004; Bernardi et al., 2001). These spiritual practices are well documented to produce equally powerful resonant breathing (i.e. RSA at 0.1 Hz) as that seen with HRV biofeedback and modern-era paced-breathing devices. Common to these practices is the use of a slightly longer exhalation in combination with normal inhalation. Prolonged exhalation immediately increases vagal tone, decreases heart rate, increases calm, prevents hyperventilation, and invites resonant breathing (see Appendix D). In this author's experience, it was found that simple long-exhalation breathing was highly effective among the chronically ill for improving emotional self-regulation and sleep as well as for reducing pain and anxiety (Stanley et al., 2011).

Given the primary importance of breathing to ANS function, health, and wholeness, the use of breathing techniques to improve health cannot be understated. Breathing is an easy, safe practice that produces an immediate impact on ANS function and consistently results in positive benefit if patients are willing to use the technique. I recommend simple long-exhalation breathing (see Appendix D) as a technique easily mastered and as a good starting point for most people interested in learning a practice to quickly calm themselves.

SIMPLE PHYSICAL MOVEMENT

A second universal spiritual practice is simple movement. The tendency in chronic illness to become rigid in both mind and body was well recognized by spiritual masters. Because activation of the sympathetic system prepares the body for active mobilization, exercise and simple physical movement are highly effective for re-establishing vagal tone and inviting calm states. Physical activity, even in small amounts such as walking pets, is relaxing and highly beneficial for reducing sympathetic overactivity and improving HRV (Motooka et al., 2006; Sakuragi & Sugiyama, 2006). Ancient healing practices took this one step further and emphasized slow, deliberate physical movement synchronized with breathing. The conscious intention to slow physical motion and focus sole attentiveness on gentle body movement significantly alters emotions and communication. Gentle mobilization strategies using slowed breathing coupled with specific physical poses, postures, and movements increase fluidity, strength, balance, and flexibility, which parallel emotional, psychological, and spiritual shifts toward wholeness. Simple movement improves vagal tone and overall HRV, allowing our gatekeeper the opportunity to reassess internal and external stimuli and re-label as needed to reset our ANS in favor of calm, restorative, maintenance functions. The most common forms of simple movement used in the treatment of chronic illness are the Eastern techniques of yoga, tai chi, and qigong, all of which come in many forms, styles, and intensities.

Clinical benefit is seen across a spectrum of chronic disease states with breathing and simple movement to restore ANS function and create calm somatic and visceral states associated with safety. HRV analysis with yoga shows significant increase in resonant breathing (i.e. RSA at 0.1 Hz innate healing frequency), reduction in sympathetic response (i.e. fight or flight), increase in vagal tone, and overall improvement in HRV (Melville et al., 2012; Santaella et al., 2011; Satyapriya et al., 2009; Jovanov, 2005; Khattab et al., 2007; Patra & Telles, 2010; Vempati & Telles, 2002; Shapiro et al., 2007; Yurtkuran et al., 2007; Wolever et al., 2012). These HRV changes are consistent with improved ANS gatekeeping and vagal tone dial control in managing sympathetic response (i.e. fight or flight). As would be expected with HRV improvement, practicing yoga improves emotional self-regulatory capacity as evidenced by significant increases in subjective positive mood (i.e., happy, relaxed, optimistic, confident, content) ratings and corresponding decreases in negative mood (i.e. stressed, sad, frustrated, irritated, depressed, anxious, blue, angry, pessimistic) ratings (Shapiro et al., 2007, Khalsa, 2007). When practicing yoga, corresponding measures of well-being (attentiveness, fatigue, alertness, overall energy, improved sleep) are also significantly improved as well. In chronic end-stage renal dialysis patients, improvements in fatigue, depression, sleep, and energy were also accompanied by improved clinical indices such as hemoglobin and electrolytes (Yurtkuran et al., 2007). Positive effects can be seen with as little as 15 minutes of chair-based yoga or with full 30–90 minute regimens (Melville et al., 2012). It has been postulated that shorter sessions are more dependent on breathing patterns, while longer yoga regimens enhance vagal tone through both breathing and extensive improvements in overall ANS function. Because ANS imbalance is found in most chronic disease states, subjective and objective improvements with yoga are rather consistent across most chronic disease states as would be expected with ANS improvement. As a result, there is a growing trend in health care to recommend some form of yoga or modified yoga regimen for reducing chronic sympathetic stimulation, improving ANS function, and increasing quality of life in chronic illness.

There are less HRV data for tai chi and qigong, but the data that exist supports the same underlying ANS mechanism for these modalities as seen with yoga. Qigong has been shown to produce resonant breathing (i.e. RSA at 0.1 Hz innate healing frequency), increase vagal tone, improve HRV, and decrease sympathetic response (i.e. fight or flight) (Sun & Yan, 1992; Lee et al., 2002, 2005a, 2005b). Much like yoga, qigong has also been shown to produce significantly higher positive emotions and self-regulatory capacity as would be expected with HRV improvement. Tai chi has been shown to improve vagal tone as well as decrease pain and emotional syndromes related to common chronic illnesses including fibromyalgia, osteoarthritis, rheumatoid arthritis, autoimmune and immune conditions, diabetes, cardiac disease, and HIV (Audette et al., 2006; Field, 2011; Chang et al., 2008; Lu & Kuo, 2003; Väänänen et al., 2002; Sato et al., 2010; Yeh et al., 2008).

To summarize, simple movement coupled with breathing is an effective way to relax the body and improve HRV and clinical outcomes related to chronic illness. This practice can be especially useful in chronic illness as an adjunct to medical therapy for reducing both emotional and physical burden of disease. Like breathing, there are no adverse effects when properly done, and benefits far outweigh any risks for those patients who wish to participate in yoga, tai chi, or qigong classes.

EMOTIONAL REFOCUS PRACTICES

A third spiritual practice used by ancient healing traditions was emotional refocus. As previously discussed, ancient healing traditions were very attuned to human negativity bias and the impact of negative emotional and thought patterns on health. Techniques to promote greater neutrality and acceptance emphasized recognition of destructive, ruminating thought and emotional patterns known to worsen chronic illness. Particular focus on poorly controlled anger, anxiety, depression (or sadness), lust, gluttony, and pride can be found across all healing traditions, suggesting a universal healing wisdom regarding destructive human perceptual tendencies and common strategies to overcome them (Cassian, 2000). The remedy for these negative patterns was to refocus emotionally by cultivating positive emotions, such as love, gratitude, or peace. The simplicity of this ancient practice is profoundly intuitive . . . we cannot hold two opposing emotions (i.e. positive and negative) at the same time (Emmons, 2007; McCraty, 1995). Emotional refocus practices re-establish a heartfelt sense of trust, safety, and security, which neutralizes fear and fosters more neutral or positive perceptions of people, circumstances, or events. The hardest part of this practice is a conscious choice to shift feelings. How does this practice affect ANS function?

As previously discussed, emotional self-regulation is critically dependent on vagal tone and our ANS gatekeeper, thus making it highly measurable with HRV. Positive heartfelt emotions such as love, compassion, peace, and appreciation improve HRV while negative emotions such as anger, hostility, anxiety, fear, and depression decrease HRV (McCraty, 1995; Rein et al., 1995; McCraty, 2006; McCraty & Childre, 2004). Myelinated vagal pathways from the heart to the emotional and cognitive centers in the brain far outweigh those going in the opposite direction. Although thoughts and emotions influence each other, emotions rather than thoughts appear to be a stronger natural preference for the ANS gatekeeper when assessing safety or danger. As organic markers of safety or danger, emotions directly impact physiologic responses, brainwave frequencies, thoughts, and behavior (i.e. approach or withdrawal). As previously noted, negative thoughts or emotions reduce vagal tone, trigger sympathetic response (i.e. fight or flight) behavior, and reduce overall emotional self-regulation. In contrast, positive emotions reverse or undo sympathetic responses (i.e. fight or flight) by re-establishing vagal dominance (i.e. reset our gatekeeper and volume dial), improving

HRV, and promoting rapid recovery from negative stimuli (McCraty, 2006; McCraty et al., 1998; Lai et al., 2005; Lane et al., 2009).

Emotional refocus practices decrease cortisol (i.e. stress hormone) and emotional arousal to stress, anxiety, anger, or fear (Emmons, 2007; Emmons and McCullough, 2004; McCraty, 2004, 2006; McCraty et al., 1998; Lai et al., 2005). Refocusing emotional energy on positive heartfelt emotions such as love, compassion, appreciation, or peace immediately improves HRV, negates "fight or flight" response, facilitates social engagement, improves critical thinking skills, and increases emotional self-regulatory capacity. These practices directly promote innate healing (i.e. 0.1 Hz frequency) and increase vagal tone (i.e. dial volume high) to suppress sympathetic response (i.e. fight or flight), both of which result in better overall coping skills, well-being, longevity, self-regulatory capacity, quality of life, cognition, memory, and word recall. The more intense and heartfelt the positive emotion, the greater improvement in HRV and likelihood of producing sustained innate healing (i.e. 0.1 Hz frequency).

In chronic disease states known to be associated with low baseline HRV, conscious cultivation of positive emotions correlates positively with sustained HRV improvement, innate healing, and clinical outcome improvements. For example, HRV improvement from emotional refocus practices resulted in reduced blood pressure in hypertensive patients (McCraty et al., 2003); improvements in glucose control and hemoglobin A1C in diabetics (McCraty et al., 2000); improvements in cognition, behavior, and attention in attention deficit disorder (Lloyd et al., 2010); reduced pain and improved emotional self-regulation, overall quality of life and optimism in breast cancer patients (Groff et al., 2010); and reduced stress burden, panic, and anxiety as well as improved cognition and overall emotional self-regulatory capacity across a variety of settings (Thurber et al., 2010; Lemaire et al., 2011; Ginsberg et al., 2010; McCraty et al., 2009; McCraty et al., 1999; Luskin et al., 2002; Hughes & Stoney, 2000; Rockliff et al., 2008). Routine use of emotional refocus practices have been correlated with reduced medical and pharmacy costs as well as increased workplace productivity, suggesting significant reductions in health-care costs when used with medical therapy (Bedell & Kaszkin-Bettag, 2010). Thus, both our body's gatekeeper and vagal tone dial are physiologically hardwired to restore and maintain an optimal balance when directed toward positive heartfelt feelings that foster a sense of safety, security, or trust. Positive emotions naturally help restore ANS adaptability and invite innate healing.

Emotional refocus practices using gratitude, in particular, have been extensively studied across the spectrum of chronic illness. People who regularly practice gratitude reported a greater sense of connectedness to others, more loving attitude, and stronger positive feelings of happiness, contentment, joy, and peace. Heartfelt appreciation resulted in robust and reproducible improvements in HRV, sustained innate healing (0.1 Hz frequency), and emotional self-regulation with regular practice. Fostering a deep sense of gratitude results in reduced morbidity, mortality, and cortisol levels; increased physical and cognitive performance and achievement; better sleep, creativity, decision making, and innovative problem solving; more flexibility; and improved memory, well-being, immunity, and hormonal balance. Gratitude practices have also been shown to be highly effective for overcoming greed, envy, resentment, anger, hostility, bitterness, anxiety, depression, victimhood, entitlement, and comparison (Emmons, 2007; Emmons & McCullough, 2004; McCraty et al., 2006). In our holistic clinic, we regularly teach gratitude practices as simple and effective starting points for learning how to refocus emotionally on the positive (see Appendix E). These practices are especially helpful to patients who are overly negative toward their disease or circumstances. It is important to focus the practice on something that engenders a true heartfelt appreciation, no matter how big or small it may seem. When combining emotional refocus techniques with simple long-exhalation breathing, 70 percent of our patients reported reductions in anxiety and stress and a third of our patients experience improved sleep and pain management. Whether alone or in combination with breathing or movement techniques, emotional refocus practices are excellent for resetting our gatekeeper and vagal tone dial and can be safely used with great benefit as adjuncts to routine medical therapy.

SPIRITUAL AND PERCEPTUAL AWARENESS

A fourth and final universal practice is spiritual and perceptual awareness techniques, the most common of which are meditation and prayer. These practices are usually considered the most obviously spiritual in nature because they bring greater awareness and integration to core beliefs, desires, perceptions, emotions, thoughts, and behaviors. The basic intentions of meditation and prayer are fundamentally different, although the practices may share common attributes and techniques. Simply stated, meditation is *cognitive awareness using the mind* and prayer is *relational awareness using the heart* (see Appendix F). Both profoundly affect our awareness of perceptions, emotions, and behavior. Meditation is cognitive by design, focusing on mindful awareness (i.e. nonjudgmental awareness of thoughts and emotions) or concentration (i.e. conscious fixed attention on sound, word, intention) to recognize thought patterns associated with suffering and fear (Henepola Gunaratana, 2011). Prayer, on the other hand, is heart-focused on relationship with creation, self, others, and the Divine (i.e. a greater "*Who*" to whom we direct prayers) and brings awareness to thoughts and emotions influencing our most significant relationships (Stanley, 2009). Meditation brings neutrality and calm while prayer fosters trust and connection with a greater "*Who*" through whom we believe neutrality, freedom, and transformation occur. Understanding this basic distinction makes it easier to see how the two practices are complementary in fostering wholeness of mind, body, heart, and spirit and also why they are more transformative in nature. In chronic illness, meditation and prayer are far more integrative than breathing, movement, or refocus exercises; therefore they are highly useful in producing significantly greater improvements in overall ANS function, HRV, and emotional self-regulation in complex pathologies.

Meditation is a self-directed practice that affects both mind and body but is uniquely and highly cognitive in nature. Calm, alert mental attentiveness is achieved through either mindful awareness or conscious concentration. Meditation practices come in many forms across a myriad of Western and Eastern religious traditions, including Judeo-Christian, Taoist, Confucianist Hindu, and Buddhist (Henepola Gunaratana, 2011; Kabat-Zinn, 2005). In chronic illness, meditation is specifically focused on awareness and freedom from destructive thought and emotional patterns leading to pain and suffering, especially where negative perceptual patterns impede healing or worsen prognosis. Because of its predominantly cognitive nature, meditation is easily taught outside of any religious context. However, because meditation fosters exploration of deep spiritual levels of the mind and consciousness, it has its most profound effect when practiced and grounded within the context of a particular spiritual foundation. Mindful and concentration forms of meditation are associated with clinical improvements in most chronic illnesses, both producing well-documented spiritual, psychological, physical, and emotional benefits (Kabat-Zinn, 2005; Kristeller, 2007; Arias et al., 2006). Since the primary purpose of meditation is to open and free the mind of unhealthy and negative perceptions, the more pervasive the opening and freedom, the more transformative the practice will be.

Mindfulness forms of meditation show strong benefit in chronic illness, with documented improvements in HRV, vagal tone, RSA, and emotional self-regulation with routine use (Kabat-Zinn, 2005; Tang et al., 2009;Wolever et al., 2012; Ditto et al., 2006; Tsunetsugu et al., 2007; Park et al., 2007; Nesvol et al., 2011; An et al., 2010; Libby et al., 2012). Correlations can be found between level of HRV improvement and direct level of clinical response. Mindfulness techniques are easily taught, with benefits seen almost immediately for improved sleep and lower perceived levels of stress, anxiety, and pain. In addition, cortisol levels (i.e. stress hormone) are lowered correlating with brain imaging consistent with increased vagal tone and decreased sympathetic response (i.e. fight or flight). In addictive behaviors, acute positive changes in HRV predict level of success or failure of meditation practices as an adjunct to treatment, highlighting the complex role of ANS mediated emotional self-regulation in addictive behavioral patterns (Libby et al., 2012). Even with a poor baseline HRV, improvements in HRV result in significant clinical improvements, reduction of addictive behaviors, and increased emotional self-regulatory capacity. Integrated mindfulness practices incorporating concentration or single focused concentration meditation techniques are extremely effective in restoring ANS balance, improving HRV, promoting 0.1 Hz innate healing frequency, increasing vagal tone, decreasing sympathetic response (i.e. fight or flight), and improving the overall efficiency of respiratory gas exchange (Phongsuphap et al., 2008; Wu & Lo, 2008; Peng et al., 1999; Kemper & Shaltout, 2011; Sebastiani et al., 2007; Patra & Telles, 2010). These forms of meditation also produce significant improvements in sleep and felt sense of stress, relaxation, and peacefulness.

Zen-based meditation incorporates the benefits of breathing, mindfulness, and focused concentration based on levels of mastery, making it one of the most popular and practical forms of meditation used in clinical practice. Zen-based meditation improves HRV, RSA, vagal tone, and emotional self-regulating capacity (Murata et al., 2004; Peressutti et al., 2010; Cysarz & Bussing, 2005; Takahashi et al., 2005; Lehrer et al., 1999). High degrees of RSA can be achieved with inexperienced meditators; suggesting early benefit from Zen-based meditations is likely due to improved breathing techniques. When comparing novice to experienced Zen practitioners, differing HRV patterns associated with ANS changes and respiratory oscillations were recorded, suggesting increasing levels of benefit beyond breathing alone in more experienced practitioners (Peressutti et al., 2010; Cysarz & Bussing, 2005). As external sensory attention increased during early meditation and then shifted to inner directed sensory attention, the magnitude of shift correlates with the degree of positive changes in HRV, emotional self- regulation, and overall ANS function. Typically seen with experienced practitioners or Zen masters, greater focused consciousness and inwardly directed concentrated attention result in significantly greater improvements in vagal tone, HRV, and emotional self-regulatory abilities. These observations make sense when viewed through the lens of gatekeeping and a vagal tone dial. The more calmly aware people become, the better the gatekeeper is at accurately assessing safety or threat and the more sensitive the vagal tone volume dial becomes. Electroencephalogram (i.e. EEG) recordings are consistent with improvements in HRV, showing higher power shifts in frontal area alpha and theta waves with corresponding increases in vagal tone (Takahashi et al., 2005). These findings are similar to those in which brain imaging showed impact of 0.1 Hz innate healing frequency on emotional and cognitive centers of the brain (McCraty et al., 2006).

Success of various forms of meditation also has been linked to baseline trait and personality levels (Murata et al., 2004; Takahashi et al., 2005). People with low trait anxiety shift more quickly and easily into calm internalized concentrative attentiveness while people with high trait anxiety depend more heavily on breathing and mindfulness to reach a calm state. These findings are consistent with observations in patients with high trait anxiety who are more prone to lower baseline HRV and find mindfulness meditation techniques easier than concentration techniques when first learning meditation. This likely explains why healing traditions typically encourage mindfulness practices coupled with breathing as initial starting points and foundations for beginning perceptual awareness practices. Mastery over time with continued practice allows deeper concentration meditation, which was recommended by healing masters for more complex pathologies. This, too, makes physiologic sense because more difficult pathologies or patterns are associated with greater impairment of ANS gatekeeping and vagal tone (i.e. dial volume low). Thus, mindfulness allows initial perceptual awareness and leads to eventual concentration, which results in deepening awareness and healing. Both forms of meditation facilitate wholeness and are extremely powerful methods for significantly improving and maintaining overall ANS function (i.e. better gatekeeping and dial function).

Many healing traditions consider cognitive awareness through meditation, especially mindful awareness, to be a precursor to prayer since prayer is more personal, intimate, and focused on relationship. Regardless of religious tradition or context of beliefs, prayer forms are universal in that they focus on the "*Who*" from whom one finds safety, security, meaning, and purpose in life. Heartfelt prayers are always relationally oriented toward a "*Who*" with whom we seek connection and trust. Just as mindfulness forms of meditation lead to deeper awareness through concentration meditation, so prayers of supplication, devotion, and intercession invite deeper relational prayers of gratitude and contemplation. As with meditation, there appears to be greater improvement in HRV with more integrated, deeper forms of prayer that focus on trust.

Prayer types that foster initial awareness of fears, intentions, desires, and needs can be broadly categorized as prayers of supplication, devotion, and intercession (Stanley, 2009). There is something inherently healing in vocalizing fears or needs, and most healing traditions have an abundance of these types of prayers to help identify negative thought and emotional patterns. Much like mindfulness meditation refocuses and quiets the mind, these prayers refocus and quiet the heart. Verbalizing one's needs to our "*Who*" positively impacts HRV and improves vagal tone (Bernardi et al., 2000, 2001). Slower, more deliberate breathing patterns and speech are accompanied by a greater felt sense of security. Personal and communal devotional prayers such as the rosary, Jesus prayer, and Lord's Prayer or mantras produce moderate degrees of HRV improvement and resonant breathing patterns of six breaths per minute. Spiritual healing masters consistently recommended these forms of prayer for chronic illness. Robust positive improvements in HRV explain, in part, the value of rote prayers and mantras across all traditions in providing immediate relief from anxiety and pain in chronic illness. Likewise, forms of intercessory prayer show drops in inflammatory cytokines (IL–6) and increases in anti-inflammatory cytokines (IL–10) corresponding to HRV improvements, innate healing (0.1 Hz frequency), increased vagal tone, better emotional self-regulation, and subjective improvement (Stanley, 2009; Kurita et al., 2011; Bernston et al., 2008; Childre & McCraty, 2001). These observations appear consistent in showing that typical prayer forms invite moderate forms of healing and subjective emotional and physical improvements by improving vagal tone (i.e. dial volume high) and overall gatekeeper function.

Prayers of gratitude and contemplation are deeper, more relational forms of prayer reflecting a significantly higher foundation of trust, love, and security in our relationship with the "*Who*" from whom we seek safety and meaning (Stanley, 2009). Also found in all healing traditions, these prayers produce significantly greater improvements in HRV and require focused inward heart attentiveness or concentration on being with our "*Who*". Much like increasing integrative levels of meditation, these prayers evolve from a relational foundation of love and trust nurtured through supplication, devotion, and intercessory prayers. Prayers of gratitude are unique because they require both an awareness of a beneficiary and a heartfelt gratefulness to receive. Increased gratitude leads to greater integration and results in a positive impact on emotional, psychological, spiritual, and physical well-being. Likewise, contemplative prayer denotes greater integration and intimate personal encounter with the "*Who*" in whom trust and security is placed. Where gratefulness is heartfelt thanksgiving to the greater "*Who*" for "doing", contemplation is simply "being" with the sacred greater "*Who*." Both "doing" and "being" can free and transform people from destructive emotional and thought patterns. Although there is obvious overlap with concentration meditation, contemplative prayer is specifically attentive to engendering heartfelt union, presence, and love with a "*Who*" as a source of transformation and healing.

A more intense shift in heart focus seen with both gratitude and contemplation prayers appears vitally important and quite powerful in terms of HRV response, suggesting that relationship is of the highest importance to our ANS, especially where love and trust are found. As social and communal beings, the need to be relationally safe and secure is paramount, and the primary focus of the ANS gatekeeper is in regulating motion, emotion, and communication. Increasing a sense of felt safety and relational security directly impacts the gatekeeper to adjust vagal tone high and to inhibit sympathetic response (i.e. fight or flight) associated with destructive emotional and thought patterns. Observations with both gratitude and contemplation show strong innate healing (i.e. 0.1 Hz frequency), improved overall HRV, increased emotional self- regulation, increased quality of life, decreased morbidity and mortality, increased coping skills, and increased positive emotions (Stanley, 2009; McCraty & Childre, 2004; Emmons, 2007). Prayers of gratitude and contemplation are very effective practices for resetting and maintaining high functionality of both gatekeeper and vagal tone dial. Comparison of prayer with mindfulness meditation techniques show that these highly integrated prayer forms are more effective in improving HRV parameters, most likely due to the strong relational safety component hardwired in the ANS (Bernston et al., 2008; Moritz et al., 2006). Even so, the heart and brain are designed to work together, so awareness practices of the mind and heart work best when used to complement each other.

Both meditation and prayer are powerful adjuncts to medical therapy. Alone or in combination, these awareness techniques offer profound benefit to patients with chronic illness. Based on personal belief systems, either can be used to facilitate improved emotional and cognitive responses to disease. Best clinical outcomes are seen in those patients who practice both meditation and prayer, with more highly integrated practice of greater benefit. Practitioners are encouraged to support patients who wish to pursue awareness techniques as a part of their medical care.

Summary

Personal perceptions, emotions, and thoughts are important modifiable factors affecting clinical outcomes and quality of life for patients with chronic illness. As such, it is the key to overall health and well-being. Ancient traditions recognized the importance spiritual integration and the role fear plays in physical, emotional, spiritual, and perceptual health. As such, these traditions concentrated healing efforts on spiritual practices fostering safety and calm, which effectively transform destructive emotional, thought, and behavioral patterns toward more neutral and positive influences. A common physical and spiritual pathway to healing can now be traced through the ANS as a pathophysiologic foundation for these anciently rooted practices. Each of these universal practices improves ANS function and draws forth the body's innate capacity for wholeness and healing within the boundaries of chronic disease. Breathing, simple movements, emotional refocus, and awareness practices can result in sustained and consistent improvements in HRV, overall ANS function, and emotional self-regulation. Subjectively, these practices foster acceptance, produce physically calm states, and shift emotional and cognitive perceptual capacity toward wholeness, safety, and trust. Objectively, these practices and states result in improved clinical outcomes, overall coping, and quality of life in chronic illness. Optimizing ANS function through regular use of these practices is safe, simple, and highly effective. As such, it seems prudent to consider incorporating these core healing practices as adjuncts to medical treatment in those patients with chronic illness who desire to use them. At minimum, these practices can be recommended with confidence to patients who wish to enhance their health and wellness in correlation with routine medical care.

APPENDIX A: ANS GATEKEEPER AND VAGAL TONE

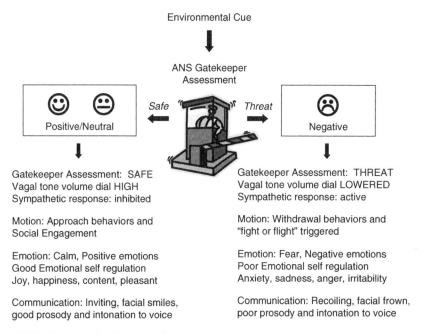

Environmental Cue

ANS Gatekeeper
Assessment

Safe   Threat

Positive/Neutral   Negative

Gatekeeper Assessment: SAFE
Vagal tone volume dial HIGH
Sympathetic response: inhibited

Gatekeeper Assessment: THREAT
Vagal tone volume dial LOWERED
Sympathetic response: active

Motion: Approach behaviors and
Social Engagement

Motion: Withdrawal behaviors and
"fight or flight" triggered

Emotion: Calm, Positive emotions
Good Emotional self regulation
Joy, happiness, content, pleasant

Emotion: Fear, Negative emotions
Poor Emotional self regulation
Anxiety, sadness, anger, irritability

Communication: Inviting, facial smiles,
good prosody and intonation to voice

Communication: Recoiling, facial frown,
poor prosody and intonation to voice

ANS: Autonomic Nervous System

APPENDIX B: HEART RATE VARIABILITY (HRV) AND INNATE HEALING

Physiologic, cognitive, and emotional correlates of 0.1 Hz innate healing frequency

Resets autonomic nervous system (ANS) gatekeeper to accurately assess positive, neutral, or negative stimuli.

Resets vagal tone dial sensitivity for optimal control of sympathetic response (i.e. fight or flight).

Maximizes emotional and cognitive self-regulatory capacity (i.e. improves critical thinking, behavioral responses). Correlates with resonant breathing frequency and respiratory sinus arrhythmia (RSA).

Fosters approach: perfect calm, sense of unity, oneness, freedom, quiet mind, very open or focused.

Triggers positive emotions: love, peace, joy, appreciation, happiness, gratefulness Other:

- Five-fold increase in alpha and theta brain waves.
- Improves neuroplasticity, perceptual capacity, cognition, word recall, memory, cognitive response time, intuition.
- Resets all neurohormonal feedback loops.
- Decreases stress hormones and boosts anti-stress hormones and immune function
- Optimizes breathing and oxygenation.
- Increases blood flow to brain and vital organs allowing more efficient oxygenation, fluid exchange, toxin filtration, and nutrient absorption between capillaries and tissues.

APPENDIX C: CHRONICALLY LOW HEART RATE VARIABILITY (HRV) AND COMMON CHRONIC DISEASE STATES ASSOCIATED WITH LOW HRV:

- Cardiovascular

  o Hypertension
  o Coronary artery disease
  o Dysrhythmias
  o Stroke and vascular disease
  o Valvular disease

- Mental health

  o Personality disorders
  o Depression
  o Anxiety
  o Panic disorder

- o Bipolar
- o Compulsive or addictive pathologies
- o Schizophrenia

- Endocrine

  - o Diabetes
  - o Thyroid
  - o Pituitary and hypothalamic disorders

- Cancer

  - o Breast
  - o Prostate
  - o Lung
  - o Lymphoma
  - o Leukemia
  - o Pancreatic

- Autoimmune disorders

  - o Arthritis
  - o Thyroid
  - o Celiac

- Pain syndromes

  - o Fibromyalgia
  - o Complex regional pain syndrome
  - o Musculoskeletal syndromes
  - o Chronic fatigue syndrome

- Infectious disorders

  - o HIV

- Pulmonary

  - o Chronic obstructive pulmonary disease
  - o Asthma
  - o Pulmonary hypertension

APPENDIX D: LONG-EXHALATION BREATHING PRACTICE

Long-exhalation breathing is a highly effective way to calm and restore balance to our bodies. Just follow these simple steps:

1) Whether sitting, standing, or lying down, keep your back as straight as possible to allow your lungs to get plenty of air.
2) If you are sitting, open your hands and lay them flat on your knees.
3) Position your head so that if you hum, you feel it in your chest.

4) Place your tongue behind your front teeth and flat against the roof of your mouth.
5) Put a smile on your face to relax your facial muscles.
6) Breathe in normally and breathe out very slow and even. It should take you about two times longer to breathe out. If you need help getting started, count to 3 or 4 when breathing in and to 6 or 7 when breathing out. The body automatically slows breathing after about 2 or 3 minutes of slower breathing.
7) Focus on exhaling slowly and evenly rather than the amount of air coming in or out. Breathing slower allows your lungs extra time to absorb the oxygen breathed in.
8) Do not hold your breath in between breaths. Do not wait until you have fully exhaled to take your next breath. Breathe in when you feel you need to, just like when you are talking with someone. Do not push or force air out of your lungs; just simply breathe out normally, only slower.

Some basic tips to foster healthy breathing:

• Practice daily. If possible, regular practice of 10–15 minutes one to three times daily is very good for your body and can be done while doing other things. If that is not possible, try using long-exhalation breathing as often as you can remember, even if only for a few breaths. You can practice anywhere or anytime and cannot overdo this practice.
• The most important thing is to SLOW your rate of breathing. The amount of air you breathe in or out is not as important as the quality with which you breathe air out slowly and evenly. Your body will usually maintain this slower pattern of breathing within a few minutes.

APPENDIX E: EXAMPLES OF GRATEFULNESS PRACTICES

Fostering gratefulness is healthy for you and everyone around you. Here are some simple ways to express gratitude.

✓ Say one thing you are genuinely grateful for today.
✓ Tell someone today how much you love them.
✓ Affirm someone today by sharing what you appreciate about them.
✓ Tell someone today how grateful you are for a kindness extended to you.
✓ Keep a gratefulness journal.
✓ Write a "thank you" note today.
✓ Keep track of the positive changes in your mood, behavior when you practice gratitude.
✓ Practice gratitude even when you don't feel particularly grateful.
✓ Give out spontaneous tokens of appreciation.
✓ Speak or sing your gratitude to a favorite melody.
✓ Express gratitude every time a recurring event happens (ie phone rings, TV commercials, email or text message, etc.).

✓ Give brief, genuine expressions of gratitude to coworkers and people you meet.

✓ Form a supportive gratitude partnership with a friend.

✓ Say "thank you" to people on a regular basis.

Appendix F: Types of Meditation and Prayer

Description

Two Major Types of Meditation (can be used alone or combined during a single session with mindfulness leading to concentration)

Mindfulness	Mindful awareness, nonjudgmental awareness of thoughts and emotions, simple body sensations, breathing patterns, attending to a particular point of awareness: The discipline is to allow thoughts and feelings to simply exist without engaging them in order to become aware of them. To do so means to grow in one's own awareness of destructive emotional, thought, and behavioral patterns. This is a very relaxing form of meditation.
Concentration	Very focused, conscious inward fixed attention on sound, word, breath, feeling, intention, or particular area of the body to cultivate an inward state and feeling of calm: This is a deeper, more healing form of meditation requiring greater discipline to focus feelings, thoughts, and body in quiet freedom with a single focal point to help clear the mind and heart in order to open oneself spiritually. This is a very healing form of meditation.

Five Major Types of Prayer (can be used alone or combined during a single session)

Supplication	Petitions for personal needs and forgiveness; focus on meeting needs and recognizing attitudes; represent initial perceptual awareness. This form of prayer is typically relaxing and reduces stress.
Devotion	Basis for mantras and represents desire to seek deeper relationship with the "who" to whom prayers are given; beginning of deliberate seeking of relationship and foundation of trust; usually focuses on love or devotion to the "who." This is a very relaxing form of prayer.
Intercession	Petitions for others and for personal transformation as reflected in more communal and mutual interaction implying some degree of listening as well as asking as foundation of trust grows. This is a relaxing form of prayer.
Gratefulness	Focused attention to gratefulness toward the "who" reflecting a more integrated faith grounded in humility, openness, and awareness. This prayer implies love and trust in the ongoing presence of the "who" in the believer's life. This is a more healing form of prayer.
Contemplative or Pure	Focused attention on cultivating awareness of a loving and trusting presence with the "who" to whom one looks for transformation and transcendence. Focus is on "being" rather than "doing" to grow in awareness and loving relationship. This form of prayer is considered paramount to healing processes and necessary for achieving more integrated faith. This is the most healing form of prayer.

REFERENCES

Adams, J., Julian, P., Hubbard, M., Hartman, J., Baugh, S., Segrest, W.,...&
Wheelan, K. (2009) A randomized controlled trial of a controlled breathing pro-
tocol on heart rate variability following myocardial infarction or coronary artery
bypass graft surgery. *Clinical Rehabilitation*, 23(9): 782–789.

An, H., Kulkarni, R., Nagarathna, R., & Nagendra, H.R. (2010) Measures of heart
rate variability in women following a meditation technique. *International Journal
of Yoga*, 3(1):6–9.

Appelhans, B.M. & Luecken, L.J. (2006) Heart rate variability as an index of
regulated emotional responding. *Review of General Psychology*, 10(3): 229–240.

Arias, A.J., Steinberg, K., Banga, A., & Trestman, R.L. (2006) Systemic review of
the efficacy of meditation techniques as treatments for medical illness. *Journal of
Alternative and Complementary Medicine*, 12(8): 817–832.

Audette, J.F., Jin, Y.S., Newcomer, R., Stein, L., Duncan, G., & Frontera, W. (2006)
Tai chi versus brisk walking in elderly women. *Age and Ageing*, 35: 366–393.

Bedell, W. & Kaszkin-Bettag, M. (2010) Coherence and health care cost—RCA actu-
arial study: A cost-effectiveness cohort study. *Alternative Therapies*, 16(4): 26–31.

Bernardi, L., Sleight, P., Bandinelli, G., Cencetti, S., Fattorini, L., Wdowczk-
Szulc, J., & Lagi, A. (2001) Effect of rosary prayer and yoga mantras on
autonomic cardiovascular rhythms: Comparative study. *British Medical Journal*,
323: 1446–1449.

Bernardi, L., Wdowczk-Szulc, J., Valenti, C., Castoldi, S., Passino, C., Spadacini,
G., & Sleight, P. (2000) Effects of controlled breathing, mental activity and mental
stress with or without verbalization on heart rate variability. *Journal of the American
College of Cardiology*, 35(6): 1462–1469.

Berntson, G., Bigger, T., Eckberg, D.L., Grossman, P., Kaufman, P. G., Malik,
M.,...& Maurits, W. (1997) Heart rate variability: Origins, methods, and interpretive caveats. *Psychophysiology*, 34: 623–648.

Bernston, G.G., Norman, G.J., Hawkley, L.C., & Cacioppo, J.T. (2008) Spirituality
and autonomic cardiac control. *Annals of Behavioral Medicine*, 35(2): 198–208.

Cassian, J. (2000). *The institutes*. Ed. Boniface Ramsey. New York: Newman Press.

Chang, R.Y., Koo, M., Yu, K.Z., Chu, I.T., Hsu, C.T., & Chen C.Y. (2008) The effect
of tai chi exercise on autonomic nervous function of patients with coronary artery
disease. *Journal of Alternative and Complementary Medicine*, 14(9): 1107–1113.

Childre, D. & McCraty, R. (2001) Psychophysiological correlates of spiritual experience. *Biofeedback*, 29(4),: 13–17.

Courtney, R., Cohen, M., & van Dixhoorn, J. (2011) Relationship between dysfunctional breathing patterns and ability to achieve target heart rate variability with
features of coherence during biofeedback. *Alternative Therapies in Health and
Medicine*, 17(3): 38–44.

Cysarz, D. & Büssing, A. (2005) Cardiorespiratory synchronization during Zen
meditation. *European Journal of Applied Physiology*, 95: 88–95.

Cysarz, D., von Bonin, D., Lackner, H., Heusser, P., Moser, M., & Bettermann,
H. (2004) Oscillations of heart rate and respiration synchronize during poetry
reading. *American Journal of Physiology and Heart Circulation Physiology*, 287:
H579–H587.

Ditto, B., Eclache, M., & Goldman, N. (2006) Short-term autonomic and
cardiovascular effects of mindfulness body scan meditation. *Annals of Behavioral
Medicine*, 32(3): 227–234.

Emmons, R. A. (2007) *Thanks: How the new science of gratitude can make you happier.* New York, NY: Houghton Mifflin Company.

Emmons, R.A. & McCullough, M.E. (2004) *The psychology of gratitude.* New York, NY: Oxford University Press.

Field, T. (2011) Tai chi research review. *Complementary Therapy in Clinical Practice,* 17(3): 141–146.

Ginsberg, J. P., Berry, M. E., & Powell, D.A. (2010) Cardiac coherence and posttraumatic stress disorder in combat veterans. *Alternative Therapies in Health and Medicine,* 16(4): 52–60.

Groff, D.G., Battaglini, C., Sipe, C., Peppercorn, J., Anderson, M., & Hackney, A.C. (2010) Finding a new normal: Using recreation therapy to improve the well being of women with breast cancer. *Annual in Therapeutic Recreation,* 18: 40–52.

Henepola Gunaratana, B. (2011) *Mindfulness in plain English.* Somerville, MA: Wisdom Publications.

Hughes, J.W. & Stoney, C. M. (2000) Depressed mood is related to high frequency heart rate variability during stressors. *Psychosomatic Medicine,* 62: 796–803.

Jovanov, E. (2005) On spectral analysis of heart rate variability during very slow yogic breathing. *Conference Procedings IEEE End Medical Biology Society,* 3: 2467–2470.

Kabat-Zinn, J. (2005) *Full catastrophe living: Using the wisdom of the body and mind to face stress, pain, and illness.* New York, NY: Bantam Bell, Random House.

Karavidas, M.K., Lehrer, P.M., Vaschillo, E., Vaschillo, B., Marin, H., Buyske, S., & Hassett, A. (2007) Preliminary results of an open label study of heart rate variability biofeedback for the treatment of major depression. *Applied Psychophysiology Biofeedback,* 32: 19–30.

Kemper, K.J. & Shaltout, H.A. (2011) Non-verbal communication of compassion: Measuring psychophysiologic effects. *BMC Complementary and Alternative Medicine,* 11: 132.

Khalsa, S.B. (2007) Yoga as a therapeutic intervention. In: Lehrer, P.M., Woolfolk, R.L., & Sime, W.E. (eds). *Principles and practice of stress management* . New York: Guilford Press, 449–464.

Khattab, K., Khattab, A., Ortak, J., Richardt, G. & Bonnemeier, H. (2007) Iyengar yoga increases cardiac parasympathetic nervous modulation among health practitioners. *eCAM,* 4(4): 511–517.

Kristeller, J.L. (2007) Mindfulness meditation. In: Lehrer, P.M., Woolfolk, R.L. & Sime, W.E. (eds). *Principles and practice of stress management.* New York, NY: Guilford Press, 393–427.

Koenig, H., McCullough, M.E. & Larson, D.B. (2001). *Handbook of religion and medicine.* New York, NY: Oxford University Press.

Kok, B.E. & Fredrickson, B.L. (2010) Upward spirals of the heart: Autonomic flexibility, as indexed by vagal tone, reciprocally and prospectively predicts positive emotions and social connectedness. *Biological Psychology,* 85(3): 432–436.

Kulur, A.B., Haleagrahara, N., Adhikary, P. & Jeganathan, P.S. (2009) Effect of diaphragmatic breathing on heart rate variability in ischemic heart disease with diabetes. *Argentine Brasilian Cardiology,* 92(6): 423–429.

Kurita, A., Takase, B., Shinagawa, N., Kodani, E., Okada, K., Iwahara, S.,... & Atarashi, H. (2011) Spiritual activation in very elderly individuals assessed as heart rate variability and plasma IL/10/IL/-6 ratios. *International Heart Journal,* 52: 299–303.

Lai, J., Evans, P.D., Ng, S.H., Chong, A., Siu, O.T., Chan, C., . . . & Chan, C.C. (2005) Optimism, positive affectivity, and salivary cortisol. *British Journal of Health Psychology*, 10: 467–484.

Lane, R.D., McRae, K., Reiman, E. M., Chen, K., Ahern, G. L., & Thayer, J.F. (2009) Neural correlates of heart rate variability during emotion. *Neuroimage*, 44: 213–222.

Lee, M.S., Huh, H.J., Kim, B.G., Ryu, H., Lee, H.S., Kim, J.M., & Chung, H.T. (2002) Effects of Qi-training on heart rate variability. *American Journal of Chinese Medicin*, 30(4): 463–470.

Lee, M.S., Kim, M.K., & Lee, Y.H. (2005a). Effects of Qi-therapy (external qigong) on cardiac autonomic tone: A randomized placebo controlled study. *International Journal of Neuroscience*, 115: 1345–1350.

Lee, M.S., Rim, Y.H., Jeong, D.M., Kim, M.K., Joo, M.C., & Shin, S.H. (2005b). Nonlinear analysis of heart rate variability during qi therapy (external qigong). *American Journal of Chinese Medicine*, 33(4): 579–588.

Lehrer, P., Sasaki, Y., & Saito, Y. (1999). Zazen and cardiac variability. *Psychosomatic Medicine*, 61: 812–821.

Lehrer, P.M. (2007) Biofeedback training to increase heart rate variability. In: Lehrer, P.M., Woolfolk, R.L., & Sime, W.E. (eds). *Principles and practice of stress management*. New York, NY: Guilford Press, 227–248.

Lehrer, P.M., Vaschillo, E., & Vaschillo, B. (2000) Resonant frequency biofeedback training to increase cardiac variability: Rationale and manual for training. *Applied Psychophysiology and Biofeedback*, 25(3): 177–191.

Lehrer, P.M., Vaschillo, E., Vaschillo, B., Lur, S.E., Scardella, A., Siddique, M., & Habib, R.H. (2004) Biofeedback treatment for asthma. *Chest*, 126: 352–361.

Lemaire, J.B., Wallace, J.E., Lewin, A.M., De Grood, J., & Schaefer, J. (2011) The effect of a biofeedback based stress management tool on physician stress: a randomized controlled clinical trial. *Open Medicine*, 5(4): e154–e163.

Libby, D.J., Worhunsky, P.D., Pilver, C.E., & Brewer, J.A. (2012) Meditation-induced changes in high-frequency heart rate variability predict smoking outcomes. *Frontiers in Human Neuroscience*, 6: 1–8. doi: 10.3389/fnhum.2012.00054.

Lloyd, A., Brett, D., & Wesnes, K. (2010) Coherence training in children with attention-deficit hyperactivity disorder: Cognitive functions and behavioral changes. *Alternative Therapies in Health and Medicine*, 16(4): 34–42.

Lu, W.A. & Kuo, C.D. (2003) The effect of tai chi chuan on the autonomic nervous modulation in older persons. *Medicine and Science in Sports and Exercise*, 35(12): 1972–1976.

Luskin, F., Reitz, M., Newell, K., Quinn, T.G., & Haskell, W. (2002) A controlled pilot study of stress management training of elderly patients with congestive heart failure. *Preventive Cardiology*, 5: 168–172, 176.

McCraty, R., Atkinson, M., & Lipsenthal, L. (2000) *Emotional self-regulation program enhances psychological health and quality of life in patients with diabetes*. Boulder Creek, CA: HeartMath Research Center, Institute of HeartMath, Publication No. 00-006.

McCraty, R., Atkinson, M., Lipsenthal, L., & Arguelles, L. (2009) New hope for correctional officers: an innovative program for reducing stress and health risks. *Applied Psychophysiology and Biofeedback*, 34: 251–272.

McCraty, R., Atkinson, M., Tiller, W.A., Rein, G., & Watkins, A.D. (1995) The effects of emotions on short-term power spectrum analysis of heart rate variability. *American Journal of Cardiology*, 76(14): 1089–1093.

McCraty, R., Atkinson, M., & Tomasino, D. (2003) Impact of a workplace stress reduction program on blood pressure and emotional health in hypertensive employees. *Journal of Alternative and Complementary Medicine*, 9(3): 355–369.

McCraty, R., Atkinson, M., Tomasino, D., & Bradley, R. (2006). *The coherent heart: Heart- brain interactions, Psychophysiological coherence, and the emergence of system-wide order.* Boulder Creek, CA: Institute of HeartMath, Publication 06–022.

McCraty, R., Atkinson, M., Tomasino, D., Goelitz, J., & Mayrovitz, H.N. (1999) The impact of an emotional self-management skills course on psychosocial functioning and autonomic recovery to stress in middle school children. *Integrative Physiological and Behavioral Science*, 34(4): 246–268.

McCraty, R., Barrio-Choplin, B., Rozman, D., Atkinson, M., & Watkins, A.D. (1998) The impact of a new emotional self-management program on stress, emotions, heart rate variability, DHEA, and cortisol. *Integrative Physiological and Behavioral Science*, 33(2): 151–170.

McCraty, R. & Childre, D. (2004) The grateful heart: The psychophysiology of appreciation. In: Emmons, R.A. & McCullough, M.E. (eds). *The psychology of gratitude.* New York, NY: Oxford University Press, 230–256.

Melville, G.W., Chang, D., Colagiuri, B., Marshall, P., & Cheema, B.S. (2012) Fifteen minutes of chair-based yoga postures or guided meditation performed in the office can elicit relaxation response. *Evidence Based Complementary and Alternative Medicine*, article ID 501986; doc:10.1155/2012/501986.

Moritz, S., Quan, H., Rickhi, B., Liu, M., Angen, M., Vintila, R.,...& Toews, J. (2006). A home study-based spirituality education program decreases emotional distress and increases quality of life: A randomized controlled trial. *Alternative Therapies*, 12(6): 26–35.

Motooka, M., Koike, H., Yokoyama, T., & Kennedy, N.L. (2006) Effect of dog walking on autonomic nervous activity in senior citizens. *Medical Journal of Australia*, 184(2): 60–63.

Murata, T., Takahashi, T., Hamada, T., Omori, M., Kosaka, H., Yoshida, H., & Wada, Y. (2004). Individual trait anxiety levels characterizing the properties of Zen meditation. *Neuropsychobiology*, 50: 189–194.

Nesvol, A., Fagerland, M.W., Davanger, S., Ellingsen, Ø., Solberg, E.E., Holen, A.,...& Atar, D. (2011) Increased heart rate variability during nondirective meditation. *European Journal of Cardiovascular Prevention and Rehabilitation*, 0(00): 1–8. DOI: 10.1177/1741826711414625.

Oveis, C., Cohen, A.B., Gruber, J., Shiota, M.N., Haidt, J., & Keltner, D. (2009) Resting respiratory sinus arrhythmia is associated with tonic positive emotionality. *Emotion*, 9(2): 265–270.

Park, B., Tsunetsugu, Y., Kasetani, T., Hirano, H., Kagawa, T., Sato, M., & Miyazaki, Y. (2007) Physiological effects of shinrin-yoko – Using salivary cortisol and cerebral activity as indicators. *Journal of Physiological Anthropology*, 26(2): 123–128.

Patra, S. & Telles, S. (2010) Heart rate variability during sleep following the practice of cyclic meditation and supine rest. *Applied Psychophysiology and Biofeedback*, 35: 135–140.

Peng, C.K., Mietus, J.E., Liu, Y., Khalsa, G., Douglas, P.S., Benson, H., & Goldberger, A.L. (1999). Exaggerated heart rate oscillations during two meditation techniques. *International Journal of Cardiology*, 70: 101–107.

Peressutti, C., Martin-Gonzalez, J.M., Garcia-Manso, J.M., & Mesa, D. (2010) Heart rate dynamics in different levels of Zen meditation. *International Journal of Cardiology*, 145(1): 142–146.

Phongsuphap, S., Pongsupap, Y., Chandanamattha, P., & Lursinsap, C. (2008) Changes in heart rate variability during concentration meditation. *International Journal of Cardiology*, 130: 481–484.

Porges, S W. (2007a) The polyvagal perspective. *Biological Psychology*, 74: 116–243.

Porges, S.W. (2007b) A phylogenetic journey through the vague and ambiguous Xth cranial nerve: A commentary on contemporary heart rate variability research. *Biological Psychology*, 74(2): 301–307.

Porges, S.W. (2009) The polyvagal theory: New insights into adaptive reactions of the autonomic nervous system. *Cleveland Clinic Journal of Medicine*, 76 (suppl 2): S86–S90.

Porges, S.W. (2011). *The polyvagal theory: Neurophysiological foundations of emotions, attachment, communication, self Regulation.* New York: W.W. Norton and Company.

Porges, S.W. & Furman, S.A. (2011) The early development of the autonomic nervous system provides a neural platform for social behavior: A polyvagal perspective. *Infant and Child Development*, 20(1): 106–118.

Rein G., Atkinson M., & McCraty, R. (1995) The physiological and psychological effects of compassion and anger. *Journal for the Advancement of Medicine*, 8(2): 7–105.

Rockliff, H., Gilbert, P., McEwan, K., Lightman, S., & Glover, D. (2008) A pilot exploration of heart rate variability and salivary cortisol responses to compassion-focused imagery. *Clinical Neuropsychiatry*, 5(3): 132–139.

Rossi-Caruso, F.C., Arena, R., Mendes, R.G., Reis, M.S., Papa, V., & Borghi-Silva, A. (2011) Heart rate autonomic responses during deep breathing and walking in hospitalized patients with chronic heart failure. *Disability and Rehabilitation*, 33(9): 751–757.

Sakuragi, S. & Sugiyama, Y. (2006). Effects of daily walking on subjective symptoms, mood, and autonomic nervous function. *Journal of Physiological Anthropology*, 25(4): 281–289.

Santaella, D.F., Devesa, C., Rojo, M., Amato, M., Drager, L., Casali, K.,... & Lorenzi-Filho, G. (2011) Yoga respiratory training improves respiratory function and cardiac sympathovagal balance in elderly subjects: A randomized controlled trial. *British Medical Journal Open*, 1:e000085. doi:10.1136/bmjopen–2011–000085.

Sato, S., Makita, S., Uchida, R., Ishihara, S., & Masuda, M. (2010) Effect of tai chi training on baroflex sensitivity and heart variability in patients with coronary artery disease. *International Heart Journal*, 51: 238–241.

Satyapriya, M., Nagendra, H.R., Nagarathna, R., & Padmalatha, V. (2009) Effect of integrated yoga on stress and heart rate variability in pregnant women. *International Journal of Gynaecology and Obstetrics*, 104(3): 218–222.

Sebastiani, L., D'Alessandro, L., Menicucci, D., Ghelarducci, B., & Santarcangelo, E. (2007) Role of relaxation and specific suggestions in hypnotic emotional numbing. *International Journal of Psychophysiology*, 63: 125–132.

Segerstrom, S., & Nes, L.S. (2007) Heart rate variability reflects self-regulatory strength, effort, and fatique. *Psychological Science*, 18(3): 275–281.

Shapiro, D., Cook, I.A., Davydov, D.M., Ottaviani, C., Leuchter, A.F., & Abrams, M. (2007) Yoga as a complementary treatment in depression: Effects of traits and moods on treatment outcome. *eCAM*, 4(4): 493–502.

Shields, R.W. (2009) Heart rate variability with deep breathing as a clinical test of cardiovagal function. *Cleveland Clinic Journal of Medicine*, 76(1): S37–S40.

Stanley, R. (2009) Types of prayer, heart rate variability, and innate healing. *Zygon*, 44(4): 825–846.

Stanley, R., Leither, T.W., & Sindelir, C. (2011) Benefits of a holistic breathing technique in patients on hemodialysis. *Nephrology Nursing Journal*, 38(2): 149–153.

Sun, F.L. & Yan, Y.A. (1992) Effects of various qigong breathing patterns on variability of heart rate. *Zhongguo Zhon Xi Yi Jie He Za Zhi*, 12(9): 527–530, 516.

Takahashi, T., Murata, T., Hamada, T., Omoris, M., Kosaka, H., Kikuchi, M.,...& Wada, Y. (2005). Changes in EEG and autonomic nervous activity during meditation and their association with personality traits. *International Journal of Psychophysiology*, 55: 199–207.

Tang, Y., Ma, Y., Fan, Y., Feng, H., Wang, J., Feng, S., & Fan, M. (2009) Central and autonomic nervous system interaction is altered by short-term meditation. *Proceedings of the National Academy of Sciences*, 106(22): 8865–8870.

Thayer, J.F., Hansen, A.L., Saus-Rose, E., & Johnson, B.H. (2009) Heart rate variability, prefrontal neural function, and cognitive performance: The neurovisceral integration perspective on self-regulation, adaptation, and health. *Annals of Behavioral Medicine*, 37: 141–153.

Thurber, M.R., Bodenhamer-Davis, E., Johnson, M., Chesky, K., & Chandler, C. K. (2010) Effects of heart rate variability coherence biofeedback training and emotional management techniques to decrease music performance anxiety. *Biofeedback*, 38(1): 28–39.

Tsunetsugu, Y., Park, B., Ishii, H., Hirano, H., Kagawa, T., & Miyazaki, Y. (2007) Physiological effects of Shinrin-yoku (taking in the atmosphere of the forest) in and old-growth broadleaf forest in Yamagata Prefecture, Japan. *Journal of Physiological Anthropology*, 26(2): 135–142.

Väänänen, J., Xusheng, S., Wang, S., Laitinen, T., Pekkarinen, H., & Länsimies, E. (2002) Taichiquan acutely increases heart rate variability. *Clinical Physiology and Functional Imaging*, 22(1): 2–3.

Van Dixhoorn, J. (2007) Whole body breathing: A systems perspective on respiratory retraining. In: Lehrer, P.M., Woolfolk, R.L., & Sime W.E. (eds). *Principles and practice of stress management* . New York: Guilford Press, 290–332.

Vempati, R.P., & Telles, S. (2002). Yoga-based guided relaxation reduces sympathetic activity judged from baseline levels. *Psychological Reports*, 90: 487–494.

Wang, S.Z., Li, S., Xu, X., Lin, G.P., Shao, L., Zhao, Y., & Wang, T.H. (2010) Effect of slow abdominal breathing combined with biofeedback on blood pressure and heart rate variability in prehypertension. *Journal of Alternative and Complementary Medicine*, 16(10): 1039–1045.

Wolever, R.Q., Bobinet, K.J., McCabe, K., Mackenzie, E.R., Fekete, E., Kusnick, C.A., & Baime, M. (2012) Effective and viable mind-body stress reduction in the workplace: A randomized controlled trial. *Journal of Occupational Health Psychology*, 17(2): 246–258.

Wu, S., & Lo, P. (2008) Inward attention meditation increases parasympathetic activity: A study based on heart rate variability. *Biomedical Research*, 29(5): 245–250.

Yeh, G.Y., Wayne, P.M., & Phillips, R.S. (2008) Tai chi exercise in patients with chronic heart failure. *Medicine and Sports Science*, 52: 195–208.

Ysauma, F. & Hayano, J. (2004) Respiratory sinus arrhythmia: Why does heartbeat synchronize with respiratory rhythm? *Chest*, 125: 683–690.

Yurtkuran, M., Alp, A., Yurtkuran, M., & Dilek, K. (2007). A modified yoga-based exercise program in Hemodialysis patients: A randomized controlled study. *Complementary Therapies in Medicine*, 15: 164–171.

CHAPTER 5

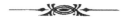

Origins and Applications of Music in Chronic Illness: Role of the Voice, Ancient Chant Scales, and Autonomic Nervous System

Ruth Stanley

Simple ancient chant scales were used prescriptively by our ancestors to treat chronic illness. These scales are remarkably similar to human vocal patterns, suggesting their healing power is related to something inherently whole already within us (Gill & Purves, 2009; Ross et al., 2007). Because we experience all of life as some form of frequency through our five senses of sight, sound, smell, taste, and touch, our body selectively uses frequencies to initiate behaviors and coordinate our well-being. The vast neural, neurohormonal, and emotional responses seen with music, a form of ordered frequencies, imply a primary role for our autonomic nervous system (ANS) in discriminating audio frequencies for the management of emotions, motion, and communication (Ellis & Thayer, 2010; Porges, 2011). Hardwired from birth, we have a predilection for vocal frequency intervals and selectively filter them to communicate our physiologic state (i.e. fear or calm) and guide overall health. Spiritual healers of diverse healing traditions appear to have keenly understood our innate preferences for precise distances between two tones (i.e. intervals) and used music to mirror these inborn audio-vocal cues for modifying ANS cognitive, physical, emotional, and spiritual states. For them, the sacred healing power of music lay primarily in the unique and ineffable supremacy of the human voice.

Ancient chant scales, the origin of music today, offer a unique and clear glimpse into underlying pathophysiologic mechanisms of music in chronic illness. Ancient cultures believed the voice held special mystical powers and

seamlessly travelled through temporal and spiritual realms to facilitate healing (Gass, 1999). Thus, spirituality was deeply intertwined with voice in the
ongoing expression and fulfillment of the deepest desires and needs of the
human condition. Vocalization served as a bridge between worlds and could
be used to directly impact mental, physical, and emotional well-being. As the
primary tool for communicating needs, vocalization lay at the heart of any
ritual involving fundamental human experiences such as healing, joy, or sadness. It is no surprise then that the oldest musical origins across all cultures
share monophonic vocal chant as a primary expression for healing, transformation, and wholeness in chronic illness. Eastern chant traditions typically
incorporate pentatonic or five note scales, melodies commonly heard today
in popular Indian raga sitar music or intoned mantras (Gardner, 1990).
Western vocal chant traditions are best characterized by Gregorian chant,
which uses eight separate heptatonic (i.e. seven note) scales or modes. These
eight scales remain the most popular recurring building blocks found in music
composition worldwide.

An excellent example of the mysterious healing power of these simple
ancient scales in our modern era was observed in a Benedictine monastery
in southern France in 1968 (Tomatis, 2005). After Vatican II, the monastery
had replaced traditional Western chant with modern polyphonic celebration
of the liturgy. Following this change, 78 percent of the monks began experiencing poor sleep, fatigue, mild depression, and interpersonal disharmony.
Dr. Alfred Tomatis, a French Ear, Nose, and Throat physician, was consulted
and he diagnosed the problem as audiologic deficits created by the loss of
healing and energizing tones found within ancient chant scales. Chant was
reinstituted and the monastery placed back on their original rhythm of chant
seven times daily with prayers. Within six months of singing and listening
to chant, 97 percent of the monks experienced complete physical and emotional healing, with significant improvements in emotional self-regulation.
Dr. Tomatis' work formed the foundation for audio-psycho-phonology
(APP) listening therapy, which includes prescriptive use of filtered frequencies of voice, classical music, and Western chant. APP has resulted in up
to 80 percent long-term improvement in some emotional, behavioral, and
communication disorders (Vervoort et al., 2007).

As can be seen in the example above, the voice, music, and chant can be
enormously beneficial for restoring or maintaining well-being. It is true that
music soothes the savage breast but how do we know which music soothes
best? Although research has primarily focused on defining neuropeptides,
regions or neural pathways in the brain affected by music, studies have, for the
most part, ignored the fact that humans process music with exactly the same
ANS pathways used to control emotion, motion, and communication. Vocal
frequency patterns appear to modify ANS control of physical, emotional, spiritual, and psychological states more powerfully than other environmental cues
(Porges, 2011). Because heart rate variability (HRV) reflects ANS function,
HRV can be both a practical and a simple measurement of any ANS change
seen with music. In particular, HRV can be an excellent tool for exploring

how ancient chant scales derived from human vocal interval templates function like encoded auditory cues to directly modulate ANS function. Since these ancient scales still form the basis of most music composition today, the positive benefits noted with music in chronic illness may ultimately be secondary to changes in ANS function and therefore very measurable with HRV. Indeed, this is an emerging field of research in music to help prescriptively guide music selection and enhance clinical outcomes in chronic illness. With the help of modern technology, we are learning how to use music to both calm and heal mind, body, and spirit. Perhaps this technology is reflective of ancient wisdom; for it seems ancient healing traditions were indeed accurate in their belief and use of the human voice to draw forth an innate capacity for wholeness, even in the midst of disease.

This chapter will explore the remarkable correlation of vocal intervals to ancient scales and how human predilection for the human voice directly impacts ANS function and healing associated with music in chronic disease. This chapter's focus will be on the universal origins of music from ancient scales using vocal interval sequences and the corresponding healing applications as related to ANS pathophysiology. Specific topics discussed are: origins of music from ancient scales and vocal intervals; physiologic hardwiring for vocal intervals and scales; relationship of vocal intervals and ancient scales to physiologic states; and practical treatment applications in chronic illness using HRV as a measure of ANS function. What follows is a description of ancient scales and their relationship to human vocal intervals.

ORIGINS OF MUSIC: ANCIENT SCALES AND VOCAL INTERVALS

Most musical compositions fall within a particular frequency range (1,000–3,000 Hz) included in the human vocal frequency range (500–4,000 Hz). Human ears can distinguish about 240 different pitches over an octave in the mid-range of hearing, theoretically allowing countless possibilities for tone combinations to create music (Gill & Purves, 2009). Despite this seemingly endless ability for note combinations, humans have a deliberate preference for specific series of frequencies or pitch intervals between notes. This is evidenced by the uncommonly universal features of musical scales incorporating five (pentatonic scale) or seven (heptatonic scale) notes. Music compositions across thousands of years are predominantly based on just a tiny fraction of pentatonic and heptatonic scales with very similar component intervals to a harmonic series (see Appendix A). Even more fascinating is that these remarkably similar recurring scales form the basis of ancient monophonic chant in healing traditions across all major Eastern and Western cultures. The discovery of almost identical scales across virtually every ancient music tradition implies a universal innate wisdom for specific harmonic frequency patterns to which the human body responds.

The mystery behind why most musical composition is predominantly based on just a small, predictable handful of pentatonic and heptatonic scales is slowly being solved. It seems more than mere coincidence that cultures distanced by time and geography, different in innumerable ways, would be so precisely alike in their musical origins, especially as related to ancient healing rituals. Interestingly, these recurring scales are nearly identical to vocal intervals or spectral patterns characteristic of typical human speech (Bowling et al., 2010; Gill & Purves, 2009; Juslin & Laukka, 2003; Ross et al., 2007; Scherer, 1986). Because these scales exactly match typical formant ratios found in human speech, it means the origin and still most common source of music are human prosodic vocal patterns. Thus, it appears that ancient humans recognized the unique power of and predilection for certain vocal intervals and developed music scales to mirror them. So, what are these scales and how do they relate to vocal intervals?

Pentatonic or five note scales are still used in Asian cultures and the folk music of Russia, India, Africa, Europe, and America (Gardner, 1990). In our Western culture, Native American chants and blues music would be the most common examples. Pentatonic scales are typically used in a more dissonant and descending fashion to create mystical melodies evoking a high to low spirituality, akin to Spirit to Earth or calling for Spirit forces to enter and intervene into physical matter for healing. As such, pentatonic melodies typically start higher and descend to lower frequencies, giving them a magical yet very earthy, humanistic quality. These scales naturally take full advantage of smaller pitch intervals (i.e. two or three notes next to each other) and the tritone to create intense emotional and spiritual effects for physiologic release during healing rituals. These scales remain prominent today in healing rituals and spirituality expressing darkness, cleansing, purification, and release.

Heptatonic or seven note scales are created by adding an additional two notes to the pentatonic scale to form a full octave for harmonic unison (Gardner, 1990). Although heptatonic melodies use both ascending and descending frequency motion to evoke various moods, ascending scales are often more prominent, especially in religions reflecting spirituality associated with ascension or transcendence of material to Spirit such as Christianity. These scales remain prominent today in healing rituals and spirituality expressing light, transcendence, freedom, and union. Since our heptatonic scales are the basis of the "sol-fa" system of modern music and a primary source of music composition worldwide, we will focus most of our discussion on Western heptatonic scales.

Western chant uses a distinct musical scale system in which the emphasis is on maintaining the quality of fixed intervals (i.e. the distance between two notes) (Apel, 1958; Demetria, 1960; Gajard, 1945; Huron & Veltman, 2006). Western chant scales, or modes as they are called, are organized around four particular fixed interval sequences called the Phrygian, Dorian, Lydian, and Mixolydian scales, which are further subdivided into eight separate modes (see Appendix B). Each mode uses a particular scale created by different final and dominant notes. The final or primary note determines the basic fixed interval pattern (i.e. Phrygian Dorian, Lydian, and Mixolydian) and is the primary pitch on which the melody ends (see Appendix C). The dominant, reciting tone or tenor note is the tone around which the melody turns, helping create a quality of consonance or dissonance within each mode.

As a result of this unique fixed interval structure, Western chant scales actually mirror the same basic vocal interval templates normally found in the human voice. As such, humans have a clear predilection and innate ability to delineate these musical scales since they are naturally used when vocalizing or listening for physiologic states. If the origin of music lies hidden in human voice, then it comes as no surprise that the Phrygian and Dorian scales (i.e. Western chant modes 1–4) rank as the most popular sources of music composition worldwide since they have the closest absolute frequency spectrum or fixed intervals to the human voice (see Appendix A). How did our ancient predecessors discover these patterns and label them?

It seems they were highly astute and intuitive listeners, who defined and experienced harmony far differently than most humans do today. For them, the primary function of harmony was for spiritual expression and healing, thus evoking desired moods by using specific vocal interval patterns (Gardner, 1990; Huron & Veltman, 2006). With ancient scales, the fundamental element of harmony is the pitch interval created between two *distinct* notes sung *separately*. Monophonic healing chants create harmony by emphasizing *single note interval sequences* which naturally accentuate consonant or dissonant intervals and invite predictable emotional, cognitive, and behavioral responses based on pitch intervals (see Appendices B, C, and D). We now understand more fully what ancient healers noticed long ago regarding vocal pitch intervals in normal human speech patterns (Bowling et al., 2010; Juslin & Laukka, 2003; Ross et al., 2007; Scherer, 1986). Larger pitch movements (i.e. three to six note intervals), even when in a descending fashion, create a consonant or pleasing sound and induce positive emotions such as joy, serenity, and happiness or a rich, controlled melancholy. Smaller pitch intervals (i.e. two note interval) or highly dissonant intervals (i.e. tritone and seven note interval) invoke negative emotions such as sadness, fright, fear, or anger or uncontrolled darkness (i.e. tritone). Thus, the prescriptive interplay of consonant and dissonant tones within these unique scales creates simple yet powerfully expressive melodies no different than human speech. In the seventeenth century, harmony took on a different meaning as the simultaneous sounding of two or more notes *together* to create *chords*. Music compositions shifted to complex harmonies using organs or orchestras, thus losing the independent nature of ancient scales as they became buried in compositions. Yet, regardless of the complexity of the musical composition, we still selectively listen for these particular recurring scales and respond to them. Why is that?

Hardwired from Birth for Vocal Intervals Found in Ancient Scales

As previously stated, our ancestors considered the voice to be a primary component of healing and spiritual experiences related to overall health. It seems their emphasis on the voice was quite accurate with regard to a human sense of safety and well-being, a fundamental precept for healthy spirituality. At birth, the ear is the only fully mature organ, and hearing the most important sense for determining well-being (Porges, 2011; Sollier, 2005; Tomatis, 2005). Because humans have an unrestricted jawbone and detached middle ear bones, we can both create and hear higher frequency airborne sounds with ease. The middle ear structure allows humans to selectively filter low-amplitude, high-frequency sounds matching the frequency of the human voice. Humans specifically discriminate vocal frequencies over other lower frequency noises in the environment because our middle ear amplifies selective vocal frequencies and dampens the acoustic energy of low-frequency sounds. This shift enabled ancient humans to easily communicate at frequencies their predators could not hear, thus providing a communal survival advantage.

The normal range for human hearing is 20–20,000 Hz. Within this wide range is a very narrow selective frequency range between 500 and 4,000 Hz, which represents the normal human vocal frequency range. Newly born infants or adults easily distinguish and seek this selective human vocal frequency band. More importantly, neonates, infants, adolescents, and adults alike are hardwired with a deliberate preference for human vocal frequencies over any other frequency range because these frequency patterns carry auditory information with specific messages to and from our ANS regarding environmental cues for safety or danger (Kinzler et al., 2007, 2009; Kinzler & Spelke, 2011; Kuhl, 2004; Porges, 2011). Infants preferentially seek social engagement and evaluate safety based on vocal interval patterns related to prosody, accent, and native language. An infant's gaze response is guided by speech patterns rather than race, with accent or prosody of vocal patterns the major determining factor dictating initial social engagement and sense of safety. Areas of the brain responsible for voice and speech processing are functionally active in newborns and infants (Dehaene-Lambertz et al., 2002; Pena et al., 2003; Winkler et al., 2003). Four-day-old neonates to 2-month-old infants are exquisitely capable of discriminating sentences and words voiced in their native language, which contributes to development of selective attention, speech perception, social skills, and memory. By three months, infants have memorized the prosodic contours of their native language even though they are unable to speak words until the age of 7 months or more. The importance of the vocal intervals as found in ancient scales can be observed in mothers of differing cultural backgrounds who sing simple chant melodies to calm babies and invite social interaction (e.g. smiling, cooing, and eye gaze) (Porges, 2011).

Both consciously and unconsciously, vocal intervals are a key component for innate ANS response and assessment of safety as well as overall health and well-being. Infants and adults process music the same way when exposed to melodic or harmonic patterns and complex metric rhythms (Trainor & Trehub, 1992; Zentner & Kagan, 1996). Much of what constitutes early and later preference for social grouping or sense of belonging may be grounded in an inherent sense of safety associated with our native language and universal vocal intervals maintained through generations (Kinzler et al., 2007; Thomson, 2006). The discovery of specific audio-vocal mirror neurons in some mammalian species also suggests primal importance of vocal patterning for ANS function (Bonini & Ferrari, 2011; D'Ausilio, 2009; Levy, 2012). Audio-vocal mirror neurons are involved in the precise recognition of species specific communicative vocal signals and subsequent goal oriented responses related to danger or safety. In general, mirror neurons may play a critical role in humans' ongoing evolutionary preference for the small number of recurring pentatonic and heptatonic scales found in all cultures. These scales likely represent encoded audio-vocal frequencies, which signal our ANS regarding safety or danger to elicit appropriate behaviors. If true, this may explain why humans gravitate both unconsciously and consciously toward the same recurring scales for music composition across countless millennia. We simply cannot *not* do it.

Dr. Alfred Tomatis, a French physician mentioned earlier, was the first person in our modern era to specifically question the relationship between vocal intervals and chronic illness (Tomatis, 2005; Sollier, 2005). He found that the quality of human voice was directly linked to the quality of human listening, both of which impact overall health, well-being, and learning capacity. Inability to discriminate sounds, in particular pitches or pitch intervals in the normal frequency range of the human voice, is associated with impaired ANS function and chronic illness. Therefore, the ability to accurately discriminate vocal frequency intervals is directly related to accuracy in assessing environmental cues for safety or danger. Inability to learn, poor self-regulation of emotions, and most chronic disease states are associated with poor listening and weak discrimination of vocal intervals. More importantly, chronic illness and certain learning disorders can be significantly affected by increasing accuracy of listening for vocal intervals and patterns. Why is that possible? To understand it requires a closer look at ANS pathophysiology to discover how human vocal patterns coordinate our well-being.

RELATIONSHIP OF VOCAL INTERVALS AND ANCIENT SCALES TO PHYSIOLOGIC STATES

The ANS functions as a master gatekeeper to control all emotion, motion, and communication (Porges, 2009, 2011; Porges & Furman, 2011). The primary focus of our ANS gatekeeper is to accurately perceive danger and detect whether another person is trustworthy. ANS response can be easily categorized as either approach (i.e. safety) or withdrawal (i.e. threat) (Porges, 2011; Porges & Furman, 2011). In order to discriminate environmental cues, the ANS gatekeeper uses vagal tone to control head, neck, facial, visual, and auditory muscles necessary for interpreting and engaging socializing behaviors (Porges, 2011). ANS neural pathways necessary for listening to and decoding the human voice are identical to those controlling eye contact, gaze, and emotional expression for effective vocalization. Therefore, the acoustic characteristics of vocal patterns are very reflective of cognitive, physiologic, emotional, and spiritual states, making human vocal interval patterns one of the most highly influential environmental cues the ANS gatekeeper uses to interpret safety or threat and respond (i.e. approach or withdrawal). Vocal patterns function much like a high-level executive, perhaps even chief executive officer, to control ANS function. Indeed, ancient healers were very aware of the power of the human voice and it is no wonder they felt that the human voice traversed temporal and spiritual realms for healing.

As previously mentioned, human vocal intervals likely represent primal acoustic codes for emotional, psychological, physical, and spiritual states (Bowling et al., 2010; Huron, 2008; Huron et al., 2009; Juslin & Laukka, 2003; Porges, 2011; Ross et al., 2007; Scherer, 1986; Tsai et al., 2010). Along with facial features, vocal pitch intervals can both communicate and invoke strong positive or negative emotions, such as anger, sadness, happiness, and pleasantness. When ANS gatekeeper perceives safety through positive vocal cues, high vagal tone produces strong vocal timbre and modulates facial expression, articulation, phrasing, intonation, and patterning of our voices to signal physiologic calm (see Appendix E). When we feel safe and engage socially, we both produce and prioritize acoustic stimuli by larger absolute pitch contours or variance, typically characterized by three to six note intervals. The increased flexibility (i.e. three to six note intervals) in prosody seems to be the strongest vocal cue for safety, happiness, and pleasantness. Wider vocal intervals using normal low vocal frequencies and rising pitch contour invite friendly social approach. Ascending pitch (i.e. especially in four and five note intervals such as a perfect fourth or fifth) typically suggests welcoming, friendly, and calming signals accompanied by facial expressions like a warm, engaging smile. Smiling actually relaxes the vocal tract and produces a quality of clean resonance and rising melodic pitch to our voice. In fact, our smile may have originated as more of a vocal tool than a visual aid in communicating safety, as manifested in infants who smile when exposed to certain vocal intervals prior to any visual ability to detect facial expression (Porges, 2011).

In contrast, if the gatekeeper interprets danger from vocal cues, vagal tone is lowered to allow for appropriate withdrawal, mobilization, or active avoidance in response to threat. Low vagal tone produces a narrow voice resulting from very small pitch intervals (i.e. two note intervals) due to neck and throat constriction, tensing, and shortening (see Appendix E). So, when frightened or aggressive, human vocal volume increases significantly and the vocal pattern becomes rigid with a very high pitch (i.e. shriek or scream in fear) or a very low pitch (i.e. growl in anger or aggression), both communicating a desire to withdraw from danger by either fight or flight. Humans also prioritize acoustic stimuli by intensity (i.e. loudness) and narrow pitch variance when frightened, so these same vocal intervals also serve to detect danger. If you have ever been frightened by someone's scream or screamed yourself, you have experienced this natural auditory survival skill. Recognition of these vocal habits and intervals are extremely important since the gatekeeper's primary responsibility is to assess imminent danger and protect from harm, for the purpose of forming symbiotic relationships. There are, however, subtle nuances to how humans respond to any negative or threatening stimuli.

When sad, vocal intervals are very similar to a minor third or minor second (Bowling et al., 2010; Curtis & Bharucha, 2010; Huron, 2008) (see Appendix D). Intervals matching the tritone (i.e. diminished fifth or augmented fourth using F sharp) convey intense sadness or anger. States of chronic sadness, such as depression, are associated with chronically low vagal tone, resulting in smaller pitch intervals in normal speech and inability to distinguish larger vocal intervals. When frightened to flee, human voice narrows as opposed to the widening that occurs with calm states. A good example is an infant's cry, in which reduced vagal tone results in a significant increase in vocal pitch, dissonance, and volume (Porges, 2011). High-frequency, nasal-like vocal patterns signal fear and are often seen in states of chronic fear or submissiveness consistent with a "whiny," childlike or infantile quality to the speech pattern. This type of narrow voice is sometimes manifested in chronic disease states such as pain syndromes, autoimmune, anxiety, depression, and other mental health disorders. Similar, but different, withdrawal with fight (i.e. hostile or aggressive) is accompanied by very low pitched sounds with little pitch variance yet often intense in volume (Huron et al., 2009; Tsai et al., 2010). Very low growling frequencies signal fighting ability while volume level indicates intention to fight. Deep harsh growls also serve a physiologic purpose to enhance spine stability and prepare for physical attack. Chronic anger or aggression results in lower pitched, narrow vocalizations consistent with deep, raspy growl-like quality also present with pain syndromes, mental health disorders, and cardiac disease. In any threatened state, vagal tone is decreased, listening ability impaired, vocal intervals reduced, and vocal volume altered to convey imminent danger or attack.

When listening to music, both infants and adults selectively focus on pitch intervals and the internal structure of music composition (i.e. tone, scale, rhythmic articulation, and harmonic intervals) as the primary determinant for physiologic response when compared to other factors such as tempo or beat (Gomez & Danuser, 2007; Huron, 2008; Khalfa et al., 2008). Thus, the natural response to various pitch intervals in music are nearly identical to ANS responses typically seen with similar vocal interval patterns (Abrams et al., 2010; Flores-Gutierrez et al., 2007; Green et al., 2008; Khalfa et al., 2005; Koelsch, 2005, 2010; Koelsch et al., 2006; Levitin & Tirovolas, 2009; Mitterschiffthaler et al., 2007; Porges, 2011). It comes, then, as no surprise that major chords mirroring excited or variable speech intervals with ascending, consonant intervals result in positive emotions such as happiness. Positive feelings triggered by listening to these compositions elicit typical ANS responses seen with any other positive environmental acoustic cue, including improved ANS function, vagal tone, emotional self-regulation, and well-being (Fredrickson et al., 2000; McCraty et al., 1998a). On the other hand, minor chords with less variable, descending or dissonant intervals result in sadness (Curtis & Bharucha, 2010; Green et al., 2008; Huron et al., 2006; Koelsch et al., 2008). Once again, ANS response to dissonant or unpleasant music results in reduced emotional self-regulation, increased negative emotions (i.e. anxiety, fear, sadness), and decreased caring, all of which are clearly consistent with reductions in vagal tone seen with negative auditory cues.

The reduction in vagal tone seen with most chronic disease states impairs normal optimal function of the head, neck, throat, and middle ear muscles.

This, in turn, leads to difficulties in both articulating and listening for vital vocal intervals with subsequent long-term erosion of emotional self-regulatory capacity (Porges, 2011). These changes usually correlate with physical and mental illness and can be measured with specialized listening tests (Sollier, 2005). Listening tests measure specific frequency intervals of the human voice in order to determine individual acoustic characteristics of the voice. Inability to appropriately listen for pitch intervals corresponds to an equal inability to produce these same intervals in our personal vocal frequency repertoire. We only speak as well as we listen, and our ability to listen is directly related to our capacity for emotional self-regulation and overall well-being, something spiritual healing traditions place great emphasis upon. Poor listening equals poor emotional self-regulation and deficits in the listening curve correlate with chronic illness. For example, depression is associated with low vagal tone, and listening tests show a significant reduction in the ability to distinguish all vocal intervals, especially ascending higher vocal frequencies. As a result, depressed patients commonly exhibit softer, slowed, decreased, whiny, or monotonous speech patterns. Thus, chronic illness can be characterized as a loss of our natural ability to both listen for and articulate vital frequency patterns necessary for health and well-being . . . a notion very familiar to healing traditions from both East and West.

Increasing the ability to both listen for and distinguish critical vocal intervals significantly improves clinical outcomes associated with most chronic illness and communication disorders (Porges, 2011; Sollier, 2005). Regardless of complexity, the human ANS relentlessly seeks vocal interval sequences buried within any given piece of music. As such, ANS discrimination of intervals and subsequent response can become a more useful guide than simple major or minor keys when choosing music to facilitate treatment of chronic illness. But how can this knowledge guide practice? Human preferences for music hold the answer and can be objectively combined with HRV to guide discovery of the most effective music for facilitating healing. There are practical treatment applications in choosing music for chronic illness.

Practical Treatment Applications in Chronic Illness

Have you ever wondered why you migrate toward certain types of music when you want to relax or feel better about something or someone? With the help of computer technology, scientists and musicians are now able to analyze music in such ways that the specific ordering of interval sequences and scales can be easily found within complex compositions of any music genre (Correa et al., 2010). How humans instinctively choose music across multiple genres appears related to preferred sets of vocal interval sequencing patterns instinctively sought in any music composition. In other words, individual preference for music is defined by favorite pitch interval patterns. Regardless of the genre, similar repeating harmonic intervals show up in an individual's personal music collection, and it is these favored harmonic intervals that either attracts to or repels from any music selection. A sense of safety naturally induced by favorite music may be one reason why humans instinctively turn to particular music selections when coping with chronic illness or any stressors. This may also shed light on why humans share a passion for certain music in common with loved ones, since choice of social grouping or sense of belonging appears to be firmly grounded in the particular vocal intervals interpreted as audio-vocal cues for safety.

Music genres can often reflect the spirituality and culture from which they emerged. As such, pitch intervals commonly associated with a music genre may represent a classic archetypal spiritual journey, which of course can easily overlap with other cultures and genres. A good example is blues music, which uses the pentatonic scale in its purest form. The cultural origin of blues music is found within a people's perception of life and love amid suffering, oppression, and spiritual redemption. As such, blues music vehemently expresses the emotional, psychological, and spiritual depths of betrayal, suffering, abandonment, sexual attraction, jealousy, and loss, thus the name the "blues" (Winborn, 2011). Easily found in blues compositions are audio cues one would expect to find in expressing such powerful emotions; these typically include dissonant vocal interval patterns such as the tritone, minor second or third. Blues music uses these intervals to access deep feelings and then almost ritually release them in safe and healthy ways through musical expression. Yet, there are many other genres of music that also use the tritone, minor second or third intervals to express these charged emotions. If a person is drawn toward these intervals as a secure space for freeing these feelings, then these intervals likely show up in other musical preferences, regardless of genre.

Therefore, no matter how vast our personal music collection may be, the basis of our choosing music boils down to something very simple; we repeatedly choose specific pitch intervals to safely express ourselves and better understand each other. This could explain why studies comparing genres of music for health are often confusing; it is not the particular genre chosen, but rather the same repeating intervals found across many genres. Innate preferences therefore reflect a natural inclination for well-being. Because we discriminate audio-vocal cues, we already have a personal music collection capable of facilitating our healing, and we need to use it regularly for best benefit. But in order to fully maximize clinical outcomes, it becomes necessary to find other less familiar forms of music which use these intervals with greater clarity and intensity. Until recently, the greatest challenge was to know where to look, and for this, HRV has become the most reliable guide.

As previously stated, the primary focus of the human ANS gatekeeper is to accurately perceive danger and detect whether another person is trustworthy. ANS gatekeeper, vagal tone, and emotional self-regulation are best measured and modified using HRV (Appelhans & Luecken, 2006; Bernston et al., 1997; ; Kok & Fredrickson, 2010; McCraty et al., 2006; Thayer et al., 2009). Chronically low HRV usually denotes low vagal tone, decreased emotional self-regulation, and poor listening ability, all of which result in significantly reduced quality of life and worsening of most chronic disease states. In contrast, normal or high HRV corresponds to excellent vagal tone, emotional self-regulation, quality of life, and clinical outcomes in chronic illness. Improving HRV with frequency patterns around 0.1 Hz is associated with high innate healing and significantly improved vagal tone regardless of disease progression (see Appendix F). Because HRV is the most consistent means for assessing and modifying ANS emotional and cognitive responses to music or vocal stimuli, it is the most rapidly growing critical index with regard to music for health and well-being (Ellis & Thayer, 2010).

Not surprisingly, positive heart-felt emotions improve HRV, produce high innate healing (i.e. 0.1 Hz), and result in significant clinical improvement in chronic illness (McCraty et al., 1995, 1998b, 2006; McCraty & Childre, 2004; Rein et al., 1995). More importantly, any music containing favored intervals for evoking positive heart-felt feelings will improve HRV, innate healing (i.e. 0.1 Hz), and increase vagal tone, all of which are associated with decreased anxiety, depression, pain, inflammatory indices, and cortisol (i.e. stress hormone) as well as improved immune function, memory, cognition, mental clarity, positive emotions, and relaxation (see Appendix F) (Chiu et al., 2003; Iwanaga et al., 2005; Kemper & Hamilton, 2008; McCraty et al., 1996, 2006, 1998a; Nakahara et al., 2009; Okada et al., 2009; Peng et al., 2009; Sokhadze, 2007; Umemura & Honda, 1998; White, 1999; Yanagihashi et al., 1997). For example, a unique HRV biofeedback system is being developed to identify music and pitch intervals that improve HRV (Ho & Chen, 2011). This system identifies HRV response to our favorite music and then designs a music repertoire to enhance overall HRV. Preliminary results show significant improvements in HRV when listening to music from the program for 15–60 minutes daily. This is a novel breakthrough and likely suggests future treatment options. Yet, without the help of such a nifty program, how might a healing musical repertoire be developed? There are three reliable types of music that may facilitate healing and improve HRV; these are chant, classical, and, to a lesser extent, some forms of designer music. Chant is the most effective of the three.

As previously stated, ancient Western chant scales are almost identical to vocal intervals and serve as building blocks for modern music composition. The simplicity and intense clarity of pitch intervals of Western chant produce remarkable HRV improvement consistent with ANS acoustic cues for safety. Much like the HRV system described above, chant is highly effective for improving HRV when listened to in 10–15 minute time periods, often producing a high degree of innate healing at 0.1 Hz (Stanley, 2006). Observations with chant show significant and rapid transitions toward innate healing frequency (i.e. 0.1 Hz) during 43–87 percent of a listening interval depending on the mode. As would be expected, varying improvements in HRV correlate with improved ANS function, emotional self-regulation, and listening ability (McCraty et al., 2006; Stanley, 2006). In our clinic, we have noted that modes 1, 2, 3, 7, and 8 produce the highest immediate innate healing response (i.e. 0.1 Hz) while modes 4, 5, and 6 produce more moderate levels of HRV response. In addition, people typically show a definitive preference for three of the eight modes, usually patterned as a preference for two of the more highly innate healing modes (i.e. 1, 2, 3, 7, or 8) and one of the other more moderate modes (i.e. 4, 5, or 6). These observations seem consistent with the natural preference for particular sequencing as noted earlier. Innate preferences appear individually hardwired and explain in part why music composition is still derived from the most commonly used ancient scales (i.e. the Phrygian and Dorian scales as modes 1, 2, 3, and 4) (Gill & Purves, 2009). So it would seem these scales likely represent specific audio-vocal cues to our ANS to which humans easily respond, with each mode having a particular purpose as yet poorly defined in our era but certainly well observed in ancient times. How can chant be used in the practical treatment of chronic illness?

Use of chant melodies in addition to favorite music produces profound benefits in chronic debilitating or terminal disease. The clarity of pitch intervals found in chant melodies significantly improve HRV, listening tests, overall communication, emotional self-regulation, and behavior (Bernardi et al., 2001, 2006; Ho & Chen, 2011; Lee et al., 2011; Okada et al., 2009; Stanley, 2006; Trappe, 2010; Vervoort et al., 2007). A good example is audio-psycho-phonology (APP), which incorporates chant melodies, maternal vocal patterns, and classical music to modify ANS response, improve listening tests, and improve cognitive, emotional, and behavioral patterns (Vervoort et al., 2007). As verified with brain mapping, APP has a remarkably high success rate at 80 percent compared to other treatment modalities for chronic disabilities associated with communication, concentration, dyslexia, speech, behavior, and language disorders. Some trained APP practitioners are offering filtered music recordings for use at home with portable devices to facilitate continued benefits after treatment. Other more common uses include sung mantras or melodies and simple listening to chant, both of which result in significant improvements in HRV as well as entrained respiration (Haas et al., 1986). HRV improvements are rapidly and easily seen with chants designed to pace breathing at around six breaths per minute, suggesting that these ancient melodies are excellent tools for inducing immediate relaxation in the face of stressors (Bernardi et al., 2001). In addition, silent pauses or silence at the conclusion of a short chant melody further improves HRV (Bernardi et al., 2006). In our clinic, we routinely test HRV response to the eight modes of chant and then suggest melodies within modes where the greatest HRV responses are noted. Typically, patients are aware of which melodies they responded to because they can feel a difference when listening; this is encouraging for anyone who wants to try chant but for whom HRV assessment is unavailable. Patients are then given a CD with chant music and asked to listen to it for 10–15 minutes one to three times daily. We have found listening regularly to chant melodies produces benefits to those with chronic illness by improving coping skills, quality of life, and overall sense of well-being. Our findings are consistent with that of Tomatis (from the late 60s) as well as more recent data noted above. Overall, patients find chant melodies relaxing and report reductions in pain, anxiety, stress, and sleep disturbances. Many people have discovered the healing power of chant on their own due to the popularity of a number of high-quality recordings.

Given the profound effects of simple chant on ANS function and emotional self-regulation, the resurgence in interest for chant is not surprising. As a simple adjunct to the treatment of anxiety and pain, chant is being utilized in hospitals, special care units, and operating rooms through live or recorded melodies. Because of the immediate ANS effects, the use of chant has grown rapidly in palliative and hospice care to comfort the dying, assist in difficult symptom management, and help patients and family members cope. Given that the human sense of hearing is both the first and the last sense used to determine sense of safety, chant naturally calms the mind, body, and spirit in the midst of debilitating disease. Music thanatologists specialize in offering music vigils originally patterned from Benedictine monastic chant rituals for the dying. Consistent with the ancient belief in the power of chant to traverse spiritual and temporal realms, the goal of these vigils is to relax patients and help give them a sense of freedom as they pass gently from this life to the next (Freeman et al., 2006; Cox & Roberts, 2012; Leach et al., 2005). These vigils typically incorporate sung chants or instrumental chant, with the harp the most frequently utilized instrument. My personal experience in these settings is that positive ANS changes elicit profound states of calm, safety, and security, regardless of severity of disease. Although chant is highly effective, some patients may be hesitant to listen to it. Given the close relationship to ancient chant, classical music is a wonderful alternative.

Ancient chant scales form the basis for our modern major and minor scales, which evolved to facilitate harmonic chords and orchestration. Classical music has its origins in the transition from chant to complex harmony, and older compositions typically contain recurring ancient scales or interval patterns around which the whole composition revolves. In fact, many classical compositions originated from simple folk or chant melodies that had been creatively rewritten for orchestration or organ (Gardner, 1990). As such, classical music improves HRV and increases vagal tone, resulting in improvements in emotional self-regulation and listening ability (Bernardi et al., 2006; Burns et al., 2001; Iwanaga et al., 2005; Lee et al., 2011; McCraty et al., 1998a; Peng et al., 2009; Sokhadze, 2007; Sollier, 2005; Stanley, 2006; Trappe, 2010; Umemura & Honda, 1998; White, 1999). Consistent with improvement in HRV, classical music neutralizes negative emotions, reduces negativity, and decreases fatigue, sadness, and tension while improving overall emotional self-regulation, calm, and vagal tone. The use of recurring scales in music is most noticeable when measuring HRV, where innate healing (i.e. 0.1 Hz) occurs simultaneously with repetition of the recurring scale throughout the composition as the body recognizes the frequency interval patterns. The end result is smaller periods of innate healing compared to chant but high overall HRV improvement throughout the composition (Stanley, 2006). Compositions by Bach, Handel, Mozart, Vivaldi, Beethoven, Corelli, Tartini, Albioni, and Debussy have been studied the most and are highly effective in conditions known to have chronically low HRV such as anxiety, depression, stress, pain, sleep disorders, or cardiovascular syndromes (Trappe, 2010). The best advice is to encourage patients to listen to composers they are most drawn to; a good place to start is Mozart. Further improvements in HRV and vagal tone can be seen when classical music is combined with essential oils or nature sounds such as birdsongs (Peng et al., 2009).

Akin to classical music, designer, natural, and new-age music are newer forms of music specifically designed to produce relaxation and alter ANS function (Sokhadze, 2007). Technology, in a sense, is helping us essentially do what great composers and spiritual healers have done intuitively. These forms of music improve HRV, neutralize negativity, increase vagal tone, and improve emotional self-regulation (Chiu et al., 2003; McCraty et al., 1996, 1998a; Yanagihashi et al., 1997). When compared to classical music, designer music appears to be an equitable alternative for improving HRV.

Just a note about other forms of popular music compared to chant, classical, and designer music. In general, pop, rock, grunge rock, and techno forms of music have limited effects on HRV outside of particular songs that hold our preferred pitch interval sequences (Bernardi et al., 2006; Gerra et al., 1998; McCraty et al., 1996, 1998a; Umemura & Honda, 1998; Urakawa & Yokoyama, 2005). In general, rock music, techno, and pop can be highly beneficial for exercise, dancing, or upbeat tempo to improve our mood. These types of music are excellent for aerobic exercise and elicit better hemo-dynamic profiles during periods of exertion beyond simple entrainment to tempo. In our clinic, we recommend these to improve exercise tolerance in patients with chronic illness. In contrast, hard or grunge rock typically has highly dissonant intervals that may significantly reduce HRV and emotional self-regulation. Because this music normally results in increased tension, anxiety, irritability, and fatigue, we discourage patients from listening to hard or grunge rock if their symptoms are poorly controlled or worsened when listening. If patients are drawn toward this music, we ask them to consider adding blues, Native American drumming and chanting, or classical melodies with more upbeat tempos for a healthier release of emotions.

Choosing music to facilitate healing in chronic illness is both simple and complex. It is simple in the sense that our bodies have chosen the pitch interval sequences we need and we already have a vast collection of these intervals in the music we know and love. The complex part is finding music that more directly uses these intervals with greater clarity and intensity to improve HRV and ANS function. Chant, classical music, and designer music appear to be the most beneficial types of music to further facilitate healing benefits in chronic illness. Listening to these types of music improve HRV, vagal tone, emotional self-regulation, listening ability, and clinical outcomes. The challenge in health care is to find simple ways to manage and expand patient preferences in order to promote optimal healing and health. A great place to start is with chant, classical, or designer music.

SUMMARY

Because the origins of music are found in human vocal patterns, the human voice has the sacred power to heal and restore ANS function in chronic illness. From birth, ANS stability appears dependent on a predilection for human vocal frequency patterns as a guide for interpreting safety and establishing health and well-being. Humans are hardwired to seek, find, and use particular frequency intervals consistent with encoded acoustic cues for determining emotional intelligence and response. Ancient spiritual traditions and healers understood the remarkable properties of vocal patterns and designed scales mirroring them to create music for healing and celebration. The popularity of classical music and growing resurgence of chant for healing and relaxation may very well be related to the primal encoding of these intervals for health and well-being. The unique relationship of the voice to the ANS suggests the presence of a healer already within us . . . our own voice. The paradox is that we already innately know what music helps us but we do not know how best to use it for optimal benefit. Some difficulty lies in identifying an individual's particular intervals or ANS cues and then maximizing music using these intervals with greater intensity and clarity. As the understanding of vocal interval patterns improves and HRV technology becomes more readily available, practitioners can more accurately prescribe music in chronic illness for maximal benefit. From a practical standpoint, we can encourage patients to use their personal collection of music favorites as they are drawn to them and add chant, classical, or designer music for greater improvement in HRV and clinical outcomes. Voice is music, and music is a timeless, universal expression of the human condition and the remarkable capacity for healing. As ancient cultures understood so well, the healing power of innate wholeness is waiting to be called forth at any given moment with something as simple as a beautiful melody . . . we have only to listen for it.

APPENDIX A: MOST COMMONLY USED ANCIENT SCALES IN MUSIC COMPOSITION*

Most Commonly Used Pentatonic Scales

1. Minor pentatonic scale
2. Ritusen scale (used in traditional Chinese and Indian music)
3. Candrika todi (Classical Indian music, raga, natural minor)
4. Asa-Gaudi (classical Indian music, raga, natural major)
5. Durga Raga (identical to the Ritusen scale except higher in pitch)
6. Major pentatonic scale

Most Commonly Used Heptatonic Scales

1. Phrygian scale (Western chant modes 3 and 4)
2. Dorian scale (Western chant modes 1 and 2)
3. Major heptatonic scale (Ionian scale)
4. Husayni scale (similar to Phrygian, used in traditional Arabic music)
5. Minor heptatonic scale (Aeolian scale)
6. Lydian scale (Western chant modes 5 and 6)
7. Kafi scale (used in classical Indian music)
8. Kardaniya scale (used in Arabic music)
9. Not any well-known musical scale
10. Mixolydian scale (Western chant modes 7 and 8)

*Note: Based on Similarity to Vocal Intervals (Gill & Purves, 2009)

APPENDIX B: WESTERN CHANT MODES

	MODE 1	MODE 2	MODE 3	MODE 4	MODE 5	MODE 6	MODE 7	MODE 8
Pseudo-Greek Naming	Dorian	Hypodorian	Phrygian	Hypophrygian	Lydian	Hyoplydian	Mixolydian	Hypomixolydian
Emotional Template (Eight Modes)	Any feeling (happy to serious)	Sad, serious, tearful	Mystic, vehement emotions	Harmonious, tender, tempers emotions, delight	Happy, pleasant	Devout, pious, tearful	Angelical, youthful, pleasure, sadness	Perfect, very happy, joy, pleasant. Serenity
Emotional Template (Four Scales)	Emotionally expressive: magical, serene, passionate, exalting Used in rituals for sharing positive and negative emotions.		Dramatic, intense, and passionate. Used in rituals to incite intense positive and negative emotions.		Pious rituals mixing joy with devotion invoking a sense of up or down spirituality.		Open, joyful, extroverted, happy for celebration	

(Continued)

Final (primary pitch)	D (re)	D (re)	E (mi)	E (mi)	F (fah)	F (fah)	G (sol)	G (sol)
Dominant* (reciting tone or tenor)	A (la)	F (fah)	C (do)	A (la)	C (do)	A (la)	D (re)	C (do)
Ambitus Category**	Authentic	Plagal	Authentic	Plagal	Authentic	Plagal	Authentic	Plagal
Note Range for Octave	D-d	A-a	E-e	B-b	F-f	C-c	G-g	D-d
Correlation to major or minor key in modern composition	Minor	Both	Major	Minor	Major	Minor	Both	Major
Rank in use for modern composition	2	2	1	1	6	6	10	10

Notes: *The fifth note of each authentic mode became the dominant or reciting note. In the plagal modes, the dominant was the second note before the dominant of its related authentic. B was considered inappropriate as a tenor tone, so it was replaced by C.

**Authentic: octave begins on the final or primary pitch; Plagal: octave begins a fourth below or fifth above the final or primary pitch.

APPENDIX C: UNIQUE FIXED INTERVAL STRUCTURE OF WESTERN CHANT SCALES*

How scales are designed:

Fixed Interval Scale: Do (C)—Re (D)—Mi (E) —Fa (F)—Sol (G)—La (A)—Ti (B)—Do (C)

↓   ↓↓   ↓↓↓↓

Steps: Whole Whole Half Whole Whole Whole Half

If B flat used on fixed interval scale: La (A)—Ti (B flat)—Do (C)

↓   ↓

Position of half step changes to this: Half Whole

How interval sequences differ between scales:

	Primary pitch ("do" or beginning note for octave of each interval sequence)	Interval sequence (W = whole step, H = half step)
Western chant scale		
Dorian (modes 1 and 2)	D	W-H-W-W-W-H-W
Phrygian (modes 3 and 4)	E	H-W-W-W-H-W-W
Lydian (modes 5 and 6)	F	W-W-W-H-W-W-H
Mixolydian (modes 7 and 8)	G	W-W-H-W-W-H-W
Modern scales		
Modern major scale	C	W-W-H-W-W-W-H
Modern minor scale	A	W-H-W-W-H-W-W

*Note: Interval is the distance in pitch between two tones or notes, with the smallest interval a half step. Present day sol-fa system or diatonic scale has its origins in the Western chant fixed interval scale, where "do" is the equivalent of the key note (i.e. normally C or A) in modern music. Western chant employs only fixed intervals of the Diatonic scale listed below and uses a unique clef positioning system to indicate pitch locations from which the other notes could be sung. The only variability to the fixed intervals is the use of B flat to change the place of the half tone between La and Do. This was most common for the Lydian (modes 5 and 6) scale. The character of each mode provided for sequencing whole and half step intervals uniquely differently, thus giving each mode its characteristic sound based on interval patterns.

Appendix D: Natural Consonant and Dissonant Harmonic Intervals

	Found in Which Scales P, Pentatonic H, Heptatonic	Where to Find It Using Modern Major Scale ("do-re-mi-fa-sol-la-ti-do," with C as "do")	Ascending or Descending Interval	Emotional Correlates
Consonant intervals				
Perfect fifth (fifth above root tone)	P, H	"sol" above/below "do" (C to G)	Both	Power, happiness, pleasantness, centeredness, sturdiness, beautiful, comfortable, complete
Perfect fourth (fourth above root tone)	P, H	"fa" above/below "do" (C to F)	Both	Serenity, clarity, openness, light, angelic
Major third (third above root tone)	P, H	"mi" above "do" (C to E)	Ascending	Sweet, glad, charming, hopeful, friendly, resolved, comfortable
Minor sixth (inverted major third)	H	"mi" below "do" (C to E)	Descending	Satisfying and pleasing, soothing, sad, delicate
Minor third	P, H	"la" below "do" (C to A)	Descending	Elated, religious, uplifting, sad, tragic, melancholy
Major sixth (inverted minor third)	H	"la" above "do" (C to A)	Ascending	Pleasing, peaceful, resolved, awakening, uplifting
Dissonant intervals				
Major second	P, H	"re" above "do" (C to D)	Ascending	Mild dissonance, melancholy, anger, tense, irritating
Minor seventh (inverted major second)	H	"re" below "do" (C to D)	Descending	Mild dissonance, suspenseful, expectant, moving, rich, unbalanced
Major seventh	H	"ti" above "do" (C to B-flat)	Ascending	Strange, eerie, discordant, frightening
Minor second (inverted major seventh)	P, H	"ti" below "do" (C to B-flat)	Descending	Sad, tense, melancholy, anger, uneasy, mysterious, anticipatory
Tritone (diminished fifth or augmented fourth)	P, H	Three whole tones up or down from fundamental tone (C to F sharp)	Both	Anger, hostility, sadness, displeasing, ugly, tense, malevolence, weird, suspenseful, deep and occult, sadness

APPENDIX E: ANS GATEKEEPER AND VOCAL CUES

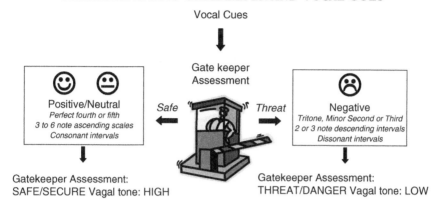

Vocal Cues

Gate keeper Assessment

Positive/Neutral
Perfect fourth or fifth
3 to 6 note ascending scales
Consonant intervals

Safe   *Threat*

Negative
Tritone, Minor Second or Third
2 or 3 note descending intervals
Dissonant intervals

Gatekeeper Assessment:
SAFE/SECURE Vagal tone: HIGH

Gatekeeper Assessment:
THREAT/DANGER Vagal tone: LOW

Motion: Approach behaviors, relaxed face, neck, and throat.

Motion: Withdrawal behaviors, tense facial, neck, and throat.

Emotion: Calm, Positive emotions
Good Emotional self regulation
Joy, happiness, content, pleasant

Emotion: Fear, Negative emotions
Poor Emotional self regulation
Anxiety, sadness, anger, irritability

Communication: Inviting, facial smiles, good prosody and intonation to voice, excellent listening ability.

Communication: Recoiling, facial frown, poor prosody and intonation to voice, poor listening ability.

ANS: Autonomic Nervous System

APPENDIX F: POSITIVE HEALING BENEFITS OF 0.1 HZ INNATE FREQUENCY

- Resets gatekeeper to accurately interpret acoustic cues for safety or threat
- Resets vagal tone higher
- Maximizes emotional and cognitive self-regulatory capacity
- Improves listening ability (i.e. ability to distinguish vocal intervals well)
- Decreases cortisol (i.e. stress hormone) levels by 25 percent
- Increases anti-stress hormones by 100 percent (i.e. DHEA)
- Increases Immunoglobulin A levels
- Fosters approach, calming, and socializing behaviors
- Produces a four- to five-fold increase in alpha and theta brainwaves
- Improves perceptual capacity and attentiveness
- Increases blood flow in the right and left hemispheres of the brain
- Improves neuroplasticity, cognition, word recall, intuition, memory (improved 12 percent), and cognitive reaction times (32 percent improvement)

- Cardiac autonomic function, cerebral blood flow, and other neurohormonal feedback loops are simultaneously optimized for more efficient oxygenation, fluid exchange, toxin filtration, and nutrient absorption between capillaries and tissues
- Experienced as clear, focused mind with extreme calm and peace

References

Abrams, D., Bhatara, A., Ryali, S., Balaban, E., Levitin, D., & Menon, V. (2010). Decoding temporal structure in music and speech relies on shared brain resources but elicits different fine-scale spatial patterns. *Cerebral Cortex, 21*(7), 1507–1518.

Apel, W. (1958). *Gregorian chant*. Bloomington: Indiana University Press.

Appelhans, B. M., & Luecken, L. J. (2006). Heart rate variability as an index of regulated emotional responding. *Review of General Psychology, 10*(3), 229–240.

Bernardi, L., Porta, C., & Sleight, P. (2006). Cardiovascular, cerebrovascular, and respiratory changes induced by different types of music in musicians and non-musicians: The importance of silence. *Heart, 92,* 445–452.

Bernardi, L., Sleight, P., Bandinelli, G., Cencetti, S., Fattorini, L., Wdowczk-Szulc, J., & Lagi, A. (2001). Effect of rosary prayer and yoga mantras on autonomic cardiovascular rhythms: Comparative study. *British Medical Journal, 323,* 1446–1449.

Bernston, G., Bigger, T., Eckberg, D. L., Grossman, P., Kaufman, P. G., Malik, M., ... & Maurits W. (1997). Heart rate variability: Origins, methods, and interpretive caveats. *Psychophysiology, 34,* 623–648.

Bonini, L., & Ferrari, P. F. (2011). Evolution of mirror systems: A simple mechanism for complex cognitive functions. *Annals of the New York Academy of Sciences, 1225*(1), 166–175.

Bowling, D. L., Gill, K., Choi, J. D., Prinz, J., & Purves, D. (2010). Major and minor music compared to excited and subdued speech. *Journal of the Acoustical Society of America, 127*(1), 491–503.

Burns, S. J., Harbuz, M. S., Hucklebridge, F., & Bunt, L. (2001). A pilot study into the therapeutic effects of music therapy at a cancer help center. *Alternative Therapies in Health and Medicine, 7*(1), 48–56.

Chiu, H. W., Lin, L. S., Kuo, M. C., Chiang, H. S., & Hsu, C. Y. (2003). Using heart rate variability analysis to assess the effects of music therapy on anxiety reduction in patients. *Computers in Cardiology, 30,* 469–472.

Correa, D. C., Saito, J. H., & Costa, L. F. (2010). Musical genres: Beating to the rhythms of different drums. *New Journal of Physics, 12,* 1–37, doi:10.1088/1367-2630/12/5/053030.

Cox, H., & Roberts, P. (2012). *The harp and the ferryman: Journeys of healing*. Melbourne, Australia: Michelle Anderson Publishing Pty Ltd.

Curtis, M. E., & Bharucha, J. J. (2010). The minor third communicates sadness in speech, mirroring its use in music. *Emotion, 10*(3), 335–348.

D'Ausilio, A. (2009). Mirror-like mechanisms and music. *The Scientific World Journal, 9,* 1415–1422.

Dehaene-Lambertz, G., Dehaene, S., & Hertz-Pannier, L. (2002). Functional neuroimaging of speech perception in infants. *Science, 298,* 2013–2015.

Demetria, M. (1960). *Basic Gregorian chant and sight reading.* Toledo, OH: Gregorian Institute of America.

Ellis, R. J., & Thayer, J. F. (2010). Music and autonomic nervous system (dys)function. *Music Perception, 27*(4), 317–326.

Flores-Gutierrez, E. O., Diaz, J., Barrios, F. A., Favila-Humara, R., Guevara, M. A., del Rio- Portilla, Y., & Corsi-Cabrera, M. (2007). Metabolic and electric brain patterns during pleasant and unpleasant emotions induced by music masterpieces. *International Journal of Psychophysiology, 65,* 69–84.

Fredrickson, B. L., Mancuso, R. A., Branigan, C., & Tugade, M. M. (2000). The undoing effect of positive emotions. *Motivation and Emotion, 24,* 237–258.

Freeman, L., Caserta, M., Lund, D., Rossa, S., Dowdy, A., & Partenheimer, A. (2006). Music thanatology: Prescriptive harp music as palliative care for the dying patient. *American Journal Hospice and Palliative Medicine, 23*(2), 100–104.

Gajard, J. (1945). *The rhythm of plainsong according to the Solesmes school.* New York: J. Fischer and Brothers.

Gardner, K. (1990). *Sounding the inner landscape: Music as medicine.* Stonington, ME: Caduceus Publications.

Gass, R. (1999). *Chanting: Discovering spirit in sound.* New York: Broadway Books.

Gerra, G., Zaimovic, A., Franchini, D., Palladino, M., Giucastro, G., Reali, N.,... & Brambilla, F. (1998). Neuroendocrine responses in healthy volunteers to 'techno-music': Relationships with personality traits and emotional state. *International Journal of Psychophysiology, 28,* 99–111.

Gill, K. Z., & Purves, D. (2009). A biological rationale for musical scales. *PloS ONE, 4*(12), e8144. doi:10.1371/journal.pone.0008144.

Gomez, P., & Danuser, B. (2007). Relationships between musical structure and psychophysiological measures of emotion. *Emotion, 7*(2), 377–387.

Green, A. C., Baerentsen, K. B., Stodkilde-Jorgensen, H., Wallentin, M., Roepstorff, A., & Vuust, P. (2008). Music in minor activates limbic structures: A relationship with dissonance? *NeuroReport, 19*(7), 711–715.

Haas, F., Distenfeld, S., & Axen, K. (1986). Effects of perceived musical rhythm on respiratory pattern. *Journal of Applied Physiology, 61*(3), 1185–1191.

Ho, T., & Chen, X. (2011). iHeartLift: A closed loop system with biofeedback that uses music tempo variability to improve heart rate variability. *Conference Proceedings: IEEE, Engineering in Medicine and Biology Society,:* 1181–1184.

Huron, D. (2008). A comparison of average pitch height and interval size in major and minor key themes: Evidence consistent with affect-related pitch prosody. *Empirical Musicology Review, 3*(2), 59–63.

Huron, D., Dahl, S., & Johnson, R. (2009). Facial expression and vocal pitch height: Evidence of an intermodal association. *Empirical Musicology Review, 4*(3), 93–100.

Huron, D., Kinney, D., & Precoda, K. (2006). Influence of pitch height on the perception of submissiveness and threat in musical passages. *Empirical Musicology Review, 1*(3), 170–177.

Huron, D. & Veltman, J. (2006). Cognitive approach to medieval mode: Evidence for an historical antecedent to the major/minor system. *Empirical Musicology Review, 1*(1), 33–55.

Iwanaga, M., Kobayashi, A., & Kawasaki, C. (2005). Heart rate variability with repetitive exposure to music. *Biological Psychology, 70,* 61–66.

Juslin, P. N., & Laukka, P. (2003). Communication of emotions in vocal expression and music performance: Different channels, same code? *Psychological Bulletin*, *129*(5), 770–814.

Kemper, K., & Hamilton, C. (2008). Live harp music reduces activity and increases weight gain in stable premature infants. *Journal of Alternative and Complementary Medicine*, *14*(10), 1185–1186.

Khalfa, S., Roy, M., Rainville, P., Bella, S. D., & Peretz, I. (2008). Role of tempo entrainment in psychophysiological differentiation of happy and sad music? *International Journal of Psychophysiology*, *68*, 17–26.

Khalfa, S., Schon, D., Anton, J., & Liegeois-Chauvel, C. (2005). Brain regions involved in the recognition of happiness and sadness in music. *NeuroReport*, *16*, 1981–1984.

Kinzler, K. D., Dupoux, E., & Spelke, E. S. (2007). The native language of social cognition. *Proceedings of the National Academy of Sciences*, *104*(30), 12577–12580.

Kinzler, K. D., Shutts, K., DeJesus, J., & Spelke, E. S. (2009). Accent trumps race in guiding children's social preferences. *Social Cognitive and Affective Neuroscience*, *27*(4), 623–634.

Kinzler, K. D. & Spelke, E. S. (2011). Do infants show social preferences for people differing in race? *Cognition*, *119*(1), 1–9.

Koelsch, S. (2005). Investigating emotions with music. *Annals of the New York Academy of Sciences*, *1060*, 412–418.

Koelsch, S. (2010). Towards a neural basis of music-evoked emotions. *Trends in Cognitive Sciences*, *14*(3), 131–137.

Koelsch, S., Fritz, T., Cramon, D. Y., Müller, K., & Friederici, A. D. (2006). Investigating emotion with music: An fMRI study. *Human Brain Mapping*, *27*, 239–250.

Koelsch, S., Fritz, T., & Schlaug, G. (2008). Amygdala activity can be modulated by unexpected chord functions during music listening. *NeuroReport*, *19*(18), 1815–1819.

Kok, B. E., & Fredrickson, B. L. (2010). Upward spirals of the heart: Autonomic flexibility, as indexed by vagal tone, reciprocally and prospectively predicts positive emotions and social connectedness. *Biological Psychology*, *85*(3), 432–436.

Kuhl, P. K. (2004). Early language acquisition: Cracking the speech code. *Nature Reviews/Neuroscience*, *5*, 831–843.

Leach, S., Cox, H., & Roberts P. (2005). *Relief of suffering at the end of life: Report from an Australian project to implement and evaluate a live harp music-thanatology program.* Australia Kings Scholarship, Geelong, Australia: St. John of God Hospital and Deakin University School of Nursing, 1–99.

Lee, Y., Lei, C., Shih, Y., Zhang, W., Wang, H., Tseng, C.,… & Huang, S. (2011). HRV response of vegetative state patient with music therapy. *Conference Proceedings: IEEE, Engineering in Medicine and Biology Society*,1701–1704.

Levitin, D. J., & Tirovolas, A. K. (2009). Current advances in the cognitive neuroscience of music. *Annals of the New York Academy of Sciences*, *1156*, 211–231.

Levy, F. (2012). Mirror neurons, birdsong, and human language: A hypothesis. *Frontiers in Psychiatry*, *2*, 1–7.

McCraty, R., Atkinson, M., Rein, G., & Watkins, A. D. (1996). Music enhances the effect of positive emotional states on salivary IgA. *Stress Medicine*, *12*, 167–175.

McCraty, R., Atkinson, M., Tiller, W. A., Rein, G., & Watkins, A. D. (1995). The effects of emotions on short-term power spectrum analysis of heart rate variability. *American Journal of Cardiology*, *76*(14), 1089–1093.

McCraty, R., Atkinson, M., Tomasino, D., & Bradley, R. (2006). *The coherent heart: Heart- Brain interactions, psychophysiological coherence, and the emergence of system-wide order.* Boulder Creek, CA: Institute of HeartMath, Publication 06–022.

McCraty, R., Barrios-Choplin, B., Atkinson, M., & Tomasino, D. (1998a). The effects of different types of music on mood, tension, and mental clarity. *Alternative Therapies in Health and Medicine, 4,* 75–84.

McCraty R., Barrio-Choplin, B., Rozman, D., Atkinson, M., & Watkins, A. D. (1998b). The impact of a new emotional self-management program on stress, emotions, heart rate variability, DHEA, and cortisol. *Integrative Physiological and Behavioral Science, 33*(2), 151–170.

McCraty, R., & Childre, D. (2004). The grateful heart: The psychophysiology of appreciation. In R. A. Emmons & M. E. McCullough (Eds.). *The psychology of gratitude.* New York, NY: Oxford University Press, 230–256.

Mitterschiffthaler, M. T., Fu, C., Dalton, J. A., Andrew, C. M., & Williams, S. (2007). A functional MRI study of happy and sad affective states induced by classical music. *Human Brain Mapping, 28,* 1150–1162.

Nakahara, H., Furuya, S., Obata, S., Masuko, T., & Kinoshita, H. (2009). Emotion related changes in heart rate and its variability during performance and perception of music. *Annals of the New York Academy of Sciences, 1169,* 359–362.

Okada, K., Kurita, A., Takase, B., Otsuka, T., Kodani, E., Kusama, Y., ... & Mizuno, K. (2009). Effects of music therapy on autonomic nervous system activity, incidence of heart failure events, and plasma cytokine and catecholamine levels in elderly patients with cerebrovascular disease and dementia. *International Heart Journal, 50,* 95–110.

Pena, M., Maki, A., Kovacic, D., Dehaene-Lambertz, G., Koizumi, H., Bouquet, F., & Mehler, J. (2003). Sounds and silence: An optical topography study of language recognition at birth. *Proceedings of the National Academy of Sciences, 100*(20), 11702–11706.

Peng, S. M., Koo, M., & Yu, Z. R. (2009). Effects of music and essential oil inhalation on cardiac autonomic balance in healthy individuals. *Journal of Alternative and Complementary Medicine, 15*(1), 53–57.

Porges, S. W. (2009). The polyvagal theory: New insights into adaptive reactions of the autonomic nervous system. *Cleveland Clinic Journal of Medicine, 76*(2), S86–S90.

Porges, S. W. (2011). *The polyvagal theory: Neurophysiological foundations of emotions, attachment, communication, self regulation.* New York: W.W. Norton and Company.

Porges, S. W., & Furman, S. A. (2011). The early development of the autonomic nervous system provides a neural platform for social behavior: A polyvagal perspective. *Infant and Child Development, 20*(1), 106–118.

Rein G., Atkinson M., & McCraty R. (1995). The physiological and psychological effects of compassion and anger. *Journal for the Advancement of Medicine, 8*(2), 7–105.

Ross, D., Choi, J., & Purves, D. (2007). Musical intervals in speech. *Proceedings of the National Academy of Sciences, 104*(23), 9852–9857.

Scherer, K. R. (1986). Vocal affect expression: A review and a model for future research. *Psychological Bulletin, 99*(2), 143–165.

Sokhadze, E. M. (2007). Effects of music on the recovery of autonomic and electrocortical activity after stress induced by aversive stimuli. *Applied Psychophysiology and Biofeedback, 32,* 31–50.

Sollier, P. (2005). *Listening for wellness: An introduction to the Tomatis method.* Walnut Creek, CA: The Mozart Center Press.

Stanley, R. (2006). Relationship of physiologic coherence to Gregorian chant, classical, and reiki music. *Abstract: Mayo Clinic End of Life Conference,* November 2006, Rochester, MN.

Thayer, J. F., Hansen, A. L., Saus-Rose, E., & Johnson, B. H. (2009). Heart rate variability, prefrontal neural function, and cognitive performance: The neurovisceral integration perspective on self-regulation, adaptation, and health. *Annals of Behavioral Medicine, 37,* 141–153.

Thomson, W. (2006). Pitch frames as melodic archetypes. *Empirical Musicology Review, 1*(2), 85–102.

Tomatis, A. A. (2005). *The ear and the voice.* (R. Prada and P. Sollier, Trans.). Lanham, MA: Scarecrow Press.

Trainor, L. J., & Trehub, S. E. (1992). A comparison of infants' and adults' sensitivity to Western musical structure. *Journal of Experimental Psychology: Human Perception and Performance, 18,* 394–402.

Trappe, H. (2010). The effects of music on the cardiovascular system and cardiovascular health. *Heart, 96,* 1868–1871.

Tsai, C., Wang, L., Wang, S., Shau, Y., Hsiao, T., & Auhagen, W. (2010). Aggressiveness of the growl-like timbre: Acoustic characteristics, musical implications, and biomechanical mechanisms. *Music Perception, 27*(3), 209–221.

Umemura, M., & Honda, K. (1998). Influence of music on heart rate variability and comfort: A consideration through comparison of music and noise. *Journal of Human Ergology, 27,* 30–38.

Urakawa, K., & Yokoyama, K. (2005). Music can enhance exercise-induced sympathetic dominancy assessed by heart rate variability. *Tohoku Journal of Experimental Medicine, 206,* 213–218.

Vervoort, J., de Voigt, M., & Van den Bergh, W. (2007). The improvement of severe psychomotor and neurological dysfunctions treated with the Tomatis audio-psycho- phonology method measured with EEG brain map and auditory evoked potentials. *Journal of Neurotherapy, 11*(4), 37–49.

White, J. M. (1999). Effects of relaxing music on cardiac autonomic balance and anxiety after acute myocardial infarction. *American Journal of Critical Care, 8*(4), 220–230.

Winborn, M. D. (2011). *Deep blues: Human soundscapes for the archetypal journey.* Carmel, CA: Fisher King Press.

Winkler, I., Kushnerenko, E., Horvath, J., Ceponiene, R., Fellman, V., Huotilainen, M., & Sussman, E. (2003). Newborn infants can organize the auditory world. *Proceedings of the National Academy of Sciences, 100*(20), 11812–11815.

Yanagihashi, R., Ohira, M., Kimura, T., & Fujiwara, T. (1997). Physiological and psychological assessment of sound. *International Journal of Biometeorology, 40,* 157–161.

Zentner, M. R., & Kagan, J. (1996). Perception of music by infants. *Nature, 383,* 29.

CHAPTER   6

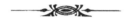

YOGA AND CHRONIC ILLNESS

Amy Holte and Paul J. Mills

Yoga is no longer a fringe, odd specter in American society, but rather so much a part of mainstream culture today that major medical centers around the country, local healthcare centers, and neighborhood Yoga centers offer Yoga as a mind–body practice to support health and healing. Although Yoga has existed in various forms for around 2,500 years, the phenomenon of Yoga for health and healing is a modern characteristic of Yoga (Alter, 2005; De Michelis, 2008; Singleton, 2008 2010). While Yoga has always offered the promise of freedom from suffering (Miller, 1995; Feuerstein, 1998), only recently has Yoga literature addressed medically defined chronic illness. We see today a field of "yoga therapeutics" in which yogic practices are pre-scribed to "heal," and sometimes "cure," specific chronic disease conditions (Swami Satyananda, 1997; Iyengar, 1979, 2001. As a health practice, it is both reflective of and a catalyst for a growing body of scientific research on Yoga that suggests a valid evidence-base for the beneficial effects of Yoga on a wide range of chronic health problems (Khalsa, 2004), including cardiovascular disease (Raub, 2002), cancer (Bower et al., 2005), diabetes (Upadhyay et al., 2008), arthritis (Haaz& Bartlett, 2011), asthma (Vempati et al., 2009), depression (Pilkington et al., 2005), and anxiety (Kirkwood et al., 2005). But scientific research on its health effects occurs against the sociocultural backdrop of Yoga schools promoting Yoga as a healing pathway in which healing is conceived of as "a holistic tool that teaches [one] how to live a better life and cope with difficulties" (De Michelis, 2008, p. 25). These two intricately interrelated contexts both shape ways in which Yoga today represents and responds to chronic illness. We examine this modern phenomenon of Yoga for its healing potential as it intersects with chronic illness, with particular consideration of the historically spiritual purpose of the Yoga traditions.

A major impetus in the acceptance of Yoga in the modern world of health-care has been a growing scientific understanding of the role of the mind in health and disease. However, while a consensus on the facticity of the mind–body connection is evident, there continues to be debate about how to theorize mind–body interrelations because the theoretical grounds on which our knowledge of cognition and the mind is based are rapidly shift-ing. A primary challenge is that theories of embodied cognition must explain interconnections between mental and physiological processes in ways that avoid reductionism (see Varela et al., 1991). In the midst of this changing paradigmatic, landscape it is no longer meaningful to conceptualize and treat chronic illness in the limited terms of the pure physicality of the body.

We analyze ways in which theories of embodied cognition might clar-ify what De Michelis (2008) calls "syncretic" theorizations in yogic milieus today, by drawing out relational and nondual realities and meanings of prac-tice that are relevant for well-being. This perspective could potentially inform our understanding of the phenomenon of alleviation of suffering through yogic practice, and specifically Yoga's process of placing attention to a spiri-tual object or reality. While different streams of yoga offer differing accounts of human nature, there is widespread agreement throughout various yoga traditions that the mind is embodied (Feuerstein, 1998). As an alternative to information processing models of mind, or theories that separate cogni-tion from physicality, embodied theories of cognition attempt to reconcile the dualism that plagues psychology and cognitive science by locating cog-nitive processes in the body, and in the body's greater physical and cultural environment (Lakoff & Johnson, 1999; Varela et al., 1991; Wilson, 2002). An embodied approach to healing, shaped by yogic knowledge, offers poten-tial for understanding chronic illness and Yoga's spiritual path for responding to it, and offers promising explanatory and predictive possibilities in both sci-entific and contemplative fields, especially on the grounds where they meet (see Varela et al., 1991; Goldberg, 2005).

While scientific studies investigate the mechanisms and health outcomes of the practice of Yoga in chronically ill populations, we analyze the meanings of health, illness, and healing in contemporary Yoga with a specific focus on how Yoga represents and responds to chronic illness. We raise specific ques-tions about the meeting between Yoga and chronic illness, and about the spiritual dimensions of Yoga's influence on health: How does Yoga's spiritual purpose translate into a valuable health practice? What kind of spirituality operates in Yoga therapeutics as a healing force? What is the role of expec-tation in curing or healing chronic illness? Why does Yoga appeal to people who are suffering from physical and mental maladies? Is there something about the spiritual purpose of Yoga that speaks to people's suffering in a way that standardized allopathic medical treatments do not? Our methodolog-ical approach engages these questions through a textual analysis of selected Yoga literatures, current popular literature on Yoga therapeutics, and relevant scholarly and scientific publications on Yoga, stress, and chronic illness. From this analysis, we suggest that modern Yoga depicts chronic illness not only as a condition of physical disease, but also as a state of suffering that can be relieved through Yoga's spiritual path as a "science of right living."

YOGA AS A SPIRITUAL PATHWAY FOR ENDING SUFFERING

Modern Yoga (Alter, 2004; De Michelis, 2004) or postural modern Yoga (Singleton, 2010) often draws on the *Yoga-Sutras* (YS) of Patanjali, widely considered to be the primary text of classical Yoga, for authority and authenticity (Singleton, 2008). While it is not our purpose to comment on the veracity of claims by modern authorizers of Yoga who maintain that modern methods are rooted in classical teachings, this linkage between today's living praxis and a classical historical text requires examination. The YS represents a major pillar of the Dharmic traditions and plays an important role in shaping the theoretical land-scape of modern Yoga as a significant religio-philosophical influence (De Michelis, 2008). In addition, classical Yoga elaborates a psychological system of the nature of suffering and pathways for alleviating suffer-ing, and this psychological process presumably operates within the body- and breath-based methodologies unique to contemporary Yoga practice (De Michelis, 2004; Alter, 2004; Singleton, 2010), as an essential means of transforming chronic illness. Therefore, we analyze the psychological aspects of suffering and its alleviation found in the YS as they relate to the body and disease conditions in order to illuminate the multidimensionality of Yoga within the context of medicine. Note that our focus on the YS is not meant to suggest that other streams of Yoga are not visible in Yoga today. Tantric and Vedantic conceptions and methods of devotional practice also remain influ-ential, for example, as do the karma (action) Yoga teachings of the Gita and even Buddhist Yoga (De Michelis, 2004; Strauss, 2005; Stern, 2006). These various approaches to Yoga each bring a different emphasis in terms of texts, theory, and methods of practice (Feuerstein, 1998). However, it is beyond the scope of this project to analyze the specific influences of each type and stream on Yoga therapeutics. Instead, we focus on the YS to draw out aspects of Patanjali's Yoga psychology of suffering and its liberation that appear to remain as elements in today's discourse of healing in Yoga therapeutics and influence how Yoga depicts itself as a pathway for healing chronic illness.

YOGA'S COGNITIVE-MOTIVATIONAL FRAMEWORK OF SUFFERING AND LIBERATION

According to classical Yoga, the most basic cause of suffering is living in spiritual ignorance (*avidya*) (YS 2.4), constituted in a distorted orientation toward self and reality, through a fundamental misidentification with the mind and one's materiality (YS 2.24). In this view, suffering is intimately tied to the Samkhya-Yoga (see Larson, 1979) theory of reality and its two principles of *purusa* (consciousness or spirit) (YS 2.18) and *prakrti* (matter, nature, or psychophysical being, which includes mind) (YS 2.19) (Whicher,

1998). *Avidya* occurs when a person identifies with *prakrti* to the exclusion of *purusa* (YS 2.4–2.5; 2.17; 2.24). From this unaware state an egoic sense of self (*asmita*) arises, in which one perceives the world through self-reference (YS 2.5–2.6; 4.4). When operating out of egotism, a person is motivated to seek pleasure because of basic attachment (*raga*) (YS 2.7) and an emotional temperament ruled by desire, and to avoid pain because of an aversion (*dvesa*) (YS 2.8) to unpleasantness, dissatisfaction, and pain, all enacted through a clinging and grasping to life (*abhinivesa*) (YS 2.9). These motivational forces are the basic causes of affliction (*kleshas*) (YS 2.3), and lead to further suffering. Moreover, suffering is endemic to the human experience because *kleshas* color the mental processes, thus making mental life largely painful (*aklista vrtti*) (YS 1.5). Yoga also suggests that past actions affect present suffering, since it presumes that the mind retains *samskaras* (impressions left by past actions) as residue of *karma* (actions) (YS 1.18; 1.50; 2.12–2.15; 4.7–4.9).

In classical Yoga, the primary motivation of Yoga practice is to overcome suffering (YS 2.2; 2.16). Actualizing this goal requires a shift in the cognitive-motivational orientation of normal waking life described above. This shift occurs through the attainment of spiritual knowledge (YS 1.3; 1.16–1.23; 1.49). YS 1.2 defines the core meaning of Yoga as a quieting of the mental fluctuations (*cittavrttinirodha*); thus, overcoming suffering requires quieting of the mind, or cessation of the afflicted mental processes (false identifications) that are associated with the samskaric mind. The samskaric mind is the accumulation of reactions and impressions from all past actions that color present moment perception and propel action. The mental quieting illuminates the cognitive realities of the samskaric self and the true self (YS 4.25). A deep understanding of the yogic path of liberation from suffering depends on one's view of self and reality, and one's relationship to reality.

Yoga's process of liberation, often described in terms of "purification" or "cleansing" of the mind, emphasizes the cognitive-motivational shifts that occur as liberation proceeds, and the shifting relational reality that occurs as self-reference changes (Mishra, 1963). In this process, mind becomes unbound by the worldly forces (*gunas*) as attention is directed inward; the self becomes liberated or free from attachments and ego boundedness. Methods of liberation mentioned in the YS include *kriya* (cleansing), *ishvara-pranidhana* (devotion), *karma* (action), and *ashtangayoga* (eight-limbed yoga).

Ultimately, practice is rooted not in striving for some goal but in attaining awareness through observation and perception. Awareness changes the relationship with pain, body, feelings, and thoughts, through a process of detachment. Awareness and detachment are freeing because they bring about a cessation of the misidentification with the material reality of body and mind, and result in a shift in one's sense of self. Spirituality is thus direct knowledge of an inner life free from egoic, samskaric, and kleshic bonds, and becomes the basis of a person's cognitive-motivational framework for acting and being in the world. The spirituality of classical Yoga is the realization of oneself as consciousness rather than solely one's psychophysical being.

Science, Yoga, and Potentials for Healing

A distinct shift has occurred in the discourse and culture of Yoga as India and the West have co-mingled in modernity. The Western intellectual streams of rationalism, positivism, and empiricism have influenced how modern authorizers of Yoga describe Yoga's purposes, purport its methods, and even interpret classical texts. Scholarship from the humanities suggests that it is out of this transnational transformation that modern Yoga has integrated the concept of healing into its discourse on suffering by tying the spirituality of Yoga to science (Alter, 2004; De Michelis, 2004; Harrington, 2008) and by situating and modifying practice within the global health context of physical culture (Singleton, 2010). This modern movement broadens and deepens the implications for the impact of Yoga in society by theoretically relocating the locus of one's spiritual reality and asserting claims about Yoga's effect on the body as well as the mind, and, consequently, its effect on health and chronic illness.

De Michelis (2004) has proposed that this modern discourse pivots on Swami Vivekananda 's (1977) interpretation of Patanjali's YS, because it was the first Yoga text to link Yoga with science, and specifically the science of healing. While Vivekananda focused on meditation, he also focused on the *prana* model of Yoga—with the concept of *prana* translated as breath, life force, or more "scientifically" as bioforce—in a way that gave new weight to the practice of *pranayama* (breath control), and therefore to the physicality of the body and its role in the spiritual purpose of Yoga (De Michelis). The idea of *prana* as a balanced or imbalanced bioforce is central to understanding health and disease from the perspective of Yoga therapeutics. This embodiment of traditionally metaphysical concepts and the secularization of Yoga's path of liberation through realization (what is now thought of as "healing," as what is being "realized" has changed over time and culture) have contributed to the rise of Yoga's use in the management of chronic illness.

A central consideration in understanding the use of Yoga to manage chronic illness is the way in which translated ideas of yogic power (such as seeing the cosmic reality of "*prana*" in physical terms of breath) problematically link metaphysics and biology. Alter (2004) focused on the work of Swami Kuvalayananda to illustrate how using science to anchor the worldview of Yoga can conflate the truths of each and thus alter the integrity of both, while simultaneously advancing the reach and utility of Yoga globally. Because the scientific method requires reliably seeing effects in the body's physicality, Swami Kuvalayananda's discussion of the scientific effects of Yoga on various medical conditions engaged analogies between the differing worldviews of Yoga and science, and involved extensive arguments presenting convergences between the two systems. However, Alter suggested that because the two systems have vastly different metaphysical understandings about human nature and reality, interpreting Yoga from the worldview of science resulted in confused translations of Yogic concepts. Specifically, this approach problematically casts the body in purely physicalistic terms in which the healing potential of Yoga is found in its apparent effect of curing physical disease.

However, the medicalization of Yoga's healing nature sets up false expectations about the therapeutic potential of Yoga, because it misplaces the value of Yoga. "Healing" is often understood as physicalistic transformation—healing signifies that the body (or mind) becomes well. Rather than seeing Yoga in terms of its potential to "cure" physical ailment, however, Yoga's healing potential should instead be viewed as experientially meaningful acts that are transformative, and thus therapeutic, through their facilitation of a perceptual shift in self-understanding. It is this esotericized view of healing (De Michelis, 2004) that potentiates Yoga's liberation as healing, where the value comes from a practitioner's direct knowledge and awareness.

It is important to recognize that this view comes close to ascribing the liberative process to the translated secularized notion of "self-realization," an approach that "ambiguously reflects many of the patterns of Yoga's textual— and 'spiritual'—popularization and medicalization as both have developed over the past seventy-five years" (Alter, 2004, p. xiii). This ambiguity arises from interpretations of contemporary Yoga literature regarding *asana* and the physical body, and modern concerns about health that link these notions with classical understandings and Patanjali's Yoga to support the theory that liberation is healing. These interpretations mistakenly attribute the notion of healing to classical Yoga; however, healing is a modern notion in the Yoga context not traceable to classical writings (Alter, 2004; De Michelis, 2004). Yet analyzing the YS's spiritual approach to suffering in terms of "therapeutics" (Fields, 2001) may still offer a useful heuristic or interpretative framework without making this erroneous assertion.

Physical ailment (YS 1.30), and unsteadiness of the body, irregular breathing, and depression (YS 1.31), are all explicitly referenced within the YS, with the implication that these conditions can be overcome through Yoga. Our assertion that overcoming these conditions is "healing," and thus that Yoga is therapeutic, considers the function of these conditions (as obstacles and distractions to liberation) in light of current theoretical propositions about the body and cognition, especially in the secularized culture of medicine today. Therefore, while we agree with the basic theory of liberation as healing, we offer instead an interpretation that considers the ongoing agency of the body as an embodied consciousness as the cause of yoga's *healing* potential.

Legitimately bringing Yoga and chronic illness together requires a careful consideration of terminology, and rethinking ways in which meanings from different Yoga traditions are linked together in theory and practice today. This approach aims toward a more solid theoretical ground for the therapeutic "healing" potential of Yoga that clarifies previously confused philosophical and biological notions without drawing its authority from the historical (religious) tradition of Yoga. We suggest that interpreting Yoga's liberation as spiritual healing from an embodied cognition perspective functions to ground yogic praxis in an emerging perspective on the mind that is theoretically syncretic. This perspective offers medicine a way of tempering the focus on physical cure by broadening the concept of suffering, and by shifting approaches toward its alleviation.

Healing Chronic Illness through Embodied Spiritual Practice

Whereas pre-modern Yoga was recognized as a meditative path of spiritual liberation, Yoga today is widely undertaken as a postural practice (Singleton, 2010) valued for its health benefits (Alter, 2004). Out of the global transformation of modern Yoga, a proliferation of Yoga practice manuals have promised health (since the 1950s) and offered explicit instructions for using Yoga to manage chronic health conditions (within the past two decades). Yoga schools promoting this health emphasis endorse the widespread practice of *asana* (translated as posture, or comfortable posture) and *pranayama* (breath control), and to a lesser extent, meditation, as therapeutic or healing pathways. Amongst Yoga authorizers in the twentieth century, the practice and teaching lineages of Krisnamacharya (1888–1989) and Swami Sivananda (1887–1963) in particular have centrally shaped the world of Yoga therapeutics and its embodied approach to Yoga (De Michelis, 2004; Strauss, 2005; Stern, 2006; Singleton, 2010) (see Appendix A for annotated list of important books and articles in the field of yoga therapeutics).

Recently, however, there have been some reversals of this secularized and medicalized trend toward seeing Yoga in physicalistic terms. Donna Farhi (2000) and others have called for Yoga teachers and students to "reclaim" the "spiritual message" (p. xvi) of Yoga that has been lost over the past several decades in the effort to popularize Yoga. Newcomb (2005) suggests that this spiritual exploration of Yoga is fairly widespread in the secularized religiosity of Yoga amongst practitioners, even amongst the most postural types of yoga such as the Iyengar school. Thus a central tension evident in modern Yoga involves the expression of the health or spiritual dimensions of Yoga, or how to integrate the two, and is variously expressed in the teaching of the body- and breath-centered innovations. We draw from the genre of contemporary writings on Yoga therapeutics to glean how modern Yoga represents and responds to chronic illness, and place its themes and meanings within the context of embodied theories of cognition as a scholarly frame of reference for understanding Yoga's potential for alleviating the suffering of chronic disease.

Chronic Illness as Relational Stress and Emotional Reactivity

Passages gathered from modern therapeutic Yoga texts suggest that emotional reactivity and stress are "primary" factors in chronic disease (Shankardevananda, 2002), and tie emotion and stress to the body. For example, Iyengar (2001, p. 160) writes, "emotional tension and muscular tension are closely related," and "turbulent emotions and physical ailments are directly connected." Furthermore, he suggests that "according to yogic science, the health of the psyche is reflected in, and partly created by, the health of the body. Affliction and sorrow are often physiologically manifested as physical pain. Psychological pressures bring stress to bear on the anatomical body, the bodily organs, and on the nervous system." Shankardevananda (2002, p. 21) echoed this view, proposing that, "every thought and emotion we have, in some way affects the body."

Modern yogic literature catalogs a range of the ways in which stress affects the body and creates conditions for disease to manifest. These all center on the effects of stress as it is processed through the nervous system and on the connection of the nervous system with the body. Most immediately, stress manifests as muscular-skeletal tension in the body's muscles, joints, etc., as "[mind-complexes] can cause great bodily changes and muscular tension" (Shankardevananda, 2002, p. 21). When people remain unaware of their emotional life, "stress will manifest itself physically and emotionally through contracted body muscles, tense facial expressions, and undesirable behavioral patterns," and stress may be felt in "stiff muscles and joints, atrophying of skeletal bones, slowing down of body systems, or sluggishness in the vital organs" (Iyengar, 2001, p. 160).

These texts suggest that chronic stress creates habits in the body that result in imbalance in bodily systems, thereby affecting their functioning. For example, stress is related to the chronic illness of asthma, in that "muscle fibers in bronchial passages constrict for several reasons, including via autonomic nervous system stimulated by tension and other stresses" (Shankardevananda, 2002, p. 12). Devi (2000) explained that "physical and mental stress accumulate" (p. 1) and that "to avoid feeling pain, our emotional hearts contract" (p. 15). She went on to suggest that "anger, hatred, and fear can be the underlying causes of many of our modern-day chronic diseases [and that] if the emotional component is not positive, it must be dealt with in ways appropriate to expression, not repression," and that "sometimes when the negative becomes in control you may rid yourself of one disease yet cause another" (p. 56). These illustrations suggest that Yoga therapeutics interprets the suffering of chronic illness in terms of stress habits. These stress habits affect the balance of the body's systems by creating tension, constriction, and contraction in any number of organs, tissues, and overall processes, the accumulation of which results in chronic disturbances.

The observation that Yoga therapeutics conceptualizes chronic illness in terms of reactions to stress may not be surprising, since stress has become of major scientific interest over the past several decades, especially as a factor in health (Antonovsky, 1979; Helman, 2000). Also, it seems inevitable that the "de-stressing" discourse of science would become a central theme in Yoga therapeutics because a characteristic feature of modern Yoga is the incorporation of the discourse of science into its own narrative (De Michelis, 2004). What is not necessarily clear, though, is the impact this narrative has made in the field of healthcare. In what ways, if at all, does (or should) the modern narrative of Yoga as therapeutic counterbalance the dominant paradigms of science and medicine in shaping today's cultural and secular norms specifically regarding conceptions of the body's relationship to suffering?

While Selye (1982) first conceptualized stress in human physiology in purely physical terms—that is, as a temporary physiological state of an organism's bodily reactions in stress-inducing circumstances—others have focused on the role of cognition in perceptual processes associated with physiological stress reactions (Lazarus & Folkman, 1984; Lazarus, 1999). Specifically, current views of stress use both of these conceptualizations of stress to frame it in terms of appraisal processes that are situationally activated in the person's mind and have neurobiological correlates. Because a basic relationality underlies appraisal, relational appraisal may be a better way of theorizing mind–body interrelations. Yoga therapeutics also represents chronic illness at a deeper level in terms of the causes of stress. The texts suggest three primary causes of stress: an individual's thoughts, modern culture, and spiritual disconnection. As Yoga therapeutics suggests that these three underlying causes of stress play a fundamental role in the suffering and healing in chronic illness, it becomes critically important to consider the way in which these three factors interrelate and affect embodied cognition (in which both the physicality of the body and lived experience constitute conditions of health and disease). It may be useful to consider both scientific and yogic conceptions of cognition, especially as cognition relates to the body, one's environment, and one's consciousness, in order to better understand these interrelationships.

A dominant theme in Yoga suggests that a person's own thoughts are a primary cause of stress: "As you think, so shall you become" is a popular saying among Yoga enthusiasts. Both Yoga therapeutics (as implied above) and health psychology suggest that thoughts may be alternatively stress-inducing or healing. For example, Lazarus (1984, 1999) suggested that the way that we appraise situations and think about them causes the experience of stress. Kendall-Tackett (2010) explained that negative emotions such as depression, anxiety, hostility, anger, shame, pessimism, and hopelessness (what Lazarus [1999] called the "stress emotions") negatively affect health by inducing the production of pro-inflammatory cytokines, which play a role in such chronic diseases as heart disease, cancer, and diabetes.

The scientific study of the role of the mind in stress and chronic illness is examined through the interdisciplinary field of psychoneuroimmunology (PNI). PNI investigates ways in which stress, especially psychological stress, triggers an inflammatory response in the body that may cause the deleterious long-term effects on the immune system that result in chronic illness (Malarkey & Mills, 2007; Kendall-Tackett, 2010). Harrington (2008) suggested that the "cure within" discourse of the role of the mind in health and disease has become assimilated into our cultural history as stories that become embodied and take on life and meaning in various ways. In fact, the discourse of the intimate connection between mind and body in health has become so much a part of the culture of yogic healing that the concept and term "psychoneuroimmunology" appear in modern Yoga literature. For example, Kraftsow expressed the basic premise of PNI that, "the link between conscious mind and unconscious body responses work in both directions: thought-emotion-body" and weaved into his Yoga writings the scientific view that "psychoneuroimmunology research points to a strong link state of mind (including habits of thought and emotional response) and physical health." Similarly, Shankardevananda (2002, p. 4–5) identified a shared perspective between the two paradigms of Yoga and science that, "the science of psychoneuroimmunology agrees with the yogic view that the mind is a more important cause of allergic diseases."

Modern Yoga literature also identifies modern culture as an overarching cause of stress, and emphasizes that how each individual perceives his or her environment determines whether that individual experiences stress. For example, Iyengar (1979, p vii) stated that "the strain of modern life can lead to physical pain and illness, as our bodies' well being is neglected in the race for material success. The stress of modern life can also lead to mental suffering like feelings of inadequacy, isolation, or powerlessness." He elaborated by suggesting that individuals' responses to cultural and environmental pressures generate (or does not) the experience of stress. By focusing on the way that people respond to these cultural and environmental problems, Iyengar illustrated how it is really the functioning of the individual's cognitive system, as it relates to the cultural, social, and physical environment, that affects one's state of suffering.

Theories of embodied mind from cognitive science also situate the mind in environment and culture. Lakoff and Johnson (1999) suggested that cognition is based in the body, by way of the sensorimotor system shaping the conceptual inferences that we make. Thus, the body and its movement in the immediate environment is the primary agent in forming how individuals think and reason about themselves and the world. Interpretive inferences are made from individual observations. The person and environment interact, and the person appraises what the situation signifies for personal well-being. But appraisals are not constituted wholly within the person and the person's reaction to situations. In Lazarus' (1999) person-in-environment view of psychological stress, appraisal is an evaluative process that occurs in the mind, in which relational meaning is constructed between goals and beliefs. Thus, the experience of stress occurs when an individual appraises a situation or environmental context as unable to support his or her goals, or as in conflict with beliefs about self or the world. From this perspective, stress can be interpreted as a kind of embodied suffering that is caused by the body's perceptual reaction to environmental pressures.

A less emphasized but discernible theme in Yoga therapeutic literature is that perception hinges on an individual's present-moment lived awareness of his or her spiritual goal or purpose (or lack thereof). Thus, spiritual disconnect is recognized as a fundamental cause of the stress that may underlie chronic illness. Using the example of chronic back pain, Devi (2000) suggested that while some may see a back pain as a simple back pain, this view is not correct, since even this seemingly simple kind of chronic condition is composed not only more broadly in term of "how we use or abuse the muscles, how we think, feel, eat, sleep, and rest," but also in terms of whether we "acknowledge the essence of who we are" (p. 5).

This discussion of the causes of stress is important because how individuals conceptualize psychological stress helps determine which scenario—health or disease—occurs in different bodies, and under what circumstances. Also important to the course stress takes in a person's life is the way in which an individual deals with stress and its effects. Understanding Yoga therapeutics' account of the causes of stress may help clarify the theoretical grounding of Yoga's embodied response to suffering, with particular consideration given to the idea embedded within the modern yogic notion of healing that managing both the causes and the symptoms of stress and emotional reactivity is what constitutes true healing. What follows is a discussion of how yogic processes may "de-stress" a person (i.e. undo the perceptual experience of stress, including relieving physically felt tensions, to the extent that stressful experience has negative consequences for the body and health) and the negative effects of previously experienced stress (in terms of undoing the damaging effects in the body and habits of mind).

Yoga as a Whole System for Healing Chronic Illness

Our analysis of contemporary writings on Yoga therapeutics suggests that Yoga's response to chronic illness involves practicing Yoga in ways that "balance" the person's "whole system," including the body, by cultivating awareness through various yogic methods. Which methods are to be employed depends on the specific chronic condition and characteristics of the individual person, but almost all texts emphasize postural movements and breathwork. Based on observations of how Yoga is "performed" today (Strauss, 2005; Singleton, 2010), it would be tempting to conclude that Yoga is solely about the physicality of the body. A purely physical perspective on health and disease necessitates medical treatment for cure of physical illness. However, many modern Yoga texts suggest that the therapeutic value of Yoga is not just physical, but mental, emotional, and spiritual, as well. From this perspective, we posit that the body is a locus of experience, experience that may be felt not only as physical sensation, but also as mental, emotional, and spiritual experiences, often simultaneously. Thus modern Yoga responds to chronic illness through postural and other yogic practices that operate on these interrelated dimensions of the human experience, through an embodied reality of self and being, Yoga therapeutics effects a remediation of stress and its causes through this multidimensional approach. As Perrson (2010) suggested, this response implicitly recognizes the coextensive phenomenological nature of interrelationship between embodied beings and the world.

In order to understand Yoga's impact on chronic illness, it is important to consider the ways in which Yoga therapeutics' interpretation of embodiment ties the body to both spirituality and healing. Our analysis suggests that body-based methods of Yoga can be understood as healing because they bring a lived spirituality into the body. This embodied spirituality occurs by practicing with (spiritual) awareness of the moment-to-moment experience of self, including body sensations, emotions, thoughts, sounds, etc. In this view, stress and related chronic illness is "healed" by reconnecting with spiritual self or center, and by reconnecting consciousness and awareness with embodied, transformed cognition. This experientially felt spiritual reconnection re-establishes an embodied equilibrium, and sometimes results in *curing* the associated physical disease. Thus, while Yoga's response to suffering has traditionally been a spiritual process, today's Yoga advocates physical practices as a way of experiencing an embodied spirituality.

Yoga, however, is more than a set of physical practices and postures. A healthy diet, ethical conduct, and service to humanity must accompany physical postural practice, and pranayama and meditation, as components of a whole system "treatment" program for specific chronic illnesses. Devi (2000) organized her chapters around these central concepts, noting, for example, that the modern diet of rich foods, high in meats and dairy products, may be linked with many chronic illnesses. Numerous texts recommend a vegetarian diet for those practicing yoga (Karmananda, 1983; Satyananda, 1997; Desikachar, 1998; Shankardevananda, 2002). Devi (2000) also emphasized how practicing the Yogic ethics of service and consideration of habits in relating to others may facilitate liberation from suffering.

Yoga's response to chronic illness brings spirituality into the body through a whole system of lifestyle transformation that links cognitive process with physical action, and associates both with the concept of "liberation from affliction" found in the YS. This linkage of spirituality to embodiment brings into focus the non-conceptual potentialities of cognition and perception. As in classical Yoga, modern therapeutic yogic texts suggest that the focus of one's attention is the key factor in the spiritual path of healing. Turning attention inwards to perceive direct experience, rather than toward some transcendent reality, has become the fundamental process of therapeutic Yoga, and this process is regarded as central to healing. Healing is dependent on the cultivation of awareness and the ability to perceive internal states—direct experience of the mind and the body. This awareness is believed to "foster awareness of emotions [and stress reactions] as they arise" (Karmananda, 1983, p. 63), which enables greater conscious control over actions, and empowers sufferers to rethink and alter harmful and unhealthy habits. Shankardevananda (2002) described awareness at "the simplest level as bare attention, the noting of events without attachment or aversion," and that success is attained when "one ceases to be 'the sufferer' and becomes 'the observer', noting bodily changes, mental states, and feelings, *without identifying with them*" (p. 42; emphasis added). Rather than being a fixed characteristic, "awareness is a skill . . . [that] must be developed" (Shankardevananda, p. 42). Karmananda (1983) explained that without developing this ability, "most of the potential of Yoga is lost" (p. 45). Explaining the healing power of awareness, McCall (2007) wrote that "students of therapeutic yoga are taught to tune in to subtle sensations of their muscles and joints, as well as the inner experience of the minds" (p. 19), and suggested that "the more we can turn our awareness inward, turn the senses internally, the more they are replenished and rejuvenated. The internalization of attention is also the bridge to the healing power of yoga" (p. 57). This cognitive-motivational framework, found in Yoga's therapeutic literature, helps explain how Yoga is valued today as a way to relieve the suffering associated with chronic illness, both physically and spiritually, and explain, in part, how Yoga has found its way into the culture of modern medicine.

Awareness may be cultivated through any number of yogic practices. In classical Yoga, the predominant methods of amplifying awareness were meditative and meditation remains a primary method of relieving suffering in Yoga today. But the same approach of inner awareness is also recommended in modern Yoga therapeutics as a way of undertaking postural practice. Perhaps the most recognized form of this mode of practice is the "mind–body" methodology of intentionally and physically moving the body with awareness of breath, in order to reestablish the body's homeostasis set point. Because the postural practice of Yoga so widely popular today is a recent innovation of methodological approach to Yoga, and because of its use in Yoga therapeutics for managing chronic illness, it is important to understand how modern authorizers of Yoga (especially those who emphasize posture in their practice) view the role of *asanas* and *pranayama* in the healing process.

The practice of *asana* corrects defects of posture and body system imbalances, but must be practiced through the focus on body awareness in order to produce the greatest effects (Satyananda, 1997). Readjustment of the physical body occurs through stimulation of the body's own regenerative processes. But *asana* also creates energy in the body. The concept of bioenergy is referenced regularly in various texts; regulating this "force" is believed to adjust organ function through the regulation of nervous impulses and blood flow, elimination of bodily disease and imbalance, and generation of "an enormous amount of energy" (Iyengar, 2002, p. 155).

A number of texts also suggest that an individual's *approach* to form, rather than focus on the form of the *asana* itself, brings awareness into the body. Inquiry, or personal reflection, into one's own physical, emotional, and psychological comfort and awareness promotes attention to the body as a whole, interconnected with mind, as an essence or being-ness: "Forms become vehicles for experiencing one's essential nature rather than goals themselves" (Farhi, 2000, p. xv). This approach treats the body holistically by integrating breath and mind into *asana* to achieve maximum therapeutic benefit. Practicing reflectively facilitates the process of Yoga practitioner meeting self.

Texts also suggest that the healing effect of Yoga may lie in controlling the senses. Practice involves drawing the five senses of perception inward, rejuvenating the body by reuniting with spiritual awareness. Controlling the senses also allows mastery of ego, as ego disconnects a person from his or her emotional center. Yoga therapeutics sees "body and mind in a state of constant interaction," and "does not demarcate where the body ends and the mind begins" (Iygenar, 2001, p. 11); therefore every aspect of the body is pervaded by consciousness. *Asana* is a way to develop the internal awareness that must permeate each movement of the *asana*, with the body as the element of cognition. The infusion of consciousness into every cell of the body occurs through focusing the mind's attention completely in the body. Perceiving clearly through the body links the embodied mind with the non-conceptual process of embodied perception, and this is why the "cure" for suffering is awareness, observation, perception, and direct experience: action follows from cognitive stance. Thus, the modern method of physical Yoga generates a clarified understanding of self, by recognizing a psychosomatic dimension of living; while one is doing a physical thing, the acting and behaving can be performed consciously, with presence and awareness.

This discussion has focused on the central theme in modern Yoga writings relating to chronic illness: the promise of a cure for a wide range of disease conditions. Shankardevananda (2002) stated that, "through Yoga and the cultivation of awareness which comes from Yoga, we are able to deal with, and occasionally remove, the sources of sickness and not just the symptoms" (p. 7). In this context, cure is defined in terms of relieving the sufferer from symptoms, eliminating the physical disease, and preventing future episodes. Cure means an end to the cycle of deep mental and emotional reactions, and freedom from drugs (since drugs are most often used to treat or manage symptoms, but do not eliminate their future occurrence, or resolve the underlying condition).

In Yoga, though, cure also involves the transformation of the chronically ill person from the position of sufferer who needs to be treated, to a position as self-healer (Harrington, 2008; Shankardevananda, 1997). In this transformation process, attitude is a prime factor in the cure, since expectations of cure can create further tensions. A positive attitude, in the yogic sense, promotes viewing situations as opportunities for learning rather than as annoyances or in terms of desired outcomes. The person seeking relief of suffering must be sincere and committed to the yogic process without becoming attached to the outcome of becoming disease-free. This interpretation of cure also identifies relaxation as the starting point for curing ailments and imbalances but not the final goal, since repressed tensions, emotions, and memories may arise in a state of relaxation. Such arisings are seen as signs of progress toward the integration of spirituality into daily being.

Attitudinal shift is seen as central to alleviation from suffering and suggests that the modern yogic notion of "cure" seems more akin to the concept of "healing" suggested in New Age alternative healing literature (Helman, 2000). In this context, biomedicine cures physical disease whereas holistic medicine heals illness (De Michelis, 2004). With this distinction, cure is a resolution of the physiological imbalance(s) whereas healing has a broader meaning that encompasses the whole person (mind, body, spirit, social, etc.). An interesting concept of healing emerges from this understanding in that "healed" could mean that the person continues to live with the physiological imbalance but is no longer suffering in an existential sense.

Thus, the Yoga therapeutic approach of grounding spirituality in the body as a pathway for healing informs a broader concept of health than typically understood in medicine today. In this approach, the concept of health is not centered on an absence of disease symptoms; rather, it involves optimizing the functioning of every body system, establishing emotional well-being, and developing spiritual resilience. As Yoga depicts the individual as more than just a psychophysical being, this view of personhood provides theoretical grounds for broadening the concept of individual health "to apply to the well-being and freedom from suffering of the whole person (De Michelis, 2004, p. 7)." De Michelis suggested that it is legitimate "to speak of health with respect to this spiritual Self, and of ultimate liberation from suffering as healing on these grounds." But Alter (2010) argued that the self-healed through therapeutic Yoga should be seen as "a field of agency" (p. 311) that exists relationally; a person is continuously engaged in environmental and cultural happenings. In this sense, Yoga depicts chronic illness not only as a condition of physical disease, but also as a state of suffering that can be healed through Yoga's spiritual path. Because it focuses on the underlying causes of ailment and suffering, Yoga as a whole system interprets disease as nature's mechanism to rebalance and heal the body.

Yoga's classical purpose of sighting the soul, which evolved into the medieval hathayoga purpose of restraining the energy, has shifted to the contemporary purpose of "healing" that draws from both and integrates each into an embodied spirituality, avoiding problematic duality between inner and outer reality. Yoga therapeutic texts present a view of Yoga as more than just a treatment (in the sense of targeting a specific illness) but as a consciousness (in the sense of transforming one's personality and character while leaving the essence through modifications of lifestyle). Thus Yoga is a transformative spiritual process. Such transformations take time, and may not immediately, or ever, cure the disease condition, but provide an avenue for liberation from the kind of mind–body suffering that comes with chronic illness. Yoga can, in fact, be understood as a way to alleviate suffering wherever it exists, including cases of chronic illness.

EMERGENCE OF YOGA THERAPEUTICS WITHIN INTEGRATIVE MEDICINE

Over the past century, Yoga has transitioned from operating as an esoteric mode for "alternative healing" to aligning with counter-culture ideology as an "alternative medicine" and finally becoming a fairly ubiquitous "complement" to standard medicine (Berliner & Salmon, 1980). The numbers of people practicing Yoga today are not insignificant. A 2001 epidemiological study counting Yoga as one of 20 CAM (Complementary and Alternative Medicine) therapies, for example, found that over two-thirds of the American adult population has used some type of CAM therapy at least once in their lives (Kessler et al., 2001). Specifically regarding Yoga, a Harris Interactive Service Bureau poll conducted in 2003 found that over 7 percent of US adults (or 15 million people) practiced Yoga regularly (Lamb, 2004). Over the past decade, Yoga has become an "integrative" component of overall treatment of illness in standard medicine within even the most elite academic medical centers and teaching facilities. The Consortium of Academic Health Centers for Integrative Medicine currently has over 50 member institutions. Yoga is taught in the vast majority of these centers. According to the National Center for Complementary and Alternative Medicine (NCCAM), the 2007 National Health Interview Study found that Yoga is one of the top ten complementary health practices used among US adults.

Chronic illness affects approximately 133 million Americans—almost 45 percent of the adult US population has at least one chronic illness (Wu & Green, 2000). People who suffer from chronic illnesses may seek out the practice of Yoga with a variety of motivations. While the traditional purpose of Yoga is spiritual liberation, De Michelis (2004) and Strauss (2005) pointed out that not everyone who practices Yoga practices it for this purpose. Many practice just for stress relief that comes with the solace of practice. Others may desire alternatives to their current lifestyle in the hope that making changes could bring about a healthier body and a greater sense of well-being. Still others may hope that Yoga can potentially cure them of their suffering and diseased condition. Literature written by modern Yoga masters and a growing evidence-base of scientific research suggests that any of these outcomes could be a possible consequence of taking up yoga in earnest. These goals could be summed up by the two main expectations of spiritual liberation or health improvement, with the main difference being the underlying motivation of the Yoga practitioner. When a person desires spiritual liberation, the motivation is to experience freedom. However, a desire for improved health involves a motivation to change and heal. This desire to change the reality at hand may function as discontentment that further contributes to suffering.

Chronic diseases are generally considered on a spectrum of "curability" from both allopathic and yogic perspectives, with some diseases considered incurable (e.g. coronary heart disease). In these cases, symptom management is the goal of treatment. For diseases considered curable (e.g. primary hypertension), there may be a standard treatment regimen given to all patients. For those diseases falling somewhere in between (e.g. asthma), there is some question about whether there can be a cure or not. Which diseases are considered curable, though, differs between these two perspectives, with Yoga therapeutics suggesting a greater potential for curability through its methods.

A measure of caution is warranted, though, when Yoga therapeutics is used to achieve health. Expectations of cure may result in harmful consequences if a Yoga teacher or a health care provider promises cure of disease through Yoga. Promises of "success" set up anticipation and belief in the patient about future outcomes, expectations that could undermine the crucial yogic process of detachment from a desire for certain results. While cure of disease through yogic processes may occur, the mindset and expectations with which one commits to the Yogic path are centrally important to attaining (or not) any goals sought with its practice. Attachment to health or to a certain state of the body can produce a seed of dissatisfaction that perpetuates suffering. Additionally, the authority of the physician or provider who recommends a

Yogic course could create expectancy that results in adverse outcomes for the patient, who might think that lack of a cure is reflective of personal fault or incorrect practice. These kinds of self-critical and doubtful thoughts are themselves symptomatic of the kind of suffering that leads to psychosomatic illness. The point of Yoga is to remain detached from the outcome so that cure or complete alleviation of the disease condition is no longer the measure of suffering or well-being. A failure of Yoga to cure may also result from limitations of the Yoga teacher or therapist. Some Yoga masters may have more knowledge of what—and *how*—to teach the sick person than the average Yoga therapist or health-care provider has. Moreover, failure to cure may be a result of timing, if therapy is started too late in the disease process. Yoga does not work overnight.

Clearly, in cases where Yoga does not cure physical disease, it can still offer significant relief from suffering, in the form of liberation from the existential suffering that occurs in spiritual disconnection or lack of awareness. Yoga can provide a different way of looking at pain and suffering, which in itself can alleviate suffering. The basic realization that "I" am not my body, or my thoughts, or my sensations of pain, is in itself healing. This perspective is what might often be considered as secular spirituality. Since spirituality is still not widely accepted within medicine, this perspective raises the question of what it means for modern medicine (especially in its secular context) to attribute a spiritual cause to chronic illness, and to offer a secularized spirituality of embodied practice as a potential treatment.

We propose that those who offer Yoga in the medical setting and elsewhere as a means to treat chronic illness temper the focus on cure of physical ailment and emphasize healing from the more holistic perspective, that fosters a non-dual, perceptual relationality to self and the world. This approach would be more meaningful, useful, valuable, and potentially more effective in promoting overall health and well-being. Rather than concentrating exclusively on eliminating disease, cultivating a basic realization of selfhood—that thoughts and pain are not the fullness or wholeness of a person's identity—offers a powerful and legitimate way to contend with the health-care crisis of chronic illness today.

Additionally, consideration of the secular culture of medicine raises the question of whether there is less alleviation of suffering if the expectation is of a cure rather than spiritual liberation. As a response, Yoga therapeutics promotes liberation as a process. In addition to a realization of wholeness and dis-identification from the illness condition, liberation involves an ongoing practice of incorporating this realization into each and every waking moment. While the former approach may offer health benefits of stress relief, the latter provides additional possibilities for those who wish to take on Yoga with a spiritual purpose. Sustaining continuous awareness is additional "healing" work. The field of palliative care provides a clear example in which movement away from an emphasis on or effort to cure opens a door for patients to potentially disassociate from identification with the disease and refocus on self, and certainly promotes healing and acceptance (in the final stages of life's experience).

While a "healing" perspective and patient-centered holistic health care is an approach widely espoused within health-care institutions, its adoption remains limited. Yoga is still seen as a culturally relative and individual practice, rather than in universal (humanistic) terms. What does liberation mean in this sense? Reflecting its adaptability to each unique historical era and cultural context, the spiritual system of Yoga has been translated into a form of practice acceptable in the secular context of medicine. What if this holistic view—that "I am not my pain"—which provides relief from existential suffering, was applied within medicine beyond the context of Yoga therapeutics, to the extent that it was taught in the health sciences and available widely in hospitals? This is one vision for integrative medicine. The growing recognition that self-knowledge is an important aspect of good health across diverse cultural contexts may lead to the promotion of this kind of knowledge in health-care settings. A holistic or whole systems approach to medicine moves consideration of health beyond physical and psychological symptoms to include the spiritual dimensions of meaning, values, purpose, connectedness, and happiness, all within culturally and environmentally situated contexts that implicitly affect quality of life (Manahan, 2011). People suffering from chronic illness who engage with Yoga in these contexts may experience relief from at least some aspects of their debilitating conditions, and gain a new perspective on an embodied reality that enriches and potentially transforms their lives in a meaningful way.

APPENDIX A

Selected annotated list of important people and works from the practice and teaching lineages of Krisnamacharya (1888–1989) and Swami Sivananda (1887–1963) that have centrally shaped the world of Yoga therapeutics:

Swami Sivananda, a former physician, became a Yoga master who wrote and traveled extensively teaching on the therapeutic functions of Yoga.

Selected list of Swami Sivananda's disciples who have made significant contributions to how Yoga is practiced and understood in its therapeutic applications:

1. Swami Satyananda Saraswati (1927–2009) founded the Bihar School of Yoga

    a. *Asana Pranayama Mudra Bandha* (first published 1969), one of the most well-known systematic yoga manuals; lists indications and contraindications regarding medical conditions, along with practice instructions of each individual practice, and contains an index of recommended Yoga practices for a number of specific health conditions.
    b. *Constipation and its Cures; Health and Diet; Practice of Nature Cure; A Boon to Diabetics.*
    c. *Yogic Management of Common Diseases; Yoga and Cardiovascular Management,* co-authored with Dr. Swami Karmananda.

    d. *Asthma and Diabetes; The Effects of Yoga on Hypertension*, Dr Swami Shankardevananda.

    e. *Yogic Management of Cancer*, Dr Swami Nirmalanada.

    f. *Yoga and Management of Back Pain Booklet*.

2. Swami Satchidananda (1914–2002) founded Integral Yoga and taught both Nischela Joy Devi and Dr. Dean Ornish. Both have gone on to play major roles in bringing Yoga into healthcare settings as part of an integrative approach to chronic illness:

    a. Nischela Joy Devi (*The Healing Path of Yoga: Alleviate Stress, Open Your Heart, and Enrich Your Life; 2000*) and

    b. Dr. Dean Ornish (Ornish, D., Brown, S. F., Scherwitz, L., W., Billings, J. H., Armstrong, W. T., Ports, T. A., McLanahan, S. M., Kirkeeide, R., L., Brand, R. & Gould, K., L. (1990). Can lifestyle changes reverse coronary heart disease? The Lifestyle Heart Trial. *The Lancet*, 336(8708), 129–133. Ornish, D., Scherwitz, L. W., Billings, J. H., Gould, K. L., Merritt, T. A., Sparler, S., Armstrong, W. T., Ports, T. A., Kirkeeide, R. L., Hogeboom, C. & Brand, R. J. (1998a). Intensive Lifestyle Changes for Reversal of Coronary Heart Disease. *JAMA*, 280(23), 2001–2007. Ornish, D. (1998b). Avoiding revascularization with lifestyle changes: The Multicenter Lifestyle Demonstration Project. *American Journal of Cardiology*, 82(10B):72T–76T).

3. Swami Vishnu Devananda (1927–1993), founder of the International Sivananda Yoga Vedanta Centres and Ashrams and wrote *The Complete Illustrated Book of Yoga: A Complete Guide to the Physical Postures, Breathing Exercises, Diet, Relaxation, and Meditation Techniques of Yoga* (first published 1959), one of the most prominent early manuals on Yoga that laid important groundwork for the understanding of Yoga as both postural and therapeutic.

Krisnamacharya revolutionized Yoga by transforming its dominant culture to postural practice, though still retaining its devotional character. His students include:

1. T.K.V. Desikachar (1938–), Krishnamacharya's son and founder of the Krishnamacharya Yoga Mandiram. Author of *Health, Healing & Beyond: Yoga and the Living Tradition of Krishnamacharya*, first published in 1998. Numerous students of Desikachar are currently leaders in the field of Yoga Therapy:

    a. Yoga Therapy: A Guide to the Therapeutic Use of Yoga and Ayurveda for Health and Fitness by A. G. Mohan, Indra Mohan, Ganesh Mohan and Nitya Mohan.

    b. Yoga for Wellness: Healing with the Timeless Teachings of Viniyoga by Gary Kraftsow (1999).

2. Pathabi Jois (1915–2009), founder of the Ashtanga Yoga Institute. Author with his son Sharath of *Yoga Mala: The Original Teachings of Ashtanga Yoga*.
3. B.K.S. Iyengar (1918–), widely viewed as the most renowned and influential authority in the world of Yoga therapeutics today, studied with Krishnamacharya in his early days.

    a. Most well-known books: *Light on Yoga: Yoga Dipika* (about *asana* or postural practice) and *Light on Pranayama: The Art of Yogic Breathing* (about yogic breathing techniques), each offering a therapeutic index identifying specific *asanas* and *pranayamas* indicated and contraindicated for a whole range of illness conditions; *Yoga: The Path to Holistic Health* specifically addresses common specific chronic illness in individual chapters.

    b. Numerous students of Iyengar are currently leaders in the field of Yoga therapeutics:Mukunda Stiles: *Structural Yoga Therapy: Adapting to the Individual* (2001); *Ayurvedic Yoga Therapy* (2008).

4. Srivatsa Ramaswami, Author of Yoga for the Three Stages of Life: Developing Your Practice as an Art Form, a Physical Therapy, and a Guiding Philosophy; The Complete Book of Vinyasa

Selected other recent publications on Yoga therapeutics:

- Healing the Whole Person: Applications of Yoga Psychotherapy by Swami Ajaya and Michael P. Butler; Yoga and Psychotherapy: The Evolution of Consciousness by Swami Rama, Swami Ajaya and Rudolpy Ballentine.
- Yoga Nidra: A Meditative Practice for Deep Relaxation and Healing by Richard Miller
- Yoga RX: A Step-by-Step Program to Promote Health, Wellness, and Healing for Common Ailments by Larry Payne, Richard P. Usatine, Merry Aronson and Rachelle Gardner.
- Yoga for Arthritis: The Complete Guide by Loren Fishman and Ellen Saltonstall.
- Yoga & Ayurveda: Self-Healing and Self-Realization by David Frawley.
- Yoga and Scoliosis: A Journey to Health and Healing by Marcia Monroe, Loren Martin Fishman and B.K.S. Iyengar.
- Cure Back Pain with Yoga by Loren Fishman and Carol Ardman.
- Yoga for Osteoporosis: The Complete Guide by Loren Fishman and Ellen Saltonstall.

REFERENCES

Alter, J. (2004). *Yoga in modern India: The body between science and philosophy.* Princeton: Oxford University Press.

Alter, J. (2005). Modern medical yoga: Struggling with a history of magic, alchemy and sex. *Asian Medicine, 1*(1), 119–146.

Alter, J. (2008). Yoga Shivir: Performativity and the study of modern yoga. In M. Singleton and J. Byrne (eds.), *Yoga in the modern world: Contemporary perspectives*. London: Routledge Hindu Series.

Alter, J. (2010). A therapy to live by: Public health, the self, and nationalism in the practice of a North Indian yoga society. *Medical Anthropology: Cross-Cultural Studies in Health and Illness, 17*, 309–335.

Antonovsky, A. (1979). *Health, stress, and coping*. San Francisco: Jossey_bass Publishers.

Berliner, H. S. & Salmon, J. W. (1980). The holistic alternative to scientific medicine: History and analysis. *International Journal of Health Services, 10*, 133–147.

Bower, J. E., Woolery, A., Sternlieb, B. & Garet, D. (2005). Yoga for cancer patients and survivors. *Cancer Control, 12*, 165–171.

De Michelis, E. (2004). *A history of modern yoga: Patanjali and Esoterism*. London: Continuum.

De Michelis, E. (2008). Modern yoga: History and forms. In M. Singleton and J. Byrne (eds.), *Yoga in the modern world, contemporary perspectives*. London: Routledge Hindu Studies Series.

Desikachar, T. K. V. (1998). *Health, healing and beyond: Yoga and the living tradition of Krishnamacharya*. New York: Aperture.

Devi, N. J. (2000). *The healing path of yoga*. New York, NY: Three Rivers Press.

Dr. Swami Karmananda. (1983). *Yogic management of common diseases*. Bihar, India: Yoga Publications Trust.

Dr. Swami Shankardevananda. (1977/2002). *Yogic management of asthma and diabetes*. Bihar, India: Yoga Publications Trust.

Farhi, D. (2000). *Yoga mind, body, & spirit*. New York, NY: Henry Holt and Company, LCC.Feuerstein, G. (1998). *The yoga tradition: Its history, literature, philosophy and practice*. Prescott, AZ: Hohm Press.

Fields, G. P. (2001). *Religious therapeutics: Body and health in yoga, Ayurveda, and Tantra*. Albany: State University of New York Press.

Goldberg, E. (2005). Cognitive science and Hathayoga. *Zygon, 40*(3), 613–629.

Harrington, A. (2008). *The cure within: A history of mind-body medicine*. New York, NY: W.W. Norton & Company.

Haaz, S. & Bartlett, S. J. (2011). Yoga for arthritis: A scoping review. *Rheumatic Disease Clinics of North America, 37*(1), 33–46.

Helman, C. G. (2000). *Culture, health and illness*. 4th ed. Oxford: Butterworth Heinemann.

Iyengar, B. K. S. (1966/1979). *Light on yoga*. New York, NY: Schocken Books.

Iyengar, B. K. S. (2001). *Yoga: The path to holistic health*. London: Dorling Kindersley Limited.

Kendall-Tackett, K. (2010). Depression, hostility, posttraumatic stress disorder, and inflammation: The corrosive health effects of negative mental states. In K. Kendall-Tackett (ed.), *The psychoneuroimmunology of chronic disease: Exploring the links between inflammation, stress, and illness*. Washington, D.C: American Psychological Association.

Kessler, R. C., Davis, R. B., Foster, D. F., Rompay, M., Walters, E. E., Wilkey, S. A., Kaptchuk, T. J. & Eisenberg, D. M. (2001). Long-term trends in the use of complementary and alternative medical therapies in the United States. *Annals of Internal Medicine, 135*, 262–268.

Khalsa, S. B. (2004). Yoga as a therapeutic intervention: A bibliometric analysis of published research studies. *Indian Journal of Physiology and Pharmacology, 48*, 269–285.

Kirkwood, G., Rampes, H., Tuffrey, V., Richardson, J., Pilkington, K. & Ramaratnam, S. (2005). Yoga for anxiety: A systematic review of the research evidence. *British Journal of Sports Medicine, 39*, 884–891.

Lakoff, G. & Johnson, M. (1999). *Philosophy in the flesh: The embodied mind and its challenge to western thought.* New York, NY: Basic Books.

Lamb, T. (2004). *Yoga statistics and demographics.* Report published by the International Association of Yoga Therapists. Prescott, AZ.

Larson, G. J. (1979). *Classical Samkhya: An interpretation of its history and meaning.* Delhi: Motilal Banarsidass.

Lazarus, R. S. (1999). *Stress and emotion: A new synthesis.* New York, NY: Springer Publishing Company.Lazarus, R. S. & Folkman, S. (1984). *Stress, appraisal, and coping.* New York, NY: Springer Publishing Company.

Manahan, B. (2011). The whole systems medicine of tomorrow: A half-century perspective. *EXPLORE: The journal of science and healing, 7*(4), 212–214.

Malarkey, W. B. & Mills, P. J. (2007). Invited review, named series: Twenty years of brain behavior & immunity—endocrinology: The active partner in PNI research. *Brain, Behavior & Immunity, 21*, 161–168.

McCall, T. (2007) *Yoga as medicine: The yogic prescription for health and healing.* New York, NY: Bantam Books.

Miller, B. S. (1995). *Yoga: Discipline and freedom: The yoga Sutra attributed to Patanjali.* Berkeley, CA: University of California Press.

Mishra, R. S. (1963). *The textbook of yoga psychology: A new translation and interpretation of Patanjali's yoga sutras for meaningful application in all modern psychological disciplines.* New York, NY: The Julian Press, Inc. Publishers.

Newcombe, S. (2005). Spirituality and 'mystical religion' in contemporary society: A case study of British practitioners of the Iyengar method of yoga. *Journal of Contemporary Religion, 20*(3), 305–322.

Ornish D. (1998b). Avoiding revascularization with lifestyle changes: The multicenter lifestyle demonstration project. *American Journal of Cardiology, 82*(10B): 72T–76T.

Ornish, D., Brown, S. F., Scherwitz, L. W., Billings, J. H., Armstrong, W. T., Ports, T. A., McLanahan, S. M., Kirkeeide, R. L., Brand, R. & Gould, K., L. (1990). Can lifestyle changes reverse coronary heart disease? The lifestyle heart trial. *The Lancet, 336*(8708), 129–133.

Ornish, D., Scherwitz, L. W., Billings, J. H., Gould, K. L., Merritt, T. A., Sparler, S., Armstrong, W. T., Ports, T. A., Kirkeeide, R. L., Hogeboom, C. & Brand, R. J. (1998a). Intensive lifestyle changes for reversal of coronary heart disease. *JAMA, 280*(23), 2001–2007.

Perrson, A. (2010). Embodied worlds: A semiotic phenomenology of Satyananda Yoga. *Journal of the Royal Anthropological Institute, 16*(4), 797–815.

Pilkington, K., Kirkwood, G., Rampes, H. & Richardson, J. (2005). Yoga for depression: The research evidence. *Journal of Affective Disorders, 89*, 13–24.

Raub, J. A. (2002). Psychophysiologic effects of Hatha yoga on musculoskeletal and cardiopulmonary function: A literature review. *Journal of Alternative and Complementary Medicine, 8*,797–812.

Selye, H. (1982). History and present status of the stress concept. In L. Goldberg and S. Breznitz (eds.), *Handbook of stress: Theoretical and clinical applications.* New York, NY: The Free Press.

Singleton, M. (2008). The classical reveries of modern yoga: Patanjali and constructive orientalism. In M. Singleton and J. Byrne (eds.), *Yoga in the modern world, contemporary perspectives.* London: Routledge Hindu Studies Series.

Singleton, M. (2010). *Yoga body: The origins of modern postural practice.* New York, NY: Oxford University Press, Inc.

Singleton, M. & Byrne, J. (eds.). (2008). *Yoga in the modern world, contemporary perspectives.* London: Routledge Hindu Studies Series.

Stern, E. (2006). The yoga of Krishnamacharya. *Namarupa, 5,* 85–93.

Strauss, S. (2005). *Positioning yoga: Balancing acts across cultures.* Oxford: Berg.

Swami, S. S. (1966/1997). *Asana, Pranayama, Mudra, Bandha.* Bihar, India: Bihar Yoga Bharati. The Complete Works of Swami Vivekananda. (1977). *Mayavati memorial edition.* Vol 1. Calcutta, India: Advaita Ashram.

Upadhyay, A. K, Balkrishna, A. & Upadhyay, R. T. (2008). Effect of Pranayama (voluntary regulated yoga breathing) and Yogasana (yoga postures) in Diabetes Mellitus (DM): A scientific review. *Journal of Complementary and Integrative Medicine, 5,* 3.

Varela, F., Thompson, E. & Rosch, E. (1991). *The embodied mind: Cognitive science and human experience.* Cambridge, MA: The MIT Press.

Vempati, R., Bijlani, R. L. & Deepak, K. K. (2009). The efficacy of a comprehensive lifestyle modification programme based on yoga in the management of bronchial asthma: A randomized controlled trial. *BMC Pulmonary Medicine, 9*(37). doi:10.1186/1471-2466-9-37.

Whicher, I. (1998). *The integrity of the yoga Darsana.* Albany, NY: State University of New York Press.Wilson, M. (2002). Six views of embodied cognition. *Psychonomic Bulletin and Review, 9*(4), 625–636.

Wu, S. Y. & Green, A. (2000). *Projection of chronic illness prevalence and cost inflation.* Santa Monica, CA: RAND Health.

PART II

CHRONIC ILLNESS: INTER-RELIGIOUS, CROSS-CULTURAL, AND NARRATIVE PERSPECTIVES

CHAPTER 7

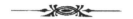

THE ZEN OF HEALING: MAKING FRIENDS WITH CHRONIC ILLNESS

Paula Arai

The crux of a Zen approach to life is to accept the present moment in its fullness.[1] When the moment is warm and sunny with a light breeze in the air, it is an enjoyable thing to do. When the moment is full of pain to perform common daily acts like walking, sitting, lying down, or standing, it is not so enjoyable. So, is Zen saying, yes, life is sometimes not very enjoyable and to just accept your pain? My in-depth ethnographic research finds that Zen offers ways of being that embed daily activities with a wisdom that understands the heart-wrenching, demoralizing, and, sometimes, infuriating challenges of living with conditions that are not desired. The key to empowering one who lives with chronic illness is a mode of healing that weaves ritualized activities into one's daily life, imbuing them with power and meaning as they help one experience one's interdependent connections to a vast web of compassion in the universe.

In a worldview where the interrelatedness of all things is the primary point of reference, healing means to be in harmony with this impermanent web of relationships that constitutes the dynamic universe. It is difficult, however, to comprehend—much less experience—the vastness of something so expansive. Interrelatedness cannot be experienced deliberately. Rituals, however, can be a conduit to an intuitive, bodily based experience of it, precisely because rituals can transport the individual to modes of being that transcend dualistic perception and rational logic by facilitating contact with the ineffable. Rituals holistically permeate the body–mind. Language and cognitive processing, on the other hand, often fall short, or even obstruct, the way to experiencing the full grandeur of one's ultimate context. Therefore, rituals that do not explicitly purport to be healing rituals can help someone heal by indirectly facilitating a fundamental dimension of Buddhist healing activity, a non-dualistic experience of reality. The Zen way of healing involves discipline, ritualized practices, and expanding one's perspective. Expanding perspective facilitates a different experience of life and transforms one's relationship with events, circumstances, and people, including oneself. These are the keys to making friends with chronic illness.

Zen is a stream within the Buddhist tradition that flourishes today in several regions of the world, especially East Asia and, increasingly, in parts of the west. It draws on the 2,500-year-old teachings that first developed in northern India with the insights of Sakyamuni, a man recognized as a Buddha or enlightened being. In short, he is recognized for finding a way to stop suffering. In his first sermon on his insights he taught the "Four Noble Truths." A medical analogy of the Four Noble Truths likens the first Noble Truth of suffering to a diagnosis. It is an observation of a condition, not a fated state. The second Noble Truth of ignorance is the cause of this condition. Ignorance of the impermanent and interrelated nature of ultimate reality is the lens through which deluded beings view things, propelling them to greed and hatred. From the Buddhist perspective humans are prone to ignorance because of experiencing life largely through the six senses of hearing, seeing, touching, smelling, tasting, and thinking. The input through these sources reinforces a distinct but false sense of being an independent self. For example, when I stub my toe, your toe does not hurt. Mine does. So, it seems like I am separate from you, no matter how much you might sympathize with me. A sense-based perspective of things leads to suffering because it frames perception to focus on experience as a matter of interacting with independent objects that, in turn, can be desired or rejected. Although conventionally distinctions can be made between this and that, ultimately everything is not separate. But when we make decisions based upon the view that things are separate, we suffer because our actions are not synchronized with the way things ultimately are: impermanent and interconnected.

The Buddhist assumption is that people are born with a longing for good things to be permanent and that people seek the fulfillment of their desires and elimination of their aversions. This is the primary condition from which people must be healed. Therefore, healing involves the transformation of habitually deluded ways of looking at the world through the lenses of attachment and aversion. The prognosis, though, could not be better. Suffering is not terminal nor is it a permanent condition. The Third Noble Truth heralds that the cessation of suffering is possible. The Fourth Noble Truth outlines guidelines for treatment: the Eightfold Path of living with awakened views, intention, speech, action, livelihood, effort, mindfulness, and concentration.[2]

Dissolving the ego through the Eightfold Path requires surgical precision to extricate the delusions that insidiously shape perception and fuel suffering. All of life can be approached as healing activity that transforms the way life is viewed and experienced. It is a way of life that emerges from a Buddhist worldview, values, and practices. The Zen concept of healing, in keeping with the larger frame of the tradition, is oriented to diminishing, and ultimately overcoming, suffering.

My theory of Zen Healing is encapsulated in the following ten activities:

1. experiencing interrelatedness,
2. living body-mind,
3. engaging in rituals,
4. nurturing the self,
5. enjoying life,
6. creating beauty,
7. cultivating gratitude,
8. accepting reality as it is,
9. expanding perspective, and
10. embodying compassion.

Each activity is distinct. Although there is overlap, there is no redundancy. Each adds a dimension to the healing paradigm. Often one element augments another, for instance interrelatedness increases one's feelings of thankfulness and heightens one's sense of beauty. This in turn commonly sharpens one's experience of fun. Performing rituals sometimes facilitates a deepening of the body–mind connection, and results in one taking better care of oneself. Indeed, any factor can initiate a heightening or enhancement of any of the other qualities. The more this happens, the more quickly and thoroughly one can experience healing.

Buddhism is an experiential tradition. It teaches that one must determine for oneself whether or not an experience or practice helps stop suffering. Nothing is taken on just faith. Therefore, Buddhism has a rather pragmatic undercurrent running through it. Likewise, healing is an experience. What works for one may not work for another, but if there are certain things that others have found to be helpful, they may be worth trying for oneself.

Implicit in the meaning of healing is the antithesis of healing: a desperate sense of loneliness where excruciating anguish is accompanied by paralytic fear and an insatiable desire for things that cannot be. Suffering arises out of a mistaken sense that one is separate, alone, and unsupported. Healing, however, is a sense of peace that does not shatter in the face of horrific events and delusional activities. Healing occurs when one has a bodily heart-felt awareness that one is integral to an all-encompassing network in which compassionate support is both given and received. In other words, healing derives from experiencing oneself as interrelated to everything in the universe.

In order to experience the universe this way, focus on desire, hatred, and fear must be dissolved. The attachments that derive out of these foci obscure interrelationships, invariably resulting in suffering. Zen healing is based on activity that loosens the grip these attachments have by fostering an experience of interrelatedness. It is a pragmatic approach. The mind cannot cut carrots and put them in the pot all by itself, no matter the level of concentration. The body must move. And the body can only move in the present. If this is the case for something as relatively straightforward as getting carrots in the soup, how much more so for things as important as healing and helping. They can only occur in the present moment.

From this non-dualistic perspective, even sickness is a Buddha. In order to heal, one must approach it as such. In other words, what is here now is what must be lived with. One cannot live later and one cannot force life to be a certain way. This healing way is based in a holistic worldview where sickness is part of the world. One must relate with sickness as an active part of one's life. In Japanese the verb used to describe this type of interaction stresses the act of two things finding common ground to enjoy meeting each other: *tsukiau*. In colloquial conversation *tsukiau* is used when one refers to interacting with people in the context of a friendship. The word suggests that you actively do things together. It would not be considered *tsukiau* if you got together with someone for tea only once a year. The word connotes a friendly familiarity between the people who get together and do things on a frequent basis such that formalities are replaced by casual comfort. Therefore, to *tsukiau* with one's sickness assumes that an active relationship exists between oneself and the sickness. How one interacts is the concern, not whether one interacts. One can be kind to one's sickness and rest when the body feels tired or refrain from foods that aggravate the sickness, or not. One woman who practices this type of healing, Gyokko Sensei, said that to *tsukiau* well involves adjusting her activity level to suit her condition. For example, before her legs began to hurt she could do eight out of ten things. Now she only does six out of ten (Gyokko, personal communication, August 13, 2003). In a similar vein, according to another woman, Honda-san, her key to a good *tsukiau* is to not strain herself unreasonably (interview, winter & spring, 1999). One can also choose to be uncaring about a condition and strain the body with overwork or partake in behaviors that are detrimental, like eating salty foods despite hypertension or ingesting large amounts of sugar despite diabetes. If one is kind to the sickness, then things often go along more smoothly. If one is unkind to the sickness, things often get worse.

In contrast to a Zen-based approach to healing, a dualistic worldview sets up an adversarial dynamic between health and sickness where sickness is something to be attacked. It is an object apart from oneself. From this perspective, sickness can be construed to be an enemy. It must be eradicated in order to get better. On the contrary, from a non-dualistic view one can experience sickness as something with which one is in relationship, not something one wishes to defeat, destroy, or conquer. *How* one relates to the sickness makes all the difference.

To *tsukiau* or relate well with a sickness, however, does not imply that the sickness will go away. Indeed, one must *tsukiau* with a chronic illness, sometimes for a long time. The question is will the relationship be open to inevitable changes or will hostility and bitterness reign. A good way to *tsukiau* or relate would involve acceptance without resentment and peace in the face of demise. Having a peaceful relationship with one's condition is the ideal of healing in a Zen mode.

Rituals can help people heal with a broad spectrum of pain, including chronic illness, times of personal emotional crisis, in the face of terminal illness, while struggling with family discord, and learning to live with loss. Rituals have this capacity, because they are a way of cultivating the heart needed to *tsukiau* or relate with illness in a healing mode, the fourth activity in the Zen way of healing. A key to being healed is to experience interrelatedness even to illness. This is not easy. Various rituals facilitate the changes in perspective needed to experience the fact that one is already embraced by the universe, aches, pains, tumors, and all. Rituals are effective in cultivating such awareness, because they involve the body. The mind alone can comprehend interrelatedness, but this knowledge does not bring about healing. A visceral experience of interrelatedness is required for the healing to occur. Some rituals are especially effective in facilitating such an experience. I should add that it is not necessarily important to be cognizant of this dimension of ritualized activity. The concern is to experience the results, but to not do the rituals *in order to* experience interrelatedness. The rituals are to be approached in order to do things like remember deceased loved ones or to mark the changes of the seasons. That is the power of rituals. They accomplish some things that are not intentionally sought after, but are nonetheless beneficial. Some things that are helpful are elusive when sought after directly. By its infinitely expansive nature, experiencing interrelatedness is a target that dissolves in the mere effort to aim at it. Through certain rituals, however, it is possible. Rituals affect the body, even if the mind is not conscious of what is going on. That is the key to their healing power.

Rituals shape, stretch, define, and re-define the identity of the participant. Engagement in rituals transforms consciousness. The power of ritual is manifest not through ability to communicate conscious knowledge, but to frame experience in such a way that it may be apprehended meaningfully. Ritual is similar to lived experience because it is performed by the body. In this way people can learn about what is important through experiencing "fresh" what others before one have experienced. Real life is very messy and organic whereas discourse about life tends to be tidier and more linear. Ritual is in between. Being in a ritual with a long tradition can make a person feel connected and as belonging. A ritual can affirm a person for being who they are.

Rituals can unite things in ways that words divide, because language is inherently dualistic. Cerebral understanding alone often does not help one feel whole and connected to the universe. Since rituals are multivalent, one can do a ritual to honor a loved one on the third anniversary of their death and not only successfully show respect, but one can also, thereby, experience being embraced by the universe. One can feel that one is not alone. This is what heals. Scholar of Ritual Studies, Tom Driver (1992), offers his insights into ritual and explains why they are effective in making one not feel alone: "Ritual ... refuses to recognize clear lines of demarcation between the psychological, the sociopolitical and the material worlds." He continues, "Ritual acts as if everything is alive and personal" (p. 174). Ritual tries to make sense out of the raw materials of lived experience. Ritual Studies scholars, Boyd and Williams (1989), amplify the significance of ritual in lived experience, and articulate why rituals are important and complex:

> Rituals aim at harmonizing disparate elements of culture and expression; they affect both our minds and hearts, rationalizing our activities and empowering us to act. And these rituals bring together diverse realms of experience—ethical, aesthetic, technical, religious—mirroring our activities and expressing our inner emotional life in voices ranging from descriptive to evaluative, worshipful, and performative, they are necessarily complex and multivalent. (pp. 30–31)

In other words, rituals help one feel connectedness through bodily action that integrates dissonant aspects of experience.

Healing is a messy matter. Engaging in rituals to heal can be especially helpful, because rituals thrive in complex and emotionally charged conditions. Competing aims, conflicting conditions, and hope for otherwise improbable results—like wanting to live long enough to see a child grow up even as the systems in one's body start shutting down—evoke intense emotions that words alone cannot convey. Rituals can heal, even in such situations, because they do not operate in chronological time. Rituals provide a space to tolerate the otherwise intolerable when they are designed and performed accordingly. A number of Buddhist rituals have helped people live with otherwise untenable conditions, because they experience themselves being in an incomprehensibly vast space. It is big enough to contain the source of angst and a peace that transcends particular conditions. Rituals are adept at working with emotions and guiding them. When emotionally upset, one's attention often becomes more narrowly focused, limiting the options that seem possible. The proper ritual can facilitate calming and expansion of perspective, thereby opening up options of response. Deep emotions become bodily embedded, so moving one's body can help shift them and guide them without needing to make a linear explanation for how one can live with the intolerable. Although meditation can help one gain a vast sense of self, time, and place, it often takes a prolonged period of practicing to experience it. Rituals, however, can help in times when sitting quietly is not possible, and they can be immediately effective. Without comparison to past events or desires for the future, the present moment can heal. In an expansive experience of the present, the ego self dissolves along with a consciousness of suffering.

Rituals work through the senses to cultivate wisdom in the bones. Unlike Buddhist discourses on wisdom, which focus on understanding the empty nature of ultimate reality—and hence are sometimes too abstract and cold to comfort someone who is experiencing excruciating pain—rituals can help one experience with one's whole body-mind that one is subtly and profoundly interconnected among, and therefore supported by, countless relationships.

Zen scholar-monk, Victor Hori (1994) notes that "Ritual formalism and mystical insight reside together" (p. 28). The typical Buddhist ritual done at home and temple altars engages all the senses. Lighting a candle provides a glow for the eyes and heat for the body. Lighting a stick of incense provides an aroma for the nose. Ringing a bell provides sound for the ear. Chanting reverberates in the body. Food offerings made will later be eaten and stir the tongue and fill the body. These typical ritual acts affirm the gift of life in concrete ways experienced by the body. It is in this way that rituals make symbols real. People can experience feelings that shift their view of life through the guidance of rituals. In the disorientation and frustration that may ensue after the loss of a basic function, capacity to care for one's own personal needs, freedom to move without pain, or any tragic event, rituals can help affirm order.

Some of the most effective rituals are "home-made," because they can be tailored to the aesthetics, fears, and hopes of the person who created them. One can draw on traditions that are creatively modified to suit personal situations. A Zen mode of healing need not be limited to Buddhist practices. The important point is to ritualize activities, because the act of ritualizing helps a person embody the ideals inherent in the ritual. In Buddhism, the focus is on awakening Buddha qualities like wisdom and compassion.

Rituals bring the mind and body together in full attention to the present moment. This capacity is why rituals are a primary resource in the quest for healing and resiliency, a staple quality in those who find happiness in adverse conditions and succeed against difficult odds. Operating from an integrated body-mind focused on the present, opens possibilities to galvanize clarity and strength. Having clarity and strength enables one to discover options and possibilities that remain faint and blurred when one is pulled in many directions at once. Ritualizing an activity raises its importance and, by extension, affirms the significance of the person who performs it. Ritualizing helps quell tortuous doubts about whether what one is doing is "good enough." Ritualizing gives little space for the erosive effects of self-doubt and lack of confidence, because ritualizing inherently embeds meaning and connections beyond oneself. One can, of course, be nervous about performing a ritual well, but the nervousness implies a respect for what is happening and thereby reinforces the importance of the act. For all these reasons, engaging in daily rituals is a way to maintain one's strength and sanity. Rituals help one nurture oneself, which in turn enhances one's ability to nurture others.

Nurturing the self is a critical component of healing in a Zen mode on two different planes. First, it is essential on a mundane level, because no matter what happens, one must eat, brush teeth and bathe, clean surroundings, launder clothes, and take out the trash. Second, skills that nurture the self affirm one's self-worth in the face of uncontrollable circumstances. After one brushes one's teeth, one not only gets clean teeth, but one also gets a sense of personal competence. This is self-affirming. Sometimes getting through a difficult situation is a matter of living with pain and loneliness, and having things to do that make a positive difference can make the time seem less intensely painful. If one does not have skills for nurturing the self, then the pain can become intractable. Taking care of basic needs like shelter and food is a source of satisfaction and gratitude. These very skills help one fare well when one needs to live with tragedy. Those who have experienced debilitating suffering know the liberating healing power of ritualized acts of self-care. They often become a lifeline to the parts of you that continue no matter what else has changed, no matter how painful or unwanted the changes are.

Another aspect of nurturing the self that is critical for this healing modality is the sense of responsibility for one's own life. Gyokko Sensei lives by the motto that "If you make something someone else's fault, you cannot be healed from the wound" (interview, June 22, 2001). It is critical to see and acknowledge responsibility for self and not blame others (including an illness) for problems. Rather than focusing on the external conditions, individuals might concentrate on their own abilities to address a situation. Maintaining awareness that no one can control other people or control circumstances puts the stress on what the individual can do. A person may choose how to act. It is important to not place future conditions on present happiness. I will be happy if the illness or pain goes away, etc. To sustain this perspective requires discipline to not lose sight of the support one receives from the universe or of the power to shape experience by how one interprets and responds to events in the present moment. Doing as many self-care acts as possible is empowering. When reliance on others is necessitated, however, opportunities to dwell in the healing balm of gratitude are made available instead.

Enjoying life is easy when things are going well, but an important aspect of this healing paradigm recognizes that there are plenty of times when there are ample things one could complain about. So, it is necessary to gain a perspective that opens up an avenue to enjoy life, pain, tubes, regular injections, and all, which is the fifth activity of Zen healing. It is a skill that many have recognized as valuable, as they have matured. Finding humor in a situation is part of transformation in which finding a different set of symbols enables one to accommodate the painful reality of loss, injury, or trauma. It is primarily in finding joy in the subtle things in daily life that is most important. Gyokko Sensei, a woman in her late 60s at the time, laughed while explaining that "suffering comes knocking even if you ignore it, so you must make a deliberate intention to invite in fun things" (interview, April 6, 1999). Whether it is collecting shells along the seashore, gazing at a wildflower by the road, or having tea with a friend, it is vital to seek ways to have fun.

Enjoying life is not about requiring entertainment from external sources. It is about realizing a supple and flexible body-mind which facilitates enjoyment of life without conditions for experiencing joy. It is the feeling that one is simply happy to be alive. Without a general sense of well-being, it would be easy to descend into a negative cycle of interpreting experiences in ways that prolong suffering and increase a sense of loneliness. Therefore, being able to adjust one's perspective to see and enjoy the beauty in what is in the present moment here and now, is an essential aspect of healing activity.

Being aware of beauty is fundamental to healing. Living itself comes from multiple elements working together to support that life. If this fundamental condition is not recognized, then one cannot see what is going on clearly. When one sees clearly, gratitude is an energizing response, because it corresponds to the activities going on in the present. Seeing beauty is based on a penetrating awareness of the fundamental nature of how things work. Umemura-san says that for her, "To think in terms of *life is a gift* is important to healing. Because you do not live on your own. You eat, and the food is supporting you. To recognize this is vital" (interview, March 30, 1999). Whether this recognition is conscious or intuitive does not matter. Seeing beauty is to be aware of and embrace how life is supported. It is an acceptance that involves seeing the beauty in events as they occur. From seeing beauty, gratitude is less than a breath away.

When one sees or creates beauty, it is not a strain to see what enormous support one receives from the universe. The fact that one is alive is proof that the universe embraces one. This awareness can sometimes make one feel connected and cared for, particularly when feeling lonely. The type of gratitude that is healing is not construed as *me* being grateful for *things*, because that sets up a dualism, which is incongruous with an interrelated worldview. If one is aware that one is already—without having to do anything special—an integral part of the world that is in a vast web of give and take, mutually influential, gratitude is a natural response.

When grateful, the individual does not have to work at seeing the good things in a situation, they just appear. Also, when in a grateful state of being, it is not an effort to avoid or to resist, restrain, or repress negative thoughts and feelings. These just do not arise in the experience of gratitude. Gratitude, the seventh principle, is, in a sense, a short cut on the path of healing. Yet, gratitude's full power to heal occurs in conjunction with the other aspects of this Zen healing mode.

To resist nothing is fundamental to healing activity, because there are no conditions on healing. Receiving everything that occurs in life, however, is extraordinarily hard. Rejecting one's actual situation and condition, however, consumes great vital energy. Wishing things were different causes suffering. Acceptance is the eighth principle in the Zen way of healing. Then, energy can be devoted to facing actual needs. If one is fighting within oneself, then relaxation is not possible. If one is not relaxed, then there is stress that taxes the immune system. A way to gain a heart that accepts reality as it is, is to treat each thing, including illness, with respect. To be aware of the value of things requires an open and accepting heart, and, in turn, one's heart becomes more accepting the more one sees the importance of things. To appreciate the value of something requires paying careful attention to it.

Healing as awareness requires acceptance of impermanence. Expanding one's sense of time is a way to help the heart become more accepting. There is a larger framework in which the significance of something can often be more easily understood, as in the greater room a person has to move around, the more options there are for action. For example, in a closet one may stand or sit. There is little room for anything else. However, in a large room, like a gym, one walk around, run in circles, or even dance. The same happens with the heart: the bigger it is, the more options there are. To not become exhausted, the heart must be made flexible and permeable to allow things in, to expand. Accepting is a matter of growing the heart bigger so everything can fit.

Cultivating gratitude, accepting reality as it is, and expanding one's perspective are critical to being able to enjoy life and are key to Zen healing activities. A narrow perspective diminishes one's ability to see things in a positive light, because the limited view diminishes fuller context and serves to distort. If decisions and actions are based on a distorted view, then actions become less and less appropriate to the situation and the situation is further complicated. On the contrary, an expansive perspective provides more information to make more informed decisions. Seeing things in their largest context diminishes distortion, situations become clearer, and decisions easier.

High levels of clarity and honesty are necessary for transforming the heart, because sometimes the apparent choices all look undesirable, like spinal surgery that could cause further nerve damage or continuing to live with debilitating chronic back pain. Recovery requires transforming experience with new symbols. When trauma, loss, and injury happen, these experiences are rendered in some fashion. The activity is to transform negatively valued metaphors into positively valued, adaptive ones. Recovery involves transforming the experience of suffering. This transformation includes cultural, social, psychological, and physiological domains. Rituals can facilitate transformation of the experience into a different set of symbols, because they have power to positively drive transformational activity. They facilitate the transformation by making metaphors internally visceral.

An expansive perspective also makes it easier to decrease cognitive dissonance like anger, frustration, or disappointment that often arises when living with chronic illness. Larger contexts tend to cultivate fewer contradictions, because contradictions often appear as a result of the distorting effects of a narrow lens. Moreover, not dividing things into subject/object dichotomies makes it easier to turn conflicts into complementary approaches. Avoiding dichotomies also enables one to see how one is interrelated with others, opening up more avenues of compassionate response, especially to difficult situations. Also, with a bigger sense of self, fewer things disrupt one's ability to maintain clarity.

What follows is an example of a ritual that healed a person through obliquely crafted mirror-image metaphors on the primary Buddhist concepts: emptiness and interrelatedness. Such expansive metaphors cannot be made directly, because the very effort to clearly delineate them will result in their failure to evoke their limitlessness. The ritual that sustained Honda-san through the worst of her incapacitating hip pain caused by nerve damage is scripture copying (interview, March 14, 1999). This ritual is often performed by very devout practitioners, but it is not formally recognized as an explicit healing ritual by the Zen tradition. The ritual, as she performs it, consists of going to the Zen nunnery in Nagoya on the third Saturday of the month and using brush and ink to copy the *Heart Sūtra*. It is a short scripture written in classical Chinese.[3] It is famous for its line, "Form is emptiness. Emptiness is form." At the end there is a place to write the prayers that the individual hopes will be answered. Indeed, it is not uncommon for people to go to the ritual only when they have problems just so they can have more efficacious prayers.[4]

Honda-san carefully brushed the strokes of each character of the *Heart Sūtra* after having arrived by taxi, a luxury that put a strain on her limited income. To even get into a taxi was a major accomplishment. She had been dragging her body with her arms through her small apartment to get herself ready to go, trying to minimize the pain that accompanies each movement of her left leg. She described the pain she had to live with in those days as even worse than if a dentist accidentally touched a nerve in a non-anaesthetized part of your mouth, because the source of her pain did not move away. It stayed in place, generating pain with each breath. She said that at times tears would quietly and uncontrollably leak out of the corners of her eyes as the pain coursed through her. And yet, she almost never failed to go to the ritualized copying of the scripture. After she recounted how the scripture copying ritual sustained her and healed her, I asked her in my most polite Japanese what I thought was a reasonable follow-up question: "At the end, if you do not mind sharing, what are the types of things you offered up in prayer?" She matter-of-factly responded that she never prayed for anything. I was shocked. "Didn't you pray for the pain in your hip to go away?" Now *she* looked surprised and confused as she sputtered, "No, I never even thought about it. It never occurred to me" (Honda-san, , March 14, 1999). Thinking that I should be a respecting ethnographer and not add any more queries that might indicate a criticism of her practice of the ritual and try to analyze what her worldview might be on my own and knowing that Japanese is such a delicate, indirect, and subtle linguistic instrument, I blurted out, "Why not?!" She was visibly uncomfortable about being pressed for a reason. She had just poured out her heart to me about how much pain she had been in—not an easy task for someone who is the epitome of politeness and master of thoughtful caring for others—and had gone on to share the beauty and joy she received from just going to the scripture copying ritual. It seemed hard for her to understand what more she could possibly explain to me. At that point I gained control of my perplexity and incredulity, and slipped in a "that's what I would have done" (referring to praying for pain to go away) and moved the conversation to another topic. It took years for me to see how the scripture copying ritual helped her with her pain if she was not even praying for her hip to stop hurting.

The key to understanding why she never prayed for her own pain to be removed lies in her confusion with why I thought she would have. At the time, I personally could not even imagine such thorough and steady acceptance of debilitating chronic pain. Honda-san does not resist her life circumstances. She does not even privately wish that things were different.

She also does not passively watch life go by without her. Honda-san has disciplined herself to perceive her situation as without fault. In fact, she claims that nothing is bad about her life. She realizes that she has the power to shape her life, and she chooses to define herself and her needs by her own standards. She does not buy into (including literally not spending a lot of money) the societal expectations of her. She did not marry, has no children, and she lives a very simple life. She has found contentment. She is a living example of medical doctor Dean Ornish's (1998) point that "The more inwardly defined you are, the less you need and the more power you retain" (p. 145). Honda-san swiftly shifted her views when her hip pain suddenly occurred one day while walking en route to work through the labyrinthine underground shopping center that winds through Nagoya's busiest district. She never felt sorry for herself. She faithfully continued her monthly visits to the temple to participate in the scripture copying ritual. Putting inked brush to paper while the incense wafts through the air of the Worship Hall with a wooden carving of Kannon-sama, the Bodhisattva of Compassion, gazing down upon all who come, she viscerally experiences being in the impermanent stream of the numberless flowing together along the way. With each intricate stroke of black ink on white *washi* rice paper, she traces the gray path of "*Form is emptiness. Emptiness is form.*" Countless people have followed this path before her, and countless more will do so in the future. In this continuous flow, each present moment is complete. In each moment there may be pain, but there is no suffering. In each moment one belongs, just as one is, in this vast and beautiful expanse. There is no need to pray for anything.

It is striking that a ritualized aesthetic activity that takes one hour to perform and occurs just once per month could have such a deep impact on someone. Honda-san's experience is so potent, though, that although she lives with often debilitating chronic hip pain, she impresses upon me how "no matter how painful it was, I went by taxi to participate in the scripture copying ritual. There were two times in 12 years that I did not go, when I threw out my back and when I had surgery" (interview, March 7, 1999). It becomes clear to me that were she not to go to the scripture-copying ritual, her pain would be unbearable.

To experience pain in this way requires focusing on the larger picture. Ritual Studies expert, Catherine Bell (1997), explains that, "the fundamental efficacy of ritual activity lies in its ability to have people embody assumptions about their place in a larger order of things" (p. xi). When people think they are not living independent lives based solely upon their own power and effort, it is easier to relax and feel grateful for what is, rather than feel strain about what is not; and to be aware that one is alive because the myriad interconnections in the universe work together to generate and support life. Buddhist teachings lend themselves to a more scientific and ecological explanation, like one offered by a Zen woman, Taniguchi-san: "Life (*inochi*) is like water which becomes fog. Fog becomes river, and so on. Nothing is lost. You cannot choose for things to be different than they are, but you can choose how they are perceived and interpreted" (interview, August 11, 2003). Whatever the metaphor used to explain, this perspective of life seems to naturally give rise to a profound sense of gratitude for all things. This ninth principle of ever adjusting one's perspective with the vicissitudes of life enables one to accept one's life into one's heart, to feel grateful for and create beauty out of what is. To do this is to embody compassion. Embodying compassion is the ultimate healing.

Compassion figures in Zen healing activity both as a source of healing and as an expression of healing. To receive compassion and to be compassionate are both part of the healing paradigm. The basis of the tenth principle of Zen healing is that one who is healed is one who is compassionate. Compassion is the alpha and the omega of healing activity. In other words, to be healed one must be a healer. When one is aware of one's interrelatedness, compassion pours in and flows out. Compassion does not come from an intellectual understanding of interrelatedness, it comes from experiencing oneself as integral to the whole. When one experiences wholeness of self, the natural response is gratitude. Gratitude opens the heart wide so that light can shine brightly onto one's interrelatedness, illuminating what compassionate activity is appropriate for the moment. From a grateful heart flows a flexibility of response that is based on an honest perspective of the big picture, that is, a view of how each event, person, or thing is ultimately part of the whole that embraces each of us. That the view is not necessarily cerebrally perceived nor is the response based on an active cognition of the dynamics of the situation is one of the main characteristics of the power of compassion. It is a response to the world that comes from the heart of impermanence, emptiness, and interrelatedness.

A Zen-based Approach to Healing with Chronic Illness

- Focus on what you can do with current conditions rather than what you cannot do with current situations.
- Design meaning-filled activities and integrate them into your daily life. Each person has this creative potential. It does not require anyone's permission, authority, or a particular educational background. In fact, the most meaningful activities are homegrown and handmade. These are the most tailored to your current and actual needs and, therefore, are the most effective.
- Breathe in and out, feeling the support of the universe providing conditions for life. Gratitude will begin to seep into the interstices of your body/mind, making you feel lighter. Even if just for the duration of the mindful breathing, a reprieve from angst, fear, anger, or frustration is worth its weight in gold.
- Expand perspective beyond the lenses of pain/no-pain, illness/no-illness, good/bad, want/not-want. Contentment, even joy, is available when you go beyond these dualistic constructs. Indeed, an awareness of beauty emerges in this expansive view that reveals how everything is cooperating in a flowing cosmic dance of interrelatedness. Even a glimmer of such

non-dualistic perception can bring an intensely relieving breath that cuts through dark despair and lonely agony.

- Acting compassionately, perhaps especially with yourself, is healing activity. Fortunately, it is not conditioned upon a certain state. In other words, there are no obstacles that cannot be dissolved by the force of your choice to be compassionate. It is always possible to make that choice. Nobody can make that choice for you. This is wonderful, because then you are not dependent on how anyone else behaves. You are in control. You may not be in control of all the conditions with which you are living, but you can always choose healing. You have the power to choose to be compassionate now.

Zen healing lies in responding to circumstances as they change and not hanging on to things that cannot be. Responsiveness to change leads to an increased awareness of vulnerability yet also a heightened sense of support from the universe. Finding balance among these ever-changing dynamics engenders a response of gratitude and compassion. To heal is to move with the changes. Healing does not occur while wishing that circumstances did not change or wanting a different kind of change. A primary strategy to employ when faced with challenge or difficulty is to hone the art of steering personal perspective. For example, from one angle a diagnosis of cancer can be devastating and debilitating, but from another angle it can be a catalyst for heightening your gratitude for life and opening unexplored avenues of trust. Seeing the universe as intimately interrelated is the key to an ability to see things from a positive view. If everything is seen in this light, then everything becomes something for which to be grateful. A line from the Zen text, *Hekiganroku*, makes the point succinctly: "Medicine and sickness cure each other, and the entire earth is medicine" (p. 117). This positive perspective is the source of a Zen-based stable centeredness. If blame for a problem is placed, then the wound will fester. Healing is possible, however, if one accepts the flow of events. Such a response requires seeing events from a vast perspective. One might say that the compass required to navigate the way of healing must be calibrated to infinite emptiness/interrelatedness, because viewing the universe as the point of reference yields the most healing results.

A wise Japanese laywoman, Umemura-san, reflected on how she would know if she were healed. Her response was simple and revealing. "I know I am healed when I am kind" (interview, March 30, 1999).

NOTES

1. This chapter draws on material from my volume, *Bringing Zen Home: The Healing Heart of Japanese Women's Rituals* (Honolulu: University of Hawaii Press, 2011).
2. In accordance with their general practice, the Japanese did not translate the *Heart Sutra* into Japanese, but retained the Chinese version.

3. See Note 2.
4. Ian Reader and George Tanabe's volume, *Practically Religious: Worldly Benefits and the Common Religion of Japan* (Honolulu: University of Hawai'i Press, 1998), offers numerous examples of this phenomenon.

REFERENCES

Bell, C. M. (1997). *Ritual: Perspectives and dimensions.* New York, NY: Oxford University Press.

Boyd, J. & Williams, R. G. (1989). Ritual spaces: An application of aesthetic theory to Zoroastrian ritual. *Journal of Ritual Studies, 3*(1), 1–43.

Driver, T. (1992). *The magic of ritual: Our need for liberating rites that transform our lives and our community* (2nd ed.). San Francisco, CA: Harper.

Hori, G. V. S. (1994). Teaching and learning in the Rinzai monastery. *The Journal of Japanese Studies, 20*(1), 5–35.

Ornish, D. (1998). *Love and survival: The scientific basis for the healing power of intimacy.* New York, NY: Harper Collins Publishers.

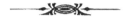

CHAPTER 8

HEARTBREAK HOTEI: SPIRITUALITY AND METABOLIC SYNDROME

Christine A. James

Clearly, only warmth and caring can motivate surrender.

(Hollis, 2012, p. 254)

Colloquially, the medical diagnosis of "metabolic syndrome" and the physical condition of obesity might not be understood as chronic illness or chronic disease. To the lay person, chronic illness often refers to something "out of the patient's control." In contrast, chronic illness such as Crohn's disease and celiac disease are not usually thought to be the result of repeated, habitual, poor dietary choices on the part of the patient; this is even less so with chronic conditions like multiple sclerosis or cystic fibrosis. Metabolic syndrome is not necessarily considered a chronic condition, because it can be remediated through lifestyle changes, healthier choices in food intake, and physical activity. Nevertheless, metabolic syndrome is directly related to chronic illness in terms of a specific set of clinical outcomes that are recognized by the Centers for Disease Control as chronic diseases, among them "heart disease, stroke, cancer, diabetes, and arthritis" (CDC, 2012). These chronic diseases are often listed in the medical diagnostic literature as clinical outcomes of metabolic syndrome, "a condition characterized by multiple risk factors" (AHA, 2004). The Mayo Clinic defines metabolic syndrome as

a cluster of conditions—increased blood pressure, a high blood sugar level, excess body fat around the waist or abnormal cholesterol levels—that occur together, increasing your risk of heart disease, stroke and diabetes. Having just one of these conditions doesn't mean you have metabolic syndrome. However, any of these conditions increase your risk of serious disease.

(Mayo Clinic, 2011)

The Mayo Clinic points to a set of possible causes of metabolic syndrome. These include insulin resistance, evidenced by elevated blood sugar in a phase known as pre-diabetes, and a lack of physical activity. One way to outline the differing opinions about the causes of metabolic syndrome is to analyze the role of inflammation in the disease; in some cases, inflammation is understood as an effect of insulin resistance, but for other researchers, inflammation is a contributing cause of the insulin resistance itself:

> The management approach in patients with the metabolic syndrome depends on the syndrome's perceived causes and the degree of risk attributed to its presence. Current general conceptual frameworks include (1) viewing the metabolic syndrome epidemic as being attributable to environmental causes (eg, the basic approach of NCEP ATP III), (2) viewing the syndrome as primarily the result of insulin resistance (eg, the WHO approach), and (3) viewing inflammation as the underlying cause of the syndrome. In the first view, the primary management approach would be lifestyle modification for reducing obesity and increasing activity. If insulin resistance is considered the underlying cause, treatment is likely to include insulin sensitizers in addition to lifestyle modifications. If inflammation is considered the underlying cause, treatment is likely to include lifestyle modification and insulin sensitizers together with other agents, such as statins, angiotensin-converting enzyme inhibitors, or angiotensin receptor blockers, depending on the presence of specific risk factors.
>
> (Haffner, 2006, p. 7A)

It is helpful to know that there is disagreement on the causes of metabolic syndrome. It is a relatively new diagnosis that is still being studied. The definition and risk factors for metabolic syndrome were first outlined in 1998, when a World Health Organization (WHO) consultation group outlined a provisional classification of diabetes that included a working definition of metabolic syndrome. Since then, the number of people diagnosed with metabolic syndrome has steadily risen, especially in the United States, according to the Centers for Disease Control and Prevention in Atlanta. In general, obesity and metabolic syndrome coexist, with obesity as one of the physical risk factors, and metabolic syndrome the name for the overall condition as defined by the diagnostic criteria: the presence of at least three of the risk factors in one patient. The increasing prevalence of metabolic syndrome is arguably due to lifestyle choices, including the fact that "more than one-third of all adults do not meet recommendations for aerobic physical activity based on the 2008 Physical Activity Guidelines for Americans, and 23% report no leisure-time physical activity at all in the preceding month" (CDC, 2007). On one level, it is a matter of eating too much and exercising too little; but there are a variety of emotional and social influences contributing to obesity as well. Some researchers, such as Steven M. Haffner (2006), note that there may be an infectious agent or inflammatory process that triggers onset of factors related to obesity before the onset of the syndrome itself.

Metabolic syndrome is apparently associated with emotional influences, which are then obvious in the patient's physical appearance. The appearance of metabolic syndrome is immediately noticeable, which is not the case with many other chronic illnesses. In their 2010 book *Savor*, Thich Nhat Hanh and Lilian Cheung argued that our society has become "obesigenic" in that we are surrounded by societal forces that drive us to eat more and move less with the result of weight gain and related health problems. In such a context, the personal decisions that result in obesity must be understood in a societal context of temptations and pressures that make us "become disassociated from what our bodies truly need and want" (Hanh & Cheung, 2010, p. 12). The interplay of inner self-understanding, and outer dialogue with others regarding food and the ethical status of over-eating, is a major theme in the popular perception of obesity among Christian and Buddhist authors.

Many lay persons, as well as spiritual and religious leaders, have written books that attempt to guide overweight people to a healthier lifestyle through a spiritual process that is intended to decrease dependence on food. The reasons people develop problematic relationships with food are complex; there are a variety of psychological and genetic tendencies that are relevant to the problem. In this literature on spirituality and diet, there is ambivalence in the interpretation of "control" and "shame." Within both Christian and Buddhist traditions, the interplay of these two concepts is the crux of understanding metabolic syndrome and obesity.

I. The Ambivalence of Largesse: Fat Body, Expanded Mind, Great Spirit?

Before discussing spirituality, obesity, and metabolic syndrome, an irony regarding obesity in many religious traditions must be acknowledged. For the Christian, Buddhist, and many philosophers, there are role models who are in tight control of their bodies and their bodies' physical desires and hungers, and there are opposite exemplar figures with bodies that are overweight. This kind of body often represents contentment and happiness, the personification and embodiment of jolly abundance. For example, a majority of Christians are raised with the concept of Santa Claus: rotund, apparently gregarious, and described as generous and physically able to give toys to girls and boys throughout the world within one night in spite of his girth. In Buddhism, the tradition of the jolly laughing Buddha is especially associated with China, and is a significant auspicious figure combining Buddhist, Zen, and Shinto wisdom. Known by the name Hotei or Pu-Tai, in China this representation of Buddha is known as the Loving One or the Friendly One. As with Santa, this incarnation of Buddha is rooted in history and a person who actually lived:

> He is based on an eccentric Chinese Ch'an (Zen) monk who lived over 1,000 years ago and has become a significant part of Buddhist and Shinto culture.

> Because of this monk's benevolent nature, he came to be regarded as an incar-
> nation of the bodhisattva who will be Maitreya (the Future Buddha). His large
> protruding stomach and jolly smile have given him the common designation
> "Laughing Buddha."
>
> (Inbasekaran, 2012)

This archetype of contentment and deep understanding, represented in an abundant figure, is also present in the history of philosophy. Richard Watson, in his book *The Philosopher's Diet* (1998), noted that David Hume was a thin and gangly youth. In today's terminology of body types, he would have been described as an ectomorph, tall and thin. But his philosophical process of skepticism on epistemological issues like cause and effect and the problem of induction, followed by the resolution of that doubt, and a variety of social engagements, soon changed his figure dramatically:

> In his twenties he had a skeptical crisis, wrote one of the classics of Western
> philosophy (*A Treatise of Human Nature*), and gained 60 pounds in six weeks
> to become a fat, jolly fellow for the rest of his life... Hume would be the first
> to suggest that the likeliest cause for weight gain is not a sluggish metabolism
> but the total intake of food.
>
> (Watson, 1998, p. 67)

Hume is indeed known as a philosopher with a sense of humor, but it is possible that his weight and the other models of girthy optimism in each of these traditions, are not the whole story.

Comedians are sometimes said to embody the Pagliacci Syndrome. This refers to the main character, Pagliacci, in Ruggero Leoncavallo's opera: a clown who appears to be happy on the surface, but who is actually hiding a much deeper sadness as a result of interpersonal communication problems and the apparent infidelity of his beloved wife (Blistein, 1964, p. 5). Although Pagliacci is not described explicitly as a "fat" clown in the libretto, one of the performers who excelled in the role, Luciano Pavarotti, was known as a man of considerable girth, and the traditional Pagliacci clown costume can be described as generously ruffled, loose-fitting, and forgiving. The perception of the overweight or obese person as happy and jolly can be like that of the clown Pagliacci, laughing on the outside and crying on the inside. Undoubtedly, persons who are obese suffer in social contexts, whether they are physically unable to engage in certain kinds of activities, or they suffer a kind of "social death" by being excluded and disinvited from social gatherings. The appearance of a jolly, happy, fat person often hides deep sorrow.

This sorrow can exist in both physical and social forms. Hanh and Cheung (2010) note that when one is overweight, one suffers a variety of pains:

> Our knees may ache, carrying too much weight, and become swollen and stiff
> with arthritis. Our heart may labor harder, our blood pressure may rise, and
> harmful plaque may build up inside the lining of our arteries, heightening the
> risk of heart attack and stroke. Our breathing itself may become a problem

around the clock as the risk of asthma, chronic obstructive pulmonary disease, and sleep apnea increases.

(Hanh & Cheung, 2010, p. 19)

The social stigma associated with weight is also a dramatic form of suffering, for obese persons of any age: "As children, they may, owing to their weight, become the target of teasing and bullying from their peers. As adults, they may be less likely to win a job or a promotion, or they may be stereotyped as lazy or less disciplined" (Hanh & Cheung, 2010, p. 19).

A related inner and outer struggle can affect those who are obese in childhood, specifically, dealing with the impression that one's parents and family did not care enough to stop the child's overeating at a young age.[1] Judi Hollis hinted at this difficulty, in her 2012 book *From Bagels to Buddha*:

> I once asked my mother about a picture of me at age five standing in the dusty, coal-covered porch on Scranton's South Side. "Why'd you let me gorge myself with a corncob in each hand?" Mom answered, "You just loved to eat. You were always hungry. I'd give you dinner and you'd say, 'Mommy, I want more.'" I know today that I was ravenously hungry for a spiritual connection not to be found in food.
>
> (Hollis, 2012, p. iv)

Many people who have been overweight as children, and who struggle with self-control as adults, wonder if their parents might have been able to give them better will power or better habits through firmer parenting in their childhood. The overweight patient's family, friends, social connections, and an environment that allows for physical activity are important influences on their attempts to lose weight and live a healthier life. Adding in the spiritual dimension might help or hinder this treatment, but there is undeniably a spiritual significance in one's relationship with food. This perception that there is a struggle for a spiritual fulfillment, or an ongoing hunger that food cannot satisfy, is a major reason why the literature on spirituality and diet continues to grow and includes texts based on many different traditions. This piece will address in turn the philosophical, Christian, and Buddhist approaches to weight loss.

II. PHILOSOPHY AND WEIGHT LOSS: CONTROL AND SHAME

Philosophers have written a variety of texts on weight loss, and the interrelationship of healthy body and healthy mind goes back to ancient Greece. Philosophers like Aristotle described the concepts of virtue and self-control that maintain a healthy balance in one's diet and physical activity. Aristotle described a character-based moral theory: one should try to become habituated into the right moral character by doing such activities that would be most likely performed by one who has a properly developed moral character. Actions have moral worth if they are done in accord with a good moral character. Moderation, as well as other virtues, are essential: one must have reason and not be too affected or misled by drives and desires. Losing control to one's drives and desires, such as hunger, would have been known as *akrasia*, acting against one's better judgment, acting without the control of reason, or incontinence. One who repeatedly overeats, then, is at the very least morally underdeveloped, and morally accountable for their apparent incontinence. This moral accountability for acting without reasoned control is why shame and guilt are directly associated with the physical state of being overweight and out of shape in a majority of Western traditions. The term for shame that is related to *akrasia* is *aischron*. The term *aischron* is especially well suited to issues of weight, as it means both *shame* and that which is *physically repelling and unattractive*. As the philosopher and psychologist Robert Metcalf pointed out, shame is "ugly." The Greek word *aischron* connotes that we only look at what is shameful "wincingly" (Metcalf, 2000, p. 3). Note that the person who winces at the shameful condition of being overweight can be both the person who is overweight (looking in a mirror) and the other who looks at them (in public). In Cheshire Calhoun's article "An Apology for Moral Shame," she stated that "in shame, we see ourselves through other's eyes, and measure ourselves by standards that we may not share" (Calhoun, 2004, p. 128). We internalize the "other" and evaluate ourselves by asking "what must they think when they see me?" This can result in a destructive cycle of self-reflexive attitudes, guilt, shame, further overeating, and another round of guilt and shame. Such a consistent and repetitive problem is both literally and figuratively "heartbreaking."

This interplay of guilt and shame is often informed by a difficult tension between the mind and the drives, desires, hungers, and inclinations associated with the body. In his article "The Genesis of Shame," J. David Velleman (2001) highlighted the importance of repeated and consistent control over one's drives and desires. Shame often involves a struggle between the mind and immediate inclinations, a struggle that shows our capacity to resist desires repeatedly, cumulatively, and consistently over time (Velleman, 2001, p. 35).

The transition between ancient Greek philosophical approaches to overeating and guilt and shame is best illustrated by Augustine's interpretation of Genesis, specifically eating the fruit of the tree of knowledge. For Augustine, shame was an internal state that originated from the struggle between the will and the body. The struggle between the will and the body began in the Garden of Eden. Before eating the fruit of the tree of knowledge, the will and the body were united, in harmony—drives and desires were never out of balance or exaggerated. After eating the fruit, Adam and Eve could see the outward results of conflict between the will and the body (for example, the outward signs of lust, on which the will did not want to act, but in which the body chose to indulge). This conflict of the body asserting its inclinations over the intentions of the will was what, for Augustine, gave rise to shame (Augustine, 1988, p. 275).[2]

Given the apparent problem in controlling drives and desires, and the resulting shame and guilt, recent philosophers have attempted to provide a solution for dealing with such temptations. The answers tend to fall into two major groups: internalized narratives regarding developing one's own moral fortitude, and externalized narratives involving pseudo-utilitarian arguments claiming that eating less will be much better for the world as a whole. In Richard Watson's book *The Philosopher's Diet*, he suggested that the diet industry is, in a way, a form of entertainment: going on a diet is like playing solitaire. But unlike playing solitaire, dieting is approved by most people as an activity requiring moral fiber (Watson, 1998, p. 5) The dieting itself is a private activity, one that involves counting calories, carbohydrates, fats, and playing an internal game with one's self; but at the same time it is a game that is seen as socially acceptable, a popular activity that leads to popularity. When one struggles with weight, one struggles with oneself.

Many philosophers have provided evidence for the internal argument to control weight. Plato posited that every individual has reason, willpower, and a set of desires. Each of us is dominated by one or another of the three. A person must be satisfied with his or her lot because there is no way of altering the proportions with which he or she was born (Watson, 1998, p. 88). But a person can exercise the will and attempt to become properly educated in use of reason and will to control the desire for food. Similarly, following Descartes, someone should change his or her opinions and desires only when the world cannot be changed to fit personal desires and opinions. It would appear then that a person can lose 20 pounds and then maintain the weight loss by responsible, free choice (Watson, 1998, p. 25). This philosophical perspective makes it seem as if weight loss is primarily an internal process, a battle that takes place primarily in one's mind. "Your strength and moral courage must come from within," says the philosophical approach to internal change. "Don't look for outside help. Human beings are capable of setting and reaching goals themselves" (Watson, 1998, p. 84).

However, there also is a set of externalized arguments for weight control and moderate eating in the philosophical canon as well. A philosopher can trace the various figures about population, nutritional requirements, and food production around the world and conclude that if all the available food in the world were shared equally, then not just some of us, but all of us, would be undernourished (Watson, 1998, p. 37). On utilitarian grounds, "the good for the greatest number," it would be immoral not to try and change a system of food production and distribution in which some are overfed while millions of others are starving. Dieting is a key part of this ethical obligation: "You can stop supporting the extravagances of the processed-food industries... You can set an example by eating less meat and less food overall" (Watson, 1998, p. 38).

One fascinating aspect of Watson's externalized argument for weight loss, the argument that one's weight loss is beneficial to humanity and the environment, is that these societal goods to the individual are also related to a more selfish good of sexual pleasure:

> People can survive without sexual satisfaction, but people cannot live without food. It seemed to me that if enough people took control of their sexual

lives and assured themselves sexual satisfaction that they don't even need, then
perhaps they could be convinced to take control of the world's food production
in order to distribute food to a billion undernourished and starving people.
                                                      (Watson, 1998, p. 79)

This concept of "taking control" of one's eating and one's sexual life is connected in multiple ways with social perceptions of obesity. On the one hand,
it can be argued that being sexually desirable is not affected by weight; on
the other hand, many argue that the social ramifications of being obese will
undoubtedly cut down on the number of sexual partners one will attract in
one's lifetime. Watson makes both arguments, simultaneously finding that
"when it comes to sexual desirability, contenders on the upper end of the
weight scale for average Americans have the edge. In our sexual fantasies
and in the flesh, we prefer someone with a little fat on his or her bones"
(Watson, 1998, p. 74), just before describing the weight loss success story of
Fats Goldberg:

> One of the greatest success stories in the diet literature is that of Fats Goldberg
> of New York City. By the time Goldberg was twenty-five years old, he had
> weighed over 300 pounds for years. For many reasons he decided to lose
> weight, but most of them can be summed up in one word: girls...Fats
> Goldberg exposed his human soul. He wanted to love and be loved. Nobody
> loves a fat man. So Fats took it off and kept it off.
>   (Watson, 1998, p. 75)

The best way to make sense of these two divergent messages, "we prefer a little fat" and "nobody loves a fat man," is to see it as a matter of rewards.
Society, and the self, gain reward for controlling and shifting drives and
desires to a focus other than food. Many diet books include a similar rhetori-
cal technique, building up the reader's confidence with the message that (s)he
need not be incredibly thin, that having some fat is acceptable as long as (s)he
is healthy; and at the same time reminding the reader that (s)he will be "loved
more" if (s)he is thinner than (s)he is. To the extent that drives and desires
are linked (in this case, sex and food), the drive for food is being replaced by
acknowledging the drive for sex and love. It is the carrot-on-a-stick approach,
with the carrot being sexual acceptance. Aligned with this shift in desire for
food and sex is the implication that the process can be fun. Watson holds
that "the crucial matter of gaining control of part of your life" can be fun,
and you won't know the enjoyment of it until you actually do it. Invoking
the Christian existentialist Kierkegaard, the process begins with a "leap of
faith" (Watson, 1998, p. 87). The efficacy of the philosophical internal and
external arguments for weight loss seems to be a bit problematic. While the
process may be "fun", lack of success produces two different kinds of guilt
and shame: the guilt of having lost the internal battle for personal control,
and the external guilt of contributing to societal problems related to world
hunger and food production. The powerful motivating force of the internal
and external arguments is a double-edged sword when we fail.

III. Christianity and Control: Powerlessness and Receiving

Christian narratives on weight loss mention the leap of faith as well; however, the leap is not toward control, but toward a special kind of powerlessness and surrendering of control. The Christian conceptual model for weight loss holds that we will learn important lessons of faith from going through the process of weight loss. One of the major lessons is the opposite of the internal arguments for control in philosophical traditions; rather than seeking to control one's drives and desires, the Christian approach often requires accepting a loss of control or acknowledging one's powerlessness in regard to food.

Like Hanh and Cheung, Matthew Anderson's *The Prayer Diet* began by acknowledging that society may "wound" those who are overweight in punishing ways: "If we remain stuck in and dominated by our society's myopic view of excess weight, we will miss one of God's most wonderful characteristics—the ability to use our wounds as windows" (Anderson, 2001, p. 14). Using "wounds as windows" refers to the concept that weight reflects certain limitations that faith in the message of Christ can correct. For Anderson, "being chronically overweight is almost always a sign of an inability to receive. It is your body's reminder to pay attention to your needs and to allow others, God included, to help" (Anderson, 2001, p. 40). So in contrast to philosophical approaches that referenced a lack of control, a lack of will, or a lack of reason in regard to drives and desires, the Christian approach suggests that chronic obesity is connected to a lack of ability to receive help from others. It is a problem in how we relate to others—we try to control what we cannot, and our frustration makes us lose control of our eating. Jesus Christ is upheld as an example of perfect powerlessness and giving up control in Claire Cloninger and Laura Barr's *Faithfully Fit*:

> The life of Jesus is a model of powerlessness. He chose to divest himself of all power to come to us as a defenseless baby. And at the end of his earthly life, he chose the cross—the ultimate picture of powerlessness. He was nailed up naked, alone, at the mercy of the Romans and the crowd—to the human eye, utterly hopeless. Although the humanity in him struggled against such submission to God's will, in the end, submission was the way he took. He chose powerlessness so that God's power could be shown through him. So many times, I realize that my struggle with overeating is really a control issue.
> (Cloninger & Barr, 1991, p. 12)

The theme of giving up control or surrendering control is evident in many Christian approaches to dieting. Matthew Anderson found control to be illusory from the outset, stating that "very little in life is a better teacher about the illusion of control than the vicious cycle of weight gain and loss" (Anderson, 2001, p. 29). These spiritual approaches to obesity emphasize that giving up control and seeking help, especially through prayer, need not be a frightening or regressive process. Surrendering in this way is a leap of faith toward a deeper way of being alive, what Anderson calls "a giant step forward on the spiritual journey and an opportunity" (Anderson, 2001, p. 27). This form of surrender is described as something that is not a battle, and that is not "suicidal"; it is merely surrendering to a more spiritual way of living (Hollis, 2012, p. vi). Surrendering in this way, and learning to "receive help" from others, may work for some people dealing with metabolic syndrome. On the other hand, offering one's powerlessness up to God as a part of spiritual growth might leave the individual feeling that they cannot do anything, or that the issue is simply out of their hands. The struggle for self-control is entirely over in this case, and many of us will resist the "deeper way of being alive." There are also many obese individuals who have formed co-dependent habits and define themselves and their vocation in terms of "being there for others" rather than being there for themselves. The shift out of that "giving" mindset will be a severe shift in personality, one that might have unexpected consequences for others in the patient's social circle. Think here of the giving mother who is constantly there for her family, who eats poorly because she does not make time for herself in terms of diet and exercise. Think of the overweight nurse working long hours in a hospital who struggles to eat nutritious regular meals and goes through regular blood sugar spikes because she must respond to patient needs before her own. A radical change in the social status quo is necessary for these individuals to truly learn to "receive."

IV. BUDDHISM: LETTING GO OF DESIRE, ACHIEVING MINDFULNESS

The Christian tradition knows it as surrender, the Buddhist tradition knows it as reducing suffering in attachment to desire. Two major Buddhist-inspired works on weight loss, Ronna Kabatznick's *The Zen of Eating: Ancient Answers to Modern Weight Problems* (1998) and Thich Nhat Hanh and Lilian Cheung's *Savor: Mindful Eating, Mindful Life* (2010) shared an emphasis on the Four Noble Truths and the Eightfold Path as a means to overcoming chronic overeating. Simply put, overeating is a disorder of desire (Kabatznick, 1998, p. 13). It is a disorder of desire that is self-perpetuating as well, since desire for food and overeating is a repetitive process that results in future suffering.

Applying the Four Noble Truths in relation to obesity, we find that: (1) There is suffering, life is unsatisfying, life is fragile, and weight and eating cannot provide lasting nourishment; (2) suffering is caused by attachment to desire, we misguidedly grasp pleasure and satisfaction, only to find that we are even more hungry and suffering more later; (3) suffering ends when we let go of attachment to desire, and we stop seeking nourishment (instead we must stay present with what is happening in the moment); (4) and the Noble Eightfold Path is the way to let go of attachments and end suffering (this form of "letting go" is not unlike the model of surrender evident in Christian approaches to weight loss).

Buddhist responses to overweight conditions also include a set of internal, individual perspectives and a set of outward, social attentions necessary for weight loss. On the individual level, Kabatznick (1998) found that the individual's feelings of satisfaction or lack of satisfaction are related to mindless chronic overeating. In a section entitled *A Closer Look at Letting Go*, Kabatznick stated that letting go of mindless eating is directly related to our feelings of deprivation, and "hatred" of feeling deprived. She advised using the Buddhist Four Noble Truths to help in the struggle to stop mindless eating: Step one involves identifying the cause of suffering (the attachment to desire). The feeling of hatred is your attachment to the desire to eat mindlessly. It is what binds you to this desire and causes suffering. The feeling of hatred is the focus of the letting-go process (Kabatznick, 1998, p. 63). Hanh and Cheung agreed that the first step is awareness of internal states and feelings: "You begin with what is already inside you, with your awareness and experience of every moment you live...mindfulness" (Hanh & Cheung, 2010, p. ix). While mindfulness begins with internal awareness of one's own feelings, the process of reducing suffering also involves outward attention. This applies to both other people and one's connectedness to other beings.

Kabatznick (1988) emphasized the role of generosity and the importance of volunteer work as a part of the process of reducing one's own suffering and feeling a lack of satiety. This reflects a renewed focus on one's interconnectedness with others, rather than the solitary feelings of hunger and solitary activities of weight loss such as counting calories:

> My enthusiasm about the nourishment that comes from helping others led me to start an organization called Dieters Feed the Hungry. The idea was to encourage people struggling with eating problems to expand the ways in which they nourish themselves by practicing generosity and feeding hungry people. I put a small ad in the local newspaper, and the program took off. I matched volunteers and their skills and interests to various soup kitchens and food giveaway programs. Some people donated eggs to a breakfast program for homeless men, and others served food or washed dishes in local soup kitchens.
>
> (Kabatznick, 1998, p. 14–15)

Involvement with others, especially others who are also on a journey of weight loss, is a common part of various weight loss companies like Weight Watchers and Metabolic Research Centers. Regular meetings are held and requirements for participation and attendance are clearly outlined. This outward attention as a step on the path to mindfulness and being present in the moment, and letting go of suffering, also relates to how we perceive our interaction with objects and food itself. Thich Nhat Hanh offered a meditation on eating an apple as an example. Often when we eat, and when we repeatedly overeat, there is a lack of mindful attention to what we are eating. Awareness of the external, and our mutual dependence on the external, reduces the suffering that comes from internal desires:

> With mindfulness, the simple act of eating an apple becomes a profound experience. It opens our awareness that the apple is a manifestation of our world and that it cannot come into being in isolation. The apple is dependent on

everything else for its existence, reminding us that we, too, are constantly
supported by the effort of many beings so that we too may enjoy the apple.

(Hanh & Cheung, 2010, p. 5)

This dichotomy between enjoyment and suffering is the core of Buddhist
approaches to obesity. In enjoying other people, and in learning to enjoy food
in a mindful way, individuals realign their perception of need. The attachment
to "needing" food in the absence of hunger, and the attachment to desiring
fullness, is the attachment that the Eightfold Path challenges. The disorder
of desire that results in obesity and the diagnosis of metabolic syndrome,
then, is a disorder of desire that comes from a lack of outward attention
to other people and to the many other beings, objects, and foods that are
supportive. There is a subtle, compelling irony in this perspective on weight
issues: In appreciating the interconnectedness and mutual dependence we
have with other beings, we become stronger in overcoming suffering. Hanh
and Cheung described it as becoming "solid and stable like an oak tree . . . not
to be blown from side to side by the emotional storm" (Hanh & Cheung,
2010, p. 16). For someone who has metabolic syndrome, there are some disadvantages to this approach as well. In becoming truly mindful, we at first
increase our stress because we become more aware of suffering and interconnectedness on a grand scale. The struggles with guilt and shame in the
philosopher's external arguments for weight loss come flooding back all at
once, and can result in a feeling of utter helplessness in the face of the world's
problems and unfairness. Becoming stable like the oak tree, in the face of suffering, can seem to be cold and unfeeling at first, and the struggle with one's
own feelings is at the heart of metabolic syndrome.

V. STOPPING THE CYCLE: UNCOMFORTABLY NUMB

Few people who have struggled with obesity would deny that emotion (inner)
and social (outer) forces are related to why they became overweight, and are
reasons why they need to overcome their dependence on overeating. Feeling
full as often as possible is pleasant because it is numbing. The inner feelings
that are numbed by overeating are replaced by a constant attempt to become
full again. When we are always thinking about how to be full again, we don't
have to think about our problems or ourselves. In not thinking about real
life, real world, real connectedness in a mindful way, we keep engaging in a
chronic, heartbreaking cycle of new emotions and new desires that mislead
us. There is a difference between being numb and being mindful.

We have to learn the art of stopping—stopping our running so that we can be
present for and embrace our habit energies of worry, blame, guilt, and fear and
calm the strong emotions that dictate us. We have to learn to live fully in the
present moment . . . we have to learn to become mindful.

(Hanh & Cheung, 2010, p. 16)

Not being numb, and not trying to control feelings and habits, are common themes in philosophical, Christian, and Buddhist approaches to the chronic illness of metabolic syndrome. Each spiritual tradition suggests ways to stop the vicious cycle of weight gain, guilt, shame, and regret, followed by more eating, weight gain, guilt, shame, and regret. In the Christian tradition, people are encouraged to surrender to these feelings and admit powerlessness in their presence. In philosophical traditions, ethical arguments are made to encourage control of these feelings, to make better choices for society, and to meet personal sexual needs. In the Buddhist tradition, individuals are encouraged to accept and embrace their feelings in order to refocus and reorder them in a way that reduces suffering.

Body weight regulation is incredibly complicated, and it involves a constellation of causes that include the biological (inflammation), the psychological (inappropriate understanding and response to hunger cues), and the emotional (seeking a feeling of calm or numbness that is associated with fullness). For those who have been diagnosed with metabolic syndrome, the implications of each spiritual and philosophical approach are confusing. The philosophical approach addresses issues of self-control, but the physical aspects of weight may be an overwhelming influence on behavior. A 2008 study found that weight loss in adults will not result in a reduction in the number of fat cells present in the body (Spalding et al., 2008, p. 785). The fat cells are replaced through normal cell-life processes, and the overall number of fat cells within the body remains constant. In the documentary film *FAT: What No One Is Telling You* (Boak & Spain, 2007), this consistent number of fat cells leads to the assumption that there will be a constant inner voice begging for more calories, no matter how diligent and disciplined the formerly fat person becomes. The struggle with shame then becomes an unwinnable situation. To the extent that both Buddhist and Christian approaches advise someone struggling with weight loss to give up certain negative emotions (by decreasing suffering in the Buddhist case, and by surrendering to God in the Christian case) the spiritual approaches do have a beneficial recommendation to break the cycle of shame, guilt, and further overeating. On the other hand, surrendering one's power seems to be inherently contradictory if one hopes to gain control over what one eats. Many eating disorders involve a problematic relationship with control; in the case of anorexia nervosa it takes the form of extreme control over one's eating as a form of defiance when there are many aspects of one's life that are out of one's own control. By overeating, one controls one's feelings by not controlling their eating, using food as a way to "eat one's feelings" rather than expressing anger or their own needs. In the case of Christian perspectives on weight loss, this is related to the "inability to receive help." In the case of Buddhist perspectives on weight loss, this attempt to control emotions leads to suffering, and the ongoing desires to control emotion and eating are what one must transcend to end suffering. For someone already in the grip of metabolic syndrome, the battle to transcend desires for food or desire to control one's feelings is a battle of life and death.

Every member of my immediate family displays at least one of the indicators of metabolic syndrome (waist measurements above 40 inches for men, above 35 inches for women, elevated blood glucose, elevated cholesterol, or elevated blood pressure). At the time my mother died of cancer in 1999, she had at least three of the indicators but was not formally diagnosed. In my father's case, he had all indicators, and has had at least three indicators since he had a heart attack and quadruple bypass in 1985, when I was in junior high school. Fat is a constant presence at our family gatherings, and in a family where food is a major part of bonding and spending time together, there is a confusing double message given to the younger members: "Getting in shape is a good thing, and you should," has a place in the same conversation as, "Make sure you try this," and "Did you have enough to eat?" The one time in my life that I lost a significant amount of weight was when I went away to college for the first time. I walked all over Northwestern's campus and the town of Evanston, Illinois, every day for hours, between class and after class. I made more friends in a few weeks than I had in my entire time in high school. I discovered dancing in clubs in downtown Chicago. I lost 60 pounds from August to November, came home for Thanksgiving, and shocked my family. To this day I am viscerally aware that I hurt my mother's feelings on multiple levels, not only through losing weight, but also by establishing a new form of independence and choosing to be different from my family, and have a life of my own. I felt healthy but deeply *disloyal*. By the time my mother died approximately eight years later, after a long and arduous battle with cancer, I had regained all the weight.

This story reflects two influences on weight that are not emphasized enough in all the philosophical, Christian, and Buddhist approaches to weight loss: the role of day-to-day family influences, emotional and habitual; and the role of physical activity on weight loss. For someone with diagnosed metabolic syndrome, physical activity and social/family connection is dramatically important. Three years ago, my father had a serious diabetic episode. He had not been monitoring his blood sugar well and was relying on oral antidiabetic medications, hoping to delay beginning insulin therapy. One day after Christmas, he did not eat, but continued to take oral Actos and Metformin. His blood glucose fell dramatically, his behavior changed, and we called an ambulance. Fortunately he was in the emergency room before it resulted in a coma. During the resulting hospital stay of three weeks, he came to the attention of a new doctor who convinced him to stop relying on medication, use insulin, and finally accept the habit of checking his blood glucose. He also began walking three times a day, often in a nearby supermarket or mall. He has lost some weight, but the way he looks at it, that isn't really the point. He feels better, of course. But more importantly, he knows he will live to spend more time with his grandchildren. He and his grandchildren need each other and enjoy each other's company. The motivating force of being a grandfather, combined with the willingness to adopt new physical activity, has been incredibly important in his treatment of metabolic syndrome. It is a shame then that many people suffering from overweight, obesity, and metabolic syndrome often do have to deal with social rejection. The social connections and the physical activity habits make a great deal of difference to the patient seeking a spiritual or philosophical understanding of weight.

NOTES

1. Questions about how parents handle overweight children are an increasingly complex issue, especially in the United States, where a variety of policies to monitor overweight children are now in place. This question of whether parents could have done something or perhaps did not have the time or energy to stop a child's weight problem is also perhaps one of the most emotionally charged issues for people who are overweight.
2. This association between erotic love (specifically the outward signs of sexual response, lust, and physical drives) and weight (as the outward sign of hunger drives controlling one's will) is a recurring theme in much of the Christian approaches to weight loss. The association can be overt or more subtle and subconscious. For example, in Matthew Anderson's The Prayer Diet, excess weight is described as a "path to self-love." Note that Watson's secular philosophical argument for weight loss involves a similar dynamic in trading food desire for sexual desire.

REFERENCES

American Heart Association. (AHA). (2004). NHLBI/AHA conference proceedings: Definition of metabolic syndrome. *Circulation, 109*(3), 433–438. January 27, 2004. Retrieved from http://circ.ahajournals.org/content/109/3/433.full#T1 and http://circ.ahajournals.org/content/109/3/433/T1.expansion.html.

Anderson, M. (2001). *The prayer diet: The unique physical, mental, and spiritual approach to healthy weight loss.* New York: Kensington Publishing Corporation.

Augustine. (1998). *St. Augustine's city of God and Christian doctrine.* Philip Schaff (Ed.), Marcus Dods (Trans.). Grand Rapids: Wm. B. Eerdmans, 1988.

Blistein, E. M. (1964). *Comedy in action.* Durham, NC: Duke University Press.

Calhoun, C. (2004). An apology for moral shame. *The Journal of Political Philosophy 12*(2), 127–146.

Boak, N. & Spain, T. (Producers), & Fredericks, A. (Director). (2007). *FAT: What no one is telling you [DVD].* United States: WGBG Educational Foundation and Twin Cities Public Television.

Centers for Disease Control and Prevention (CDC). (2007). Prevalence of self-reported physically active adults—United States, 2007. *Morbidity and Mortality Weekly Report 2008, 57,* 1297–1300. Retrieved from http://www.cdc.gov/mmwr/preview/mmwrhtml/mm5748a1.htm.

Centers for Disease Control and Prevention (CDC). (2012). Chronic diseases and health promotion. Retrieved from http://www.cdc.gov/chronicdisease/overview/index.htm.

Cloninger, C. & Barr, L. (1991). *Faithfully fit: A 40-day devotional plan to end the yo-yo lifestyle of chronic dieting.* Nashville, TN: Thomas Nelson.

Haffner, S. M. (2006). The metabolic syndrome: Inflammation, diabetes mellitus, and cardiovascular disease. *The American Journal of Cardiology, 97*(2A), 3A–11A.

Hanh, T. N. & Cheung, L. (2010). *Savor: Mindful eating, mindful life.* New York: HarperOne.

Hollis, J. (2012). *From bagels to Buddha: How I found my soul and lost my fat.* Las Vegas: Central Recovery Press.

Inbasekaran, J. (2012). *History and significance of laughing Buddha explained.* Retrieved from http://www.ijeyanthan.com/blog/archives/history-and-significance-of- laughing-buddha-explained.

Kabatznick, R. (1998). *The Zen of eating: Ancient answers to modern weight problems.* New York, NY: Penguin.

Mayo Clinic. (2011). *Metabolic syndrome: Definition.* Retrieved from http://www.mayoclinic.com/health/metabolic%20syndrome/DS00522.

Metcalf, R. (2000). The truth of shame-consciousness in Freud and phenomenology. *Journal of Phenomenological Psychology, 31*(1), 3.

Spalding, K. L., Arner, E., Westermark, P. O., Bernard, S., Buchholz, B. A., Bergmann, O., Blomqvist, L., Hoffstedt, J., Naslund, E., Britton, T., Concha, H., Hassan, M., Ryden, M., Frisen, J. & Arner, P. (2008). Dynamics of fat cell turnover in humans. *Nature, 453*(7196), 783–787.

Velleman, J. D. (2001). The genesis of shame. *Philosophy and Public Affairs, 30*(1), 27–52.

Watson, R. (1998). *The philosopher's diet: How to lose weight and change the world.* Boston, MA: Nonpareil Books.

CHAPTER 9

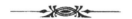

THE ROLE OF RELIGIOUS BELIEFS, PRACTICES, AND METAPHORS IN THE COPING STRATEGIES OF RARE DISEASE PATIENTS IN ROMANIA

Salomea Popoviciu, Ioan Popoviciu, Delia Birle, Serban Olah, and Paul Negrut

Most rare diseases are chronic and some are life threatening, and as a consequence their impact on the lives of patients and their families is significant. Also, rare diseases are really not that rare. Some studies have estimated that as many as 25 million North Americans and 30 million Europeans are affected by one of the 5,000–6,000 types of rare diseases identified by that time, most of which are of a genetic origin (Haffner et al., 2002; Haffner, 2006). In Romania, unofficial reports suggest that around 1,300,000 individuals suffer from rare diseases (approx. 6–8 percent of the entire population), many of whom are lacking a correct diagnosis or adequate treatment and care (National Plan for Rare Diseases in Romania 2010–2014).

Considering the total number of affected individuals, and the limited number of studies in Romania, there is a gap in the literature in areas of interest related to rare disease such as the mode in which common religious beliefs and practices, symbols and metaphors might impact the affected individual or his/her family. Schumm and Stoltzfus (2011) argue that the way a religion interprets, theorizes, and responds to illness plays an important role in how that illness is understood and also determines how persons affected by a disease are (mis)treated in a given context. Moreover, the metaphorical representations of illness often set the stage for further social implications, oftentimes functioning to shape and reflect the values of a particular community (xii). For example, Biblical studies scholar Renite Weems (as cited in Koosed & Schumm, 2011, p. 88) argues that metaphors matter as they are sometimes the very first lessons that human beings learn in prejudice, bigotry, stereotyping, and marginalizing others—be it in deed or thought.

This chapter will explore the role of religious beliefs and practices, symbols and metaphors on the coping strategies of rare disease patients in Romania. While there are studies that have examined the influence of spirituality and religion on coping with disability and chronic illness, there is a research gap in regard to the relationship between rare disease patients' coping skills and their religious or spiritual beliefs and practices. The main objective of this chapter is to contribute to the dialogue regarding illness and religious beliefs from the perspective of rare disease patients in Romania. For this purpose the chapter will be structured into three main sections: (1) an overview of the Romanian Orthodox context; (2) an exploration of the patterns of religious beliefs and practices of 599 rare disease patients or their caregiver and how they correlate with self-reported life satisfaction, optimism, and overall quality of life; and (3) an analysis of how illness narratives employ religious symbols and metaphors.

BEING RELIGIOUS: THE ROMANIAN ORTHODOX CONTEXT

In Romania, after the fall of the Communist Ceausescu regime in 1989, state support for religion was enthusiastically welcomed by a large majority of the population. After many decades of religious repression, the turn toward renewed religious vigor "was radical but somewhat expected" (Sandor & Popescu, 2008, p. 172). In Romania, religion is supported by the state, meaning that central or local governments pay for church personnel and that religion is part of public school curricula, Orthodox churches are built using both public money and private donations, and public displays of religious symbols are present in many state institutions (Sandor & Popescu, 2008).

Understandably, not all are content with the status quo. For example, the claim that the Orthodox Church is the "national church" is somewhat of a national debate, often leading to confrontations between the majority church and minority groups (Bria, 1999). The Orthodox Church argues, however, that state sponsorship of a "national church" does not equate to discrimination against the rights of religious minorities. The religious freedom of all denominations is protected by the Romanian Constitution and, in theory; the state assures the freedom and justice of all recognized religious groups in Romania.

Regardless of these debates, the emerging picture is that of a nation deeply rooted in the Orthodox tradition. In this context, the majority of Romanians report that they are religious people and that they participate in collective religious behaviors and rituals. For example, some polls note that up to 91 percent of Romanians are religious and as many as 96 percent believe in God, with less than 1 percent openly declaring themselves "atheist"

(Public Opinion Barometer, 2005). In addition, using measures of attendance at religious services and frequency of prayers, Romania ranks near countries like Ireland, United States, Uganda, Philippines, and Iran (Norris & Inglehart, 2003).

Explaining the Eastern Orthodox faith, with its icons, liturgy, symbols, and mystical-historical interplay, to other religious traditions is challenging. Romanian Orthodox theologian Ion Bria (1991) stated:

> Efforts to describe Orthodoxy often resemble a monk trying to live outside the monastery or a prophet trying to cultivate the mystery of the living God in the dry mountains of history. Rather than a precise definition or simple descriptive explanation of Orthodoxy, there is a symbolic language that throws up a barrier to meaningful interpretation by many other confessions. (p. 1)

Instead of a systematic doctrinal description of the relationship between humanity and God, the Orthodox Church takes a more mystical approach, focusing on aspects such as "the deification of man [sic]" or "the mystical union with God through the uncreated energies of God" (Lossky, 1978, pp. 13–31; Payton, 2007, pp. 74–78).

The Church's responses to suffering and disease are diverse, but the Orthodox Christian usually views them as consequences of sin—first Adam's and then one's own (Negrut, 1996). The Orthodox Church teaches that humanity sinned by misusing its freedom; therefore, the appropriate relationship with God, fellow human beings, the self, and the rest of the created world was violated (Harakas, 1999). For example, Archpriest Chad Hatfield (2006) observes, "it is sin that deprived us of Paradise, leaving us in the hands of death and suffering." However, Orthodoxy also views suffering as redemptive, if it is understood and accepted as serving a pedagogical purpose such as "the spiritual growth toward God-likeness" (p. 210). Hatfield points out that

> Orthodox Christians recognize this connection between sin, suffering, and salvation, finding it expressed in the prayers of the Orthodox Church. Sickness and suffering are understood to be avenues of salvation and a participation in the glory and joys of the resurrection of Christ and life in the Kingdom of God. This is why the Orthodox Church teaches Her faithful to accept suffering as something that has the potential of bringing them further along in the process of *theosis*. (p. 202)

Theosis is understood as a process of Deification, which is seen as the final purpose (*skopos*) of the entire creation (Payton, 2007, pp. 146–151; Mantzaridis, 1984, pp. 26–38). Also, Orthodox believers may look at the suffering of Christ or the saints and martyrs as models of salvific suffering. From an Orthodox perspective, salvation is understood in terms of God's grace, followed by a human response. This leads to a union between the believer and Christ appropriated in the Church, often articulated as the Ark of Salvation. Thus, it is noteworthy that the Church plays the most important role as a mediating agency toward the saving grace, understood in terms of uncreated divine energies. This "saving grace" is offered by Christ in the Holy Spirit, and with the help of liturgical reading of Scriptures, the mysteries of the sacraments, saints, relics, icons, and the prayers of the believers.

Icons play a large role in the religious rituals of believers, both abled and disabled, and are seen as windows on heaven. They are considered as means through which the Orthodox Christian may "commune with the person or event represented on it" (Harakas, 1999). Icons can represent Christ, Mary, the Mother of Christ (*Theotokos*), or a patron saint. Believers may pray daily before icons, and touch them and kiss them in a reverent manner. Some additionally use prayer books or prayer cards. Also, the Orthodox Christian understands healing as encompassing body and soul. As such, the religious suffering body will make use of the resources of both the medical community and the Church.

As the majority of Romanians participate in these collective religious behaviors and rituals, it can be argued that this behavior is sustained by more than an individual desire for self-transcendent experiences (Haidt et al., 2008) or a "quest" to find one's own understanding of the divine (Batson, 1976). To better grasp Romanian religious beliefs and behaviors, it is critical to look beyond the individual to the wider social and cultural context.

With the risk of oversimplifying, there are three main observations that may explain the Romanian Orthodox context. First, Remond argues that predominantly Orthodox countries from the East witnessed a delay in secularization that might be due to the long Ottoman Empire domination (as cited in Voicu, 2007). Second, the majority of these states (except Greece) had been, for at least half a century, under atheist Communist regimes that placed restrictions on religious faith and practice. In Romania, the Communist ideologues and bureaucrats, in their desire for expedient social secularization, succeeded in expelling religion from the public sphere but not from the private sphere. However, since this public secularization was not accompanied by social modernization—Romania remained one of the least developed countries in Eastern Europe—after the fall of Ceausescu's regime in 1989, private religious behaviors and rituals invaded the public sphere (Gog, 2006). Third, in Romania, religious affiliation is typically associated with a distinct cultural tradition, and therefore used as an ethnic marker. Thus, most ethnic Romanians identify themselves as Orthodox, while minority ethnic Hungarians typically identify as Reformed, and the minority ethnic Germans typically identify as Lutheran. It becomes important to note that religious affiliation does not necessarily reflect a particular religious perspective or behavior, and for some Romanians the religion with which they identify does not translate into religious beliefs or practices that revolve around God.

ENACTING RELIGIOUS BELIEFS: QUALITY OF LIFE AND THE SUFFERING BODY

In Romania, as everywhere else, the individual suffering from a rare disease must develop coping strategies in order to reduce the impact of his or her illness. Thus, the individual's subjective outlook in the presence of chronic or life-threatening illness is highly significant regarding his or her perceived quality of life (Burckhardt & Anderson, 2003). In the context of illness and suffering, quality of life is a multidimensional, dynamic, and subjective perspective of health-related satisfaction. Research shows that this health-related satisfaction is connected with spiritual and religious well-being (Bishop, 2005; Koenig et al., 1988; Mickley et al., 1995; Sawatzky et al., 2005), which in turn can be shaped by the suffering body's social culture.

Empirical studies often approach religiosity as a rigidly defined set of beliefs that individuals have about God. These belief-centered approaches may minimize the importance of religious practices and rituals.

This individual belief-focus is apparent in the division between "intrinsic" and "extrinsic" religiosity. Thus, the label "intrinsic religiosity" is understood as the commitment and importance an individual assigns to religion (Allport & Ross, 1967; Kelly, 1995), and "extrinsic religiosity" encompasses the comfort and social connections people find in their religious practices (Mickley et al., 1995). An alternative conception of religiosity is posed by Graham and Haidt (2010). The authors put forward a group-focus approach to religion that, while placing God at the center of the action, considers the action itself as the "creation, enacting, and maintaining of an emergent community by the collective behaviors taking place all around it" (Graham & Haidt, 2010, p. 142). In other words, the group rituals function to instill belief in God and commitment to a series of religious practices; rather than belief generating adherence to ritual.

Spirituality, on the other hand, may be expressed in religion but may also be expressed outside of religion as part of a person's culture or philosophy of life (Tanyi, 2002). But even in the most religious landscapes one can find a number of individuals who may not identify with a particular religious tradition or ideation, so it becomes important to examine spirituality as distinct from religion (Peterman et al., 2002). As such, "spirituality is not a homogenous practice, but reflects individual expressions of being" (Adegbola, 2006, p. 44).

In a recent study, survey data were collected from 599 participants who either had a rare disease diagnosis or were caregivers for someone with a rare disease diagnosis.[1] This study was part of a larger study funded by The Norwegian-Romanian Partnership for Progress in Rare Diseases that involved an extensive survey investigating the quality of life of rare disease patients in Romania. This chapter includes only that data related to the religious and spiritual dimension of the quality of life of rare disease patients in Romania.[2]

Access to patients was initiated through the Romanian Prader Willi Association, a patient–parent advocacy group founded in 2003. Although not all study participants were members of this group, it is the only such organization in Romania, and the authors felt that a large number of patients with rare diseases could be reached through it via snowballing and word-of-mouth. E-mails were sent to all county representatives of the National Alliance for Rare Diseases who identified patients and their families. These patients and their families were asked to forward it to other patients suffering from a rare disease. Surveys were collected in 2010–2011 from all 44 Romanian counties. The 599 respondents were aged 14–81 years ($m = 34.00$; $sd = 12.96$), 47 percent were male, 53 percent female, representing over 40 types of rare diseases.

The study yielded four important results, which will be briefly discussed here. First, this study indicated that the respondents were deeply religious people. Over 80 percent reported belonging to the Romanian Orthodox Church, and none identified as atheist or "without religion." The remainder were mainly Protestant, Roman Catholic, or Greek Catholic (see Appendix A).

While it is evident that factors other than religious beliefs are important in the quality of life of suffering bodies, religious beliefs seemed to be an important coping strategy in experiences of illness. While it should not be assumed, even in a "Christian nation" such as Romania, that all are indeed Christians, care-providers or counselors need to be willing to address issues related to religion and spirituality (Spitznagel, 1997). Providers of health or mental care have, at times, tried to avoid religious and spiritual issues, categorizing them as personal beliefs with little therapeutic value (Koenig & Larson, 2001). However, a careful assessment of the cultural variables that affect rare disease patients could lead to the development of appropriate goals that incorporate clients' religious and spiritual beliefs (or lack thereof) into intervention plans.

Second, the study also indicated that rare disease patients who perceived lower health levels were more willing to attend religious services (see Appendix B).

It is highly possible that participation in religious services could provide social support and create a context for significant interactions with others. Such interactions have the potential to enrich life and provide a sense of new meaning in the face of suffering (Sermabeikian, 1994). Research suggest that actively belonging to a religious group may offer a spiritual basis for life meaning and a place for receiving support from others—factors known to potentially reduce and protect against depression (McCullough & Larson, 1999). Studies also show that it might be the religious behavior of the tightly bound community that explains the benefits of participation in religious congregations, and not the religious congregations themselves. Wiltermuth and Heath (2009), in a rare experimental study of religious behavior (rather than religious belief), demonstrated that groups of study participants who sang or moved their arms in synchrony with each other showed greater cooperation, trust, and self-sacrifice compared to groups engaging in the same behaviors but not in synchrony. Such collective and harmonious behavior—often found in religious ritual—might function to instill belief and then bind people together in that belief.

Third, higher levels of spirituality and meaningful life positively correlated with optimism (see Appendices C and D).

Facing an illness that magnifies the fragility of existence can lead suffering bodies to question the purpose of life. Spirituality and the sense that life has meaning can provide rare disease patients with the opportunity to develop a personal symbolic visualization of a higher power. This manifestation of spirituality has the potential to help them look beyond their immediate circumstances and find optimism and courage in dealing with the painful emotions that often accompany illness (Bormann et al., 2006; Gordon et al., 2002). Sometimes, spirituality needs to be examined alone, so that those who do not subscribe to denominational religious beliefs, but who have spiritual beliefs and practices are not excluded (Peterman et al., 2002); but in the present study spirituality coexisted with religiosity, as all respondents belonged to a religious tradition.

Finally, results show that belief in heaven, afterlife, and/or God can lead to greater life satisfaction (see Appendix E).

While some people suffering from a chronic illness may have anger toward God, or may view their illness as a form of punishment (Weaver et al., 2006), others may derive hope and strength from their religious beliefs. For example, Koenig and Larson (2001) found that religious beliefs centering on compassion, caring, hope, forgiveness, and transcendent meaning provided an optimistic worldview and a better perception of well-being in the midst of illness symptoms. Thus, when religious views begin to hinder the ability to cope with illness, a suffering body may need assistance in order to challenge or redirect his or her reasoning. Other times, a suffering body may need sensitive and non-indoctrinating spiritual or religious guidance in order to find ways to enhance spiritual balance and improve his or her overall quality of life (Adegbola, 2006).

However, a word of caution is in order: religious beliefs might not give us the whole story when it comes to optimism or life-satisfaction. For example, Brooks reported that religious practice (i.e. religious attendance or prayer) and not religious affiliation (i.e. specific doctrines or beliefs) better explained the consistent research findings across numerous studies regarding the robust relationship between religiosity and self-reported happiness, optimism, or life-satisfaction (as cited in Graham & Haidt, 2010, p. 145). Also, specific research evidence presented by Graham and Haidt showed that social religious practices (i.e. attendance at communal worship) were better predictors for attitudes and behaviors than were individual practices (i.e. individual prayer). As a result, when individuals are confronted with threats such as chronic or life-threatening illness, the source of life-satisfaction may come from the benefits of group membership. Consistent with this line of argument, Diener and Seligman (2002) found that when social relationships were controlled for, religiosity showed no unique prediction of well-being.

ILLNESS NARRATIVES: HOW RELIGIOUS SYMBOLS AND METAPHORS EXPLAIN AND SHAPE PERCEPTIONS OF SUFFERING

In addition to the survey, 25 respondents were asked to write a personal illness narrative. No instructions were provided regarding the expected form, length, or content of these narratives; thus participants were completely free to take any approach deemed appropriate. An analysis of these narratives indicated that rare disease patients often use religious symbols and metaphors in describing their experiences of suffering and illness. While some symbols and metaphors served to reinforce widely shared values of the community regarding illness and health, others challenged the uncritical acceptance of messages about the suffering body.

The most common religious symbols used by rare disease patients or their caregivers in describing experiences and perceptions of suffering were: "the cross," "rainbow," "angel," "saint," "miracle," and "prayer." Also, the most common metaphors used were: "rebirth," "seeing the light," "the Author of my life," "a test from God," "fight for your soul," and "only God can keep the torch of hope alive." Overall, the illness narratives illustrate the role of religious language on the coping strategies of patients and their power in shaping and perpetuating perceptions of illness.

ILLNESS NARRATIVES AS ILLUSTRATIONS OF SOCIAL PERCEPTIONS OF HEALTH AND ILLNESS

Regarding social perceptions of health and illness there were three main findings that emerged from the narratives. First of all, respondents suggested that the problem of disability might be primarily in the perceptions of the viewer or the eye of the beholder. Contemporary disability studies scholars argue that "the stare" or the intrusive gaze of a viewer often objectifies the person being stared at (Belser, 2011, p. 5). For example, the mother of a child suffering from a rare skin condition called epidermolysis bullosa, a connective tissue disease that causes blisters in the skin and mucosal membranes, notes:

> It is very sad when you walk on the street and people stare at him like he's some kind of freak. Why is it that man is judged by his appearance and not his soul?...Why are we afraid and pity the one who's body is covered in horrible blisters, when we should fear and pity those [that stare]...I believe that without God we can do nothing. Each person, at birth, receives a cross, and the moment I realized that this was my cross I began to carry it with hope and now I just keep moving forward.

Although the mother suggested that it was the "visible flaws" that were considered unacceptable or undesirable by an "ableist" visual culture, she also felt that it was her "cross" to bear, choosing a religious symbol of suffering and redemption in explaining her experience with suffering. Another example of how "the stare" creates what Garland-Thomson (2000) calls a ritual of exclusion is given by a respondent suffering from a rare skin condition called hereditary angioedema:

> The hardest times were, and still are, when my face and neck start swelling. Ever since I was little, I had to deal with this hardship. I often missed school, and when I became a young lady I rarely left the house due to my swelling ... I didn't even dare to find a job...This illness has affected my entire life, and

even now when I'm 50 years old, I stay isolated when my face is swollen so that no one will stare at me.

What becomes evident in "the stare" is that the suffering body itself is not the main source of the problem, but the disabling gaze of the community forces the disabled body to bear the emotional burden with the real-life consequences of exclusion:

> My school teacher once hit me because she didn't know what was happening to me, she was probably frightened by my symptoms. Ever since then, I began to be ashamed of my illness, and I'm still ashamed at the age of 48. They never knew what treatment to give me, and every time I was admitted to the hospital, they tried a different medication. I gave up going to the doctor, knowing that I have no chance of getting better. [The illness] affected my life greatly as I never had a job, I was sick on a weekly basis, and because of my face swelling I had to hide. I could not allow anyone to see me, because they would laugh. Someone once saw me and said that I have leprosy, a very shameful disease, and so I am very embarrassed of my appearance. I no longer have hope of ever healing, especially since they haven't discovered the type of illness I have...

It is possible that the respondent equated leprosy with "a very shameful disease" because of the longstanding link between divine punishment and visible physical suffering. For example, traditionally lepers were cast out of society and expected to repent for the sins believed to be the cause of the illness. Thus, the internalization of this discourse by a suffering body serves to further reinforce the widely shared religious values of the community regarding visible signs of illness as markers of sin.

The second finding regarding illness narratives as illustrations of social perceptions of illness and health was that suffering was seen to emerge either as a result of divine punishment for the sins of the sufferer (or his/her parents) or as a test of one's faith. For example, a parent recalled how a doctor assumed that the newborn's disease of hypotonia, a genetic disease involving decreased muscle tone, was a consequence of the "sin" of an unsuccessful abortion:

> Two days after I gave birth, the pediatrician came to ask me if I've done something wrong during pregnancy, by which he meant if I've tried to have an abortion. When he understood that I certainly did not, he said: "Mother dear, the child has problems, he has muscular hypotonia, he will never walk and will end up eating from garbage cans!" When I heard him, I froze, and then I fainted. Later I talked to my husband and we decided to look for a specialist in genetics as soon as I will leave the maternity hospital.

> Some parents suggested that the illness was "decided" by God, and as such any attempt in finding a cure was futile: " ...all around us, society tries to blame us, the parents because they don't understand... that what God decided not to provide at conception, no one can go back and correct." Others questioned this discourse, wondering if there was indeed a divine Author of one's life: "When

he [the doctor] showed me the papers [with the diagnosis]...I went numb, and then I began to wonder: 'Who is the Author of my life?' "

In some narratives, parents described the experience of having a healthy child as "a great joy" or "beautiful dream" that becomes a "nightmare" after finding out about the illness. The condition was not seen as simply an expression of the various possibilities inherent in a physical body, and as a result, respondents often tried to find some reason or purpose for the suffering such as "a test from God":

> Ten years ago there was great joy in our family. Through providence we were given a second child. We already had a 5 year old girl and we felt so proud as parents. That beautiful dream turned into a nightmare .... We didn't know why our child suffered from this disease .... It's probably a test from God, or a genetic accident.

Only as a last possibility was the illness perceived as an "accident" and rarely as a positive gift from God, which introduces the third finding from the illness narratives. In some cases, symbols and metaphors served to challenge the uncritical acceptance of messages about the suffering body. Some of these examples emerged as participants began to describe in great detail the disturbing odyssey through the Romanian health-care system. For example, the mother of a child diagnosed with Prader–Willi Syndrome—a rare genetic disorder accompanied by a chronic feeling of hunger that can lead to excessive eating and life-threatening obesity—painfully described the sudden death of her daughter. In her narrative she argues that the death of her "angel" was an unfortunate consequence of late diagnosis (at the age of 28) and inadequate medical care. She described the experience as follows: "That night, with me next to her pillow, Maria died. I tried to resuscitate her, I begged all the saints not to take her away, but it wasn't so. The angels took my angel away..."

A common complaint was that the health-care system functioned as an authoritarian institution with a patronizing attitude. Some respondents critiqued the common perceptions of suffering bodies, defiantly maintaining that "there is more than one way to be whole" (Koosed & Schumm, 2011, p. 91). Some examples of narratives that used metaphorical language to challenge common and stereotypical perceptions of illness:

> I am a normal individual. I am already 40 years old, I look normal, go to work, socialize, walk in the rain, laugh, cry, and all this until a new attack...then I'm back into the hospital.... For three years I've been a "rare" human being diagnosed with acute intermittent porphyria [a rare metabolic disorder], an illness that I spent hours researching on the internet.... On the [hospital's] staircase a little boy tells his mom: "When we get home, I can have chicken nuggets with fries, right?"... He also has a peripheral cannula in his hand ... like the rest of us... In the hospital special friendships are weaved with SPE-CIAL, EXTRAORDINARY [respondent's emphasis] people... some suffering from cirrhosis, others from cancer... We talk and joke about all of us being on

a diet but dreaming of cake "hhmmm"... In the hospital yard there is a small wooden church... On a Sunday, during the Holy Service... during a hospital stay... I managed to attend ... I will never forget it... Half of those present in church were dressed in hospital gowns, with cannullas in their hands... Some with a headscarf... they lost their hair during chemo... I also lost a lot of hair... just like them, I don't know how long I've got left... Any attack could be fatal... I have been able to trick death for three years now... I trick the illness and the hospital, too... I don't like that I have my own hospital bed on reserve, I just have to call and there it is ... my bed... I don't like and I don't want to see the pity in my family's gaze... but for now I'm busy living... until one day... And that's my illness narrative. I still hope that the Romanian health care authorities will realize that we are just another distinct color of the rainbow, and that we are a normal part of earthly life's décor.

Another said,

I want to talk about social integration, or rather about the way that people and doctors treat those that are different from what is considered "normal" due to an illness that you are not responsible for or that you haven't chosen at birth, but one that was set apart for you ... It's important to be mentally tough and to demonstrate through your will power that we are all equal and able to achieve the same things in life only some of us need a little more attention and care [until we get there]. I believe that all those that are disabled in some way have very sensitive souls that find it hard to step upon others for personal gain. I think it is an irony of chance that my childhood dream was to become a doctor. I probably imagined that I would be better equipped to treat myself efficiently and competently.

Many participants stressed that "normal" does not equate "able" and that the "disabled" should not be "pitied" but accepted as normal but "extraordinary" just like "another distinct color of the rainbow"—a religious symbol of God's faithfulness.

The Religious Language of Coping Illustrated by Illness Narratives

Religious symbols and metaphors were also used by participants to illustrate ways of coping with illness and suffering. Many participants used religious language to describe how grateful they were to find encouragement through support groups:

As time passed, year after year the illness progressed causing greater suffering, and so my feelings of helplessness in front of this uncaring fate intensified... Until one day when all seemed brighter, the sky looked cloudless and fate proved more generous. I was lucky to meet other parents experiencing similar situations, people that shared some of the same feelings and hardships as me. It was like a rebirth, a relief, a starting point in the healing process.... [With encouragement] I decided to try different treatment plans... It was almost

impossible, terribly difficult financially and practically, and when I was on the
verge of giving up, we began to see results. It was for the first time in many years
filled with hardship and suffering . . . The joy of salvation was a new feeling for
our family that has stopped hoping for miracles.

It was evident that support groups helped foster interpersonal bonding and
provided hope and direction to participants; to the point that sometimes the
experience is described in religious terminology as "rebirth." Also, symptomatic or pain control treatment was seen as "miraculous," by those who
had to survive many years without adequate medical care or even a correct
diagnosis. Miracles were oftentimes reinterpreted as states of mind such as joy
or "being at peace with oneself" or "having a thankful attitude" or "keeping
the torch of hope alive." Thus, miracles were no longer perceived as extraordinary divine acts that defied natural laws and were beyond human control,
but rather as daily experiences, reachable and attainable by all those who
"know where to look." Consider, for example, the following extract from an
illness narrative:

All miracles that happen in daily life are under God's control. There is happiness
inside all of us, and it is up to us to know where to look and learn to keep it!
To be happy, you need to know how to fight for your soul and also forgive
because hate will destroy your soul! To know how to rejoice in all that you
have, and consider that others have less than you do, and learn to be at peace
with yourself and those around you . . . . and above all thank the Good Lord
for only God can keep the torch of hope alive!

Many participants believed that happiness did not depend on "outside circumstances" but on "inside interpretations." This belief was sometimes
characterized by religious and spiritual metaphors such as "the light of day"
or "my angel among the starry night":

When I gave birth to Dany, I felt as if the world collapsed and that no one will
be able to push away the clouds of sadness and despair from my life! I was so
unhappy that I used to walk around random streets with tears streaming down
my cheeks, and I couldn't stop them. But God, in his power allowed me to
finally discover happiness. She was in my reach, but I didn't notice before: [hap-
piness was] MY CHILDREN [respondent's emphasis] . . . Having my beautiful
and smart children around me made me happy. I'm happy that I can see the
light of day every morning and that I'm able to say my prayers at night, all the
while searching for my angel up in the starry night.

Only four out of the 25 participants regarded suffering as a positive experience. Sometimes the illness was perceived to serve some useful pedagogical
purpose. For example, a sufferer of myasthenia gravis, an autoimmune neu-
romuscular disease leading to fluctuating muscle weakness and fatigability,
believed that illness helped make her stronger:

I am a normal human being, not more special than the next person. I help others as much as I'm able, without making a big deal of it. The fact that I've been through many tribulations in life has helped make me stronger. At 50 years old I feel young and open to new experiences. I feel that I am able to start over and over again and although life has not given me the chance to do all I wanted, I did what I could, as well as I could. I can now say that I feel complete and able.

Others noted additional benefits of "befriending" the disease such as: the opportunity of meeting "special people," learning to be kind to oneself, being more patient, and better equipped to understand other sufferers:

I finally got to the point that I learned to befriend my disease. I know my disease and I no longer fight my disabled body. When I have difficult days, I rest and I'm kind with myself... My disease has taught me to be patient and to better understand those that are sick. I am glad that my parents have not allowed me to despair and they literally pushed me outside, didn't allow me to stay isolated, and made me socialize as much as I could. My family supported and helped me. My friends were tested, and only the true ones remained. Because of my disease I got to know special people. Looking back I can say that illness has brought me good things and not only suffering. And suffering can be forgotten when you have good people close by and when you find a treatment to control the pain.

While experiencing suffering some tried to find comfort in their religious faith, hoping for a "visible" divine reward of one's faith: "The Bible says that to have faith means to believe in what you don't see, and I hope that the reward for this faith will be to see what you believe."

Others seem content only with finding some meaning or purpose to the illness, as the grandmother who concludes her narrative in the following way:

It's not easy, but with a sustained social effort, love, and understanding we might find that drop of satisfaction and fulfillment, that I believe signifies true happiness... with the help of God Almighty we might one day come to think that all of this was worth it.

Conclusion

This chapter explored how common religious beliefs and practices, symbols and metaphors impacted the coping strategies both of individuals with rare diseases and of their families.

First, an analysis of survey responses showed that the religious beliefs of Romanian rare disease patients seemed to be an important coping strategy in their experiences of suffering. For example, those respondents who perceived lower health levels were more willing to attend religious services. This participation could be explained as a coping strategy that provided suffering bodies with needed social support and a context for significant interactions with others. More research is needed to determine if patients who are less religious may find that same benefit in support groups or other meaningful social connections. Also, participants who believed that spirituality and life-meaning could provide them with a better understanding of illness reported more optimism toward the future. Survey results also indicated that participants who reported believing in heaven, afterlife, and God showed greater life satisfaction.

Second, analysis of illness narratives revealed that rare disease patients often used religious symbols and metaphors when describing their experiences of suffering. While using religious language, some respondents internalized and reinforced the widely shared values of the community regarding illness and health. Others challenged the uncritical acceptance of messages about the suffering body, choosing to argue that "normal" is not synonymous with "able" and that the "disabled body" should be perceived as "normal" but "distinct" just like another "color of the rainbow." A person's interpretation of his or her own illness narrative played an important role in how suffering is conceptualized, understood, and experienced. Furthermore, societal perceptions of illness and health can determine how persons affected by chronic disease are treated or mistreated by the larger society and how people with chronic disease perceive their treatment by others. Most importantly, the metaphorical representations of illness often set the stage for further social implications, functioning to shape and reflect the values of a particular community, which had real-life consequences regarding social labeling and self-exclusion.

As a final word, we do not view this chapter as a comprehensive representation on the role of religious beliefs, rituals, and metaphors on the coping strategies of rare diseases patients in Romania. Rather, this study should be understood as a first attempt to bring the voices of the Romanian rare disease patients to the table, in the hope that future dialogue will help expand our understanding of this important subject.

APPENDIX A: RELIGIOUS AFFILIATION OF STUDY PARTICIPANTS

	Frequency	%
Orthodox	480	80.13
Neo-Protestant	55	9.18
Roman Catholic	26	4.34
Greek Catholic	16	2.67
Reformed	8	1.33
Jehovah's Witness	2	.33
Muslim	1	.16
Total valid answers	588	98.16
Missing responses	11	1.83
Total	599	100.0

Appendix B: Church Participation and Subjective Perception of Health

		Frequency of church participation					
		Not at all	Yearly	Monthly	Weekly	Multiple times a week	Total
Perceived health*	Excellent	0	1	2	0	1	4
	Very good	0	4	6	3	0	13
	Good	6	18	34	20	8	86
	With ups and downs	32	70	87	48	9	246
	Poor	30	80	81	41	5	237
Missing responses							13
Total		68	173	210	112	23	599

*Due to a high number of null responses, a frequency analysis was preferred. The data indicates that most respondents (35.8 percent) fall into the category of the "church-goers," meaning that they were present in church for at least once a month at the time of the study. Also, those who participated in church services perceived their health as being "with ups and downs" (41.4 percent) or poor (38.6 percent).

**Even though all respondents were diagnosed with a rare disease, and as such their health was not "objectively" excellent or very good, some reported perceiving such great levels of health. These answers, however, should be understood as meaning "the absence of symptomatic pain" or a "disease that does not interfere with daily activities/overall functioning" and not "the absence or denial of illness."

Appendix C: Spirituality and Self-reported Optimism of Study Participants

		Spirituality as coping strategy in illness					Total
		Very high	High	Moderate	Low	Very	
Self-reported optimism	Very high	36	24	4	2	3	69
	High	43	52	23	5	3	126
	Moderate	40	74	43	7	1	165
	Low	18	67	87	10	3	185
	Very low	5	7	4	2	2	20
Missing responses							34
Total		142	224	161	26	12	599

Appendix D: Perception of Meaningful Life and Self-reported Optimism of Study Participants

		Meaningful life					Total
		Very high	High	Moderate	Low	Very	
Self-reported optimism	Very high	39	26	1	1	1	68
	High	45	62	19	0	1	127
	Moderate	22	81	48	10	0	161
	Low	11	61	97	10	2	181
	Very low	2	7	5	5	1	20
Missing responses							42
Total		119	237	170	26	5	557

The association between the optimism and meaningful life is significant, with the value of Somers' d coefficient of 0.421, at a significance level of $p < 0.01$. Regarding the association between optimism and spirituality as a coping strategy in illness, the value of Somers' d coefficient is 0.279, and the level of significance $p < 0.01$.

APPENDIX E: BELIEF IN HEAVEN, AFTERLIFE, AND/OR GOD, AND SELF-REPORTED LIFE SATISFACTION OF STUDY PARTICIPANTS

		Belief in heaven		Total	Belief in afterlife		Total	Belief in God		Total
		yes	no		yes	no		yes	no	
Self-reported life	Very high	18	4	22	18	4	22	20	2	570
satisfaction	High	172	7	179	165	14	179	179	2	22
	Moderate	145	6	151	139	12	151	153	1	570
	Low	124	13	137	108	23	131	135	1	22
	Very low	68	16	84	63	20	83	83	1	570
Total valid answers		527	46	573	493	73	566	570	7	577
Missing responses				26			33			22
Total				599			599			599

The contingency coefficients gave statistically significant values. First, for the association between the belief in heaven and perceived life satisfaction, the contingency coefficient value was 0.208 ($p < 0.01$). Second, for the association between the belief in an afterlife and perceived life satisfaction, the contingency coefficient value was 0.184 ($p < 0.01$). Finally, for the association between belief in God and perceived life satisfaction, a contingency coefficient of 0.145 ($p < 0.05$) was obtained.

NOTES

1. The results reported in this section are based on a research published in 2012. For a more in-depth presentation of the study, including more detailed statistical analysis, see Popoviciu, S., Birle, D. Olah, S., & Popoviciu, I. (2012). The role of religious beliefs and spirituality on the quality of life of rare disease patients. *Review of Research and Social Intervention* 36, 144–161.
2. The research project that is reported in this chapter was funded by the Norwegian-Romanian Partnership for Progress in Rare Diseases; research contract No._197_/07.05.2010. The authors would also like to thank Ms. Dorica Dan, founder and president of Prader Willi Association, for the invaluable help in granting access to patients and their families.

REFERENCES

Adegbola, M. A. (2006). Spirituality and quality of life in chronic illness. *Journal of Theory Construction & Testing*, 6(2), 42–46.

Allport, G. W., & Ross, J. M. (1967). Personal religious orientation and prejudice. *Journal of Personality and Social Psychology*, 5, 432–443.

Batson, C. D. (1976). Religion as prosocial: Agent or double agent? *Journal for the Scientific Study of Religion*, 15, 29–45.

Belser, J. W. (2011). Reading Talmudic bodies: Disability, narrative, and the gaze in Rabbinic Judaism. In D. Schumm & M. Stoltzfus (Eds.), *Disability in Judaism, Christianity, and Islam: Sacred texts, historical traditions, and social analysis*. New York: Palgrave MacMillan, 5–27.

Bishop, M. (2005). Quality of life and psychosocial adaptation to chronic illness and disability: Preliminary analysis of a conceptual and theoretical synthesis. *Rehabilitation, Counseling Bulletin, 48,* 219–231.

Bormann, J. E., Gifford, A. L., Shively, M., Smith, T. L., Redwine, L., Kelly, A., & Belding, W. (2006). Effects of spiritual mantram repetition on HIV outcomes: A randomized controlled trial. *Journal of Behavioral Medicine, 29,* 359–376.

Bria, I. (1991). *The sense of ecumenical tradition. The ecumenical witness and vision of the Orthodox.* Geneva: WCC Publications.

Bria, I. (1999). Evangelism, Proselytism, and religious freedom in Romania: An orthodox point of view. *Journal of Ecumenical Studies, 36,* 163–176.

Burckhardt, C. S., & Anderson K. L. (2003). The quality of life scale (QOLS): Reliability, validity and utilization. *Health and Quality of Life Outcomes, 1*(60). doi: 10.1186/14777525-1-60.

Diener, E., & Seligman, M. E. P. (2002). Very happy people. *Psychological Science, 13,* 81–84.

Garland-Thomson, R. (2000). Staring back: Self-representations of disabled performance artists. *American Quarterly, 52*(2), 334–338.

Gog, S. (2006). The construction of the religious space in post-socialist Romania. *Journal for the Study of Religions and Ideologies, 15,* 37–53.

Gordon, P. A., Feldman, D., Crose, R., Schoen, E., Griffing, G., & Shankar, J. (2002). The role of religious beliefs in coping with chronic illness. *Counseling and Values, 46*(3), 162–174.

Graham, J. & Haidt, J. (2010). Beyond beliefs: Religions bind individuals into moral communites. *Personality and Social Psychology Review, 14*(1), 140–150.

Haffner, M. E. (2006). Adopting orphan drugs: Two dozen years of treating rare diseases. *The New England Journal of Medicine, 354,* 445–447.

Haffner, M. E., Whitley, J., & Moses, M. (2002). Two decades of orphan product development. *Nature Reviews Drug Discovery, 1,* 821–825.

Haidt, J., Seder, J. P., & Kesebir, S. (2008). Hive psychology, happiness, and public policy. *Journal of Legal Studies, 37,* S133–S156.

Harakas, S. (1999). The orthodox Christian tradition: Religious beliefs and heathcare decisions. In *Religious traditions and healthcare decisions.* Chicago, IL: Park Ridge Center for the Study of Heath, Faith and Ethics.

Hatfield, C. (2006). Sin, sickness, and salvation. *Christian Bioethics, 12,* 199–211.

Kelly, E. W., Jr. (1995). *Spirituality and religion in counseling and psychotherapy: Diversity in theory and practice.* Alexandria, VA: American Counseling Association.

Koenig, H. G., George L. K. & Siegler, I. C. (1988). The use of religion and other emotion-regulating coping strategies among older adults. *The Gerontologist, 28,* 303–310.

Koenig, H. G., & Larson, D. B. (2001). Religion and mental health: Evidence for an association. *International Review of Psychiatry, 13*(2), 67–78.

Koosed, J. L., & Schumm, D. (2011). Out of the darkness: Examining the Retoric of blindness in the Gospel of John. In D. Schumm & M. Stoltzfus (Eds.), *Disability in Judaism, Christianity, and Islam: Sacred texts, historical traditions, and social analysis.* New York: Palgrave MacMillan, 77–92.

Lossky, V. (1978). *Orthodox theology: An introduction.* New York: St. Vladimir's Seminary Press.

Mantzaridis, G. I. (1984). *The deification of man.* New York: St. Vladimir's Seminary Press.

McCullough, M. E., & Larson, D. B. (1999). Religion and depression: A review of the literature. *Twin Research*, *2*, 126–136.

Mickley, J. R., Carson, V., & Soeken, K. L. (1995). Religion and adult mental health: State of the science in nursing. *Issues in Mental Health Nursing*, *16*, 345–360.

National Plan of Rare Diseases in Romanian (2010–2014). Online at: http://nestor.orpha.net/EUCERD/upload/file/Docs/ROPlan_ro.pdf (Retrieved on October 12, 2011).

Negrut, P. (1996). *Revelatie, Scriptura, Comuniune*. Oradea: Editura Cartea Crestina.

Norris, P., & Inglehart, R. (2003). *Sacred and secular*. Cambridge: Cambridge University Press.

Payton, J. R., Jr. (2007). *Light from the Christian East. An introduction to the orthodox tradition*. Illinois: IVP Academic, Downers Grove.

Peterman, A. H., Fitchett, D. G., Brady, M. J., Hernandez, L., & Cella, D. (2002). Measuring spiritual well-being in people with cancer: The functional assessment of chronic illness therapy-spiritual well-being scale (FACIT-Sp). *Annals of Behavioral Medicine*, *24*(1), 49–58.

Public Opinion Barometer (2005). Religiozitate si relatia cu Dumnezeu. Fundatia Pentru o Societate Deschisa. Online at: http://www.soros.ro/ro/fisier_publicatii.php?publicatie=12 (Retrieved on: December 21, 2011).

Sandor, S. D. & Popescu, M. (2008). Religiosity and values in Romania. *Transylvanian Review of Administrative Sciences*, *22*(E), 171–180.

Sawatzky, R., Ratner, P.A., & Chiu, L. (2005). A meta-analysis of the relationship between spirituality and quality of life. *Social Indicators Research*, *72*, 153–188.

Schumm, D. & Stoltzfus, M. (Eds.). (2011). *Disability in Judaism, Christianity, and Islam: Sacred texts, historical traditions, and social analysis*. New York: Palgrave MacMillan.

Sermabeikian, P. (1994). Our clients, ourselves: The spiritual perspective and social work practice. *Social Work*, *39*, 178–183.

Spitznagel, R. J. (1997). Spirituality in work adjustment: A dimension to be considered. *Vocational Evaluation and Work Adjustment Bulletin*, *30*, 111–117.

Tanyi, R. A. (2002). Towards clarification of the meaning of spirituality. *Journal of Advanced Nursing*, *39*, 500–509.

Voicu, M. (2007). *Romania religioasa*. Iasi: Editura Institutului European.

Weaver, A. J., Pargament, K. I., Flannelly, K. J., & Oppenheimer, J. E. (2006). Trends in the scientific study of religion, spirituality, and health: 1965–2000. *Journal of Religion and Health*, *45*, 208–214.

Wiltermuth, S. S., & Heath, C. (2009). Synchrony and cooperation. *Psychological Science*, *20*, 1–5.

CHAPTER 10

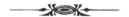

NATIVE AMERICAN ISSUES INVOLVING DIABETES AND BALANCE

Lavonna L. Lovern and Danielle R. Costello

According to the United Nations and the International Diabetes Federation, "50% of Indigenous adults over 35 have type 2 diabetes" (United Nations, 2010;). The American Diabetes Association (1995–2012) confirms the concerns with statements claiming that rates of diabetes are four times higher among Indigenous demographics than non-Indigenous. According to the Indian Health Services (IHS) "Facts At-a-Glance," American Indian and Alaska Natives between 10 and 19 years of age were nine times more likely to be diagnosed with type 2 diabetes than their non-Hispanic White counterparts (Department of Health and Human Services, 2012). Additionally, the IHS points out that the incidence of kidney failure is 1.9 times higher and the death rate due to diabetes is 1.6 times higher for American Indians and Alaska Natives compared to the general American population (Department of Health and Human Services, 2012). Indeed a good deal of diabetes research has focused on the Pima, who have been given the title of "the most diabetic demographic in the world" (Centers for Disease Control, 2011; United Nations, 2009; Smith-Morris, 2006). As indicated by these statements, type 2 diabetes has become an epidemic in Indigenous populations and, as a chronic illness, brings with it not only the daily challenge of stabilizing blood glucose, but also the threat of coma, blindness, amputations, heart attack, kidney failure, and stroke among other conditions. The cost of this epidemic, in terms of wellness and economics, continues to deplete the resources of both individuals and communities. The historic trajectory of the diabetes epidemic, in the United States, has a striking correlation to timelines reflecting the destruction

of Indigenous communities as a result of colonization and assimilation practices. In order to better explain the correlation, this chapter will be divided
into three sections representing the loss of balance, the continued imbalance,
and the potential of returning to balance; representing the past, present, and
future, respectively. This chronology has been used to reveal an aspect of diabetes care, and indeed chronic illness care in general, that is often overlooked
by Western medical practitioners. The overlooked aspect of care is that along
with the loss of traditional communities, the Native American people experienced a loss of self. The importance of the relationship involving the self
and the community is more significant than is often understood, when considering the loss of heritage or traditions, from a Western perspective. As
will be explored in the chronologically organized past, present, and future
sections of this chapter, the unraveling of community and self has devastating
effects on the wellness of both. For wellness to occur in the self, the element
of community must be present. In the case of chronic illnesses such as diabetes, community becomes even more essential. The emphasis of this chapter
is on discussing the interwoven nature of community and individual as they
function to define the self and are required for wellness.

METHOD

A reference as to the method involved in this chapter is required. This project
began with typical academic research, the searching of libraries and scholarly
articles. The search, of official national and international governmental sites,
was conducted to glean relevant information. However, what surfaced immediately was the one-sided nature of this research. The numbers, "officially
recorded" history, and academic/governmental opinions were easy enough
to find, but what was missing were the voices of the Indigenous people.
The more research was done, the more glaring the problem became. In an
effort to rectify what appeared to be an outsider's perspective of the diabetic epidemic in Indigenous cultures, contact was made with various Native
Americans by phone and email. Originally, the idea was to create a formal
structure of questions in an academic model. However, the conversations
became a narrative in themselves. So, setting aside any standard "academic
research model," the discussion was simply allowed to grow in the form of
fluid narrative. The first contacts were with people known to have worked in
Native American health and rehabilitation programs for most of their adult
lives. The idea was to ask these people to assist in the collection of relevant
data. However, it was readily evident that these people were themselves the
wealth of knowledge and experience necessary to understand the impact of
chronic illness in Native American communities, as well as the frontlines in
the battle against the epidemic. Reflected in this chapter is then a selection
of comments from those conversations, some of which were individual and
others in groups. The names and tribes have been left out in order to allow
the respondents to continue their work. The first contacts then went into various communities and gained further information through discussions. This

information was reported back without the identifying features. While only a beginning, it is hoped that this chapter will offer a glimpse into the lives of those devoted to assisting Native Americans with chronic illnesses such as type 2 diabetes.

During these discussions, one individual, who dedicated her life to the people and to health-care issues, succumbed to the effects of type 2 diabetes. It is to Mittie Wood (Mvskoke) that this work is dedicated. Her dedication to the health and well-being of her community and to those in need reflect the balance that will be discussed later. While she dealt with the challenges of type 2 diabetes, she remained an inspiration to others. A discussion of her passing and the beauty that surrounded her life began many of the conversations represented in this narrative. Thanks should also be given to Carol Locust (Eastern Cherokee), Mekko Jerry Lang (Mvskoke), and the dozens of Indigenous people who offered their wisdom to this project. These comments involved individuals in communities that include and were identified as being members of the following; Hopi, Navajo, Apache, Pima, Yaqui, Tohono O'odham, Seminole, Cherokee, Mvskoke, Akwesasne Mohawk, Tobique, Maliseet, Micmac, and Penobscott. Many of the dialogues involved Carol Locust and/or myself at various times. Interestingly, once the initial calls and emails were put out, the discussion took on a life of its own and spread from community to community, bringing together the voices of concern about diabetes in Native American communities It appears that while they are rarely asked their opinions regarding type 2 diabetes and other chronic illness, the Indigenous people have valuable experience and knowledge about it.

BALANCE

Before moving to the participants' discussions of diabetes, a brief review of basic Indigenous cosmologies is necessary. While cosmology in the United States primarily devotes itself, since the enlightenment, to a mechanistic model, Indigenous models require the elements of spirit and community. Additionally, in establishing these as present and significant elements within the universe, Indigenous cosmologies do not partition the non-mechanistic and the mechanistic aspects of existence. Instead, the sacred and the secular are intertwined in such a way as to be separable only in an abstract manner. For this reason, all things participate in both the sacred and the secular, which is especially important for the maintenance of balance. In fact, the concept of "balance" involves just that, the balancing of all elements into a harmonious state. This harmonious state is then represented as "wellness." What follows in this section is a very brief and limited discussion of balance. The discussion is no more than an introduction of basic concepts that would require additional study for a complete understanding. However, establishing some basic ideas involving cosmology is essential in order to understand the diabetes epidemic that is occurring in Indigenous communities. It must be noted that any cosmological information or discussions of wellness and balance are generalized. Given the number of global Indigenous communities and the inability to represent each one individually, generalizations are made with the understanding that generalizations should never be considered universals. Additionally, each community has a specific history, culture, and set of sacred beliefs, meaning that what is represented here should not be taken as a descriptor of any specific Indigenous community. Each community is unique and therefore may or may not fall within the realm of these generalizations. Moreover, within each community, clans and individuals differ on perspectives and opinions. Issues of assimilation as well as reservation verses non-reservation status add complexity to differences of understanding. Indeed, much discussion, both internally and externally, surrounds the question of descent. These issues, while recognized here, do not fit within the parameters of this project and so will be left to other venues. Additionally, the terms "Native American" and "Indigenous" will be used, with the understanding that these terms carry with them a plethora of unresolved issues. These terms will refer to pre-contact people, and their descendants, within North America, again with the understanding of the terminological issues involved in doing so. The concepts of balance to be discussed are therefore a compilation of ideas generalized from discussions and research, which represent a family of concepts rather than a detailed description of any one specific family member.

To begin, the reason for discussing "balance" is the place the term holds in Indigenous cosmologies. While the term "spirituality" is not unheard of in Indigenous cultures, it is not used in the same way as it is used in the communities that focus on the religions of Abraham. Spirituality, in Indigenous cosmologies, is not a duality of body and soul, nor does it involve only an internal or other-worldly human aspect. Indigenous cosmologies require the entire human to be whole, which requires the balance of all aspects of the individual. The individual self is then constructed of body, mind, and soul, but these are incomplete. The fourth aspect of the self is community. Instead of using the term "spirituality," with all the attached Western constructs, the term "balance" is more fitting for discussions of wellness. One should be cautioned in using the terms interchangeably since the Western and Indigenous cosmologies are not interchangeable. However, given the project of this text, one would certainly be encouraged to keep the two terms in mind as they function in their respective cosmologies.

Discussions involving concepts of balance can be found in readings including Cajete (2000, 2004), Basso (2000), and Mankiller and Wallis (1993) among others. The understanding of balance itself is both vastly complex and comparatively simple as is the case with most theories. The sentiment can be stated in phrases such as "living in harmony with all my relations" or "living in peace and beauty." However, as anyone who has tried to analyze these statements can attest, such statements represent unfathomable depths that one could spend a lifetime pondering. Indeed, among the Indigenous participants in this discussion, spending a lifetime pondering balance, and attempting to come to balance, should be the focus of life itself, both for the individual and for the community.

There are many ways to discuss balance depending on the context. The context of this discussion involves coping with chronic illness, specifically type 2 diabetes. For this reason, the aspects of balance to be discussed will involve the self, as that is where diabetes manifests. However, one must refer back to the statement that Indigenous cosmologies necessitate the involvement of the spirit and so the self becomes defined as the interweaving of body, mind, and spirit. Each element must be harmonized, one with the other, to create a balance. This definition, however, is incomplete. There is a fourth element of the self, which in Indigenous cosmologies is also interwoven, and that is community. The understanding is that for balance to occur in the individual, the community must be present. So, community becomes the fourth dimension of the self and if the community is damaged or not present, an imbalance of the self can result.

This aspect of community is understood here to include the broader cosmological concept involving humans and non-humans, ancestors and descendants, members of one's own community and those in other communities as well as entities involving realms such as the spirit. As stated earlier, the ideal of bringing all these aspects together into a tapestry of balance is, at least initially, not a difficult concept to grasp. However, establishing the actuality of the ideal is indeed vastly complex. Balancing the four dimensions of self requires the placing of the self within a network of community members in such a way as to create a positive interconnection among all community members. What may appear to be an impossible ideal or a paradoxical situation, may be better explained by an understanding that the manner in which these elements interact involves a concept of energy and energy transference.

Consider that the relationship among all elements is one of energy. The interaction of the elements then creates positive and negative situation forces, or energies, and these energies impact the balance and therefore the wellness of the self. Given the intricacies of relationships, of all things to all things, care must be given to every action and thought as these create energy that transfers from one relation to another (Cajete, 2000). A seemingly insignificant facial movement or word, of one relation, may have vastly significant consequences for another. Indigenous communities tend to require great care over actions and thoughts because of the potential consequences, both foreseen and unforeseen. The complexity and significance of energy interaction and interdependence are handled in more detail in other works (Cajete, 2000; Lovern & Locust, 2013).

Additionally, balance is not understood as something to be achieved as a final destination. It is not reaching a state of "perfection," but a process. Again, cosmology is significant here in that Indigenous cosmologies do not establish a fixed or static universe. Instead, the universe is in a state of continuous flux, balance is then itself in a constant state of flux (Cajete, 2000). Being able to achieve and maintain balance is often referred to in Indigenous communities as being the companion of wisdom and, in many cases, requiring the benefits of age and experience. Efforts to balance take time and careful attention before they can become "habitual." Indeed, it is often the complexity of constant shift that unmasks those outsiders who usurp Indigenous practices of balance. For those individuals, balance is considered to be a final and continuous state of existence. Cases involving the usurpation of an act, without the understanding of the spirituality or the knowledge behind the act such as a sweat, have proven not only to fail in the achievement of an idyllic state, but also have resulted in tragedy as some recent events illustrate. The Native Americans in this project were clear that no ceremony or ritual can magically catapult an individual into a state of blissful balance. Their position, across the board, was that achieving balance requires efforts that may involve ritual, but requires that these be done in the right way, with the right knowledge. In the case of chronic illness, the need for continuous effort is especially true. Each day, each hour, and even each minute represents a change in the four dimensions of self. As the individual participates in the world, the elements of self, including community, are constantly shifting and energies are constantly changing. The relationships are complex and can on the slightest event throw either the individual or the community, or both, into chaos from which balance must be rebuilt. As can be seen, there is no perfect end state of balance to be achieved and then in which to exist. Instead, the instant that balance is achieved is in the very process of falling away, requiring the self to resume the quest. This chapter focuses on the four-dimensional relationship among mind, body, spirit, and community, all of which are contained within the Indigenous self, as a means to understand wellness. The community element within the self symbolizes what could be considered the potentially paradoxical nature present when visualizing the fourth dimension, a challenge that also exists in Western cosmologies.

Given this concept of balance, wellness in the Indigenous worldview is part of the ebb and flow of balance requiring both individual and community efforts. The need to balance using mind, body, spirit, and community is a concept that tends to diverge from Western descriptions of health, which often leave out the elements of spirit and community. In this Western sense, health is an absence of illness in the body and mind. In an Indigenous sense, wellness allows for the state of living in balance with the illness rather than the elimination of illness, which in the case of chronic illness is not possible. It is not uncommon to hear the phrase "living in harmony with one's illness or disability" as a mode of wellness in Indigenous communities. Illness or disability becomes an aspect of the individual, not the defining factor. These aspects become a part of a person's existence that need to be attended to, but which do not need to consume or overwhelm the self. A chronic illness may even be viewed as an opportunity for the advancement of knowledge and wisdom. As one participant explained, "people of difference are often asked what they learned from the experience to help themselves or others. Or how having a person of difference in your life has taught you great lessons you would not have learned without this person."

In addition to frequently omitting the spiritual aspect of illness, Western communities often place illness in the realm of the individual requiring that person to overcome her illness individually as a show of strength and independence (Marcus & Kitayama, 1991; Thompson, 1997; Wendell, 2008). Indeed, phrases emphasizing "fighting the good fight" or "overcoming the situation" are common in Western communities. In many cases, this individualistic view requires the person with chronic illness to "deal with it in private" or to feel a need to "hide" the situation from others. The Native American participants, in this discussion, talked about the difference in terms of "not hiding away those who have a chronic illness." Some talked of the "shame factor" seen in Western communities if one's body or mind was experiencing a difference. For those "hiding" a situation, the fear of discovery adds additional anxiety, making balance even more elusive. One participant put it in the following terms.

> In the Native community it is known, even if it is not openly discussed, who is having difficulties with health or mind. The members of the family and the neighbors then support the person in ways that do not add to his burden by causing embarrassment, but that give comfort. If the person needs good food, or someone to listen you just do it without calling attention to yourself. Helping each other quietly helps the person find balance.

Another participant stated that

> We need each other, all things, Mother Earth, people, spirit and Creator. All have to work together to help anyone out of sorts or the whole thing is out of whack. So each part has to work to balance itself and the whole has to work together. "All for one and one for all" kind of thing.

The above discussion of the four-dimensional self, as it relates to wellness, sets the stage for the following tripartite exploration of type 2 diabetes in Native American communities. The history of conquest and assimilation fractured the balance of the four dimensions to the point that these communities have yet to recover. The fracturing of the dimensions has splintered individuals and communities like shards from a broken mirror. Unable to reassemble the shards, the communities remain splintered and separated, allowing imbalance to further fracture the four dimensions. The individuals and communities attempting to look into the broken mirror then often see only disconnected beings, images that continue to splinter with each generation. The challenge remains in the attempts to reconstruct some form of the original mirror, or four-dimensional self. Because of lost pieces and "powdered" fracturing, it may not be possible to reassemble the original Native American structures. However, as will be discussed in the last section of this chapter, attempts at reassembly are multiplying in Indigenous tribes/nations.

Paradise Conquered: The Loss of Balance

In point of fact, Indigenous life prior to European contact in North, Central, and South America was not a perfect paradise. People lived, died, and suffered. The general experiences of life were known, but the way of life differed significantly from the way of life brought by Europeans. The paradise remembered by Native Americans is not one of perfection, but one in which they were allowed to live according to their own ideals, standards, and knowledge base. The failure and refusal on the part of the Europeans to recognize the sophisticated ontology and epistemology of Native American communities inhibited understanding between Native Americans and Europeans and led to the willful destruction of Native American communities. Communication difficulties and misinformed judgments, on the part of European conquerors, led to a well-documented time of colonization and assimilation practices that have been described as advancement or destruction, depending on which side of the colonization effort one occupied. For the Indigenous of the Americas, it can be said that the efforts of colonization and assimilation have not been met with overwhelmingly positive feelings. Indeed, many Indigenous refer to these events in terms of "cultural and physical genocide." Setting aside the details of these historic events, the significance for this discussion is the effect that conquering efforts have had on the lives of those suffering from chronic illness, specifically type 2 diabetes.

In researching the appearance of type 2 diabetes in Native American communities, the decade surrounding 1940 was often discussed as the general time in which documented cases of diabetes were noted in Native Americans. This time frame may represent no more than when Western medical personnel noticed or confirmed cases of diabetes, or it may be a matter of when specific symptoms were connected to a diagnosis of what was to be called diabetes. While this research was expansive and fascinating, it painted a picture of the sudden onslaught of diabetes in Indigenous communities within a single decade. When put to the participants of this study, they questioned the 1940s appearance of diabetes. One participant noted the following.

> It may be the case that diabetes was first seen in the 1940's in places like Oklahoma or in the Eastern tribes, but in New Mexico and Arizona and places like that, it didn't really show up until the 1960s or even on some reservations until the 1980s because these places were completely cut off from the outside world. There was no traveling on some of these reservations and certainly no outside contact. So these people remained in their traditions and didn't experience the white man's disease until much later that the 1940's.

The following are some additional responses as to when diabetes entered into the Native American experience.

> Diabetes came from the boarding schools. The meals there were mostly carbs and fried. There wasn't much meat or fruits or vegetables. There was a lot of oatmeal or mush. A lot of times salt was added. There were times that sugars were used as treats or as bribes, but mostly a lot of flour, potatoes and corn stuffs. I think it depended on which part of the country the school was in. But it wasn't a traditional diet for most of the children. It changed their taste and made them want unhealthy foods.

> I remember my father saying that when he came down from the mountains for the first time and found himself in the military during World War II. He said that the food they gave him over there was really different. The one thing he remembered was the sweetened condensed milk. Even when he came back that was the one thing he just wanted. He would put it in his coffee or eat it on foods. We would get some of it and it was sure good. We developed a taste for that sweet too.

> The commodity boxes they sent had everything that we didn't eat; flour, sugar, milk, cheese and lard. So, when you cook with these, you change your diet from the healthy things we traditionally ate to things that our bodies couldn't use. It made people unhealthy. Our people started to get the white man's illnesses like diabetes, not just our old people, but our children, too.

The participants' narratives differed on the specifics of times and events, but generally agreed that the loss of traditional foods as a result of the loss of land and freedoms led to the increase in chronic illnesses such as diabetes. What these participants shared was an agreement that the movement away from the traditional ways of gathering what was "close at hand," or that which was specifically given by Mother Earth to the people of that place, led to the introduction of imbalances which in turn led to unwellness. The introduction of Western-style diets was significant in the fracturing of communities and individuals.

> When we no longer could travel to get the food from certain areas or hunt in the traditional ways, we stopped moving. We sat and waited for food to come to us. We weren't allowed to search out the traditional foods that made us healthy. We ate the foods we were given because it was all we had, but it didn't stop death it only brought it in a different form. We didn't die of starvation; we died of bad hearts, bad blood and other things from the food.

One participant recounted the history of the government slaughter of sheep on the Navajo reservation. According to this participant, the government believed that the sheep were too plentiful and were damaging the desert. So, the government sent people in to kill 70 percent of the sheep, claiming they had a venereal disease that could harm the people. The tribal people had no indication that the sheep were sick and had not suffered any negative effects from eating or being around the sheep. Nonetheless, the destruction of the sheep disrupted the lives of the people on multiple levels. Certainly food was now destroyed, but so was the wool used in clothing as well as the other products given by the sheep. The restructuring of lives forced a reliance on government and Western commodities that were foreign and disruptive.

A good deal of discussion centered on the contents of both commodity rations and local stores. The consensus was that both represented a shift to fats, carbohydrates, and dairy products, which the participants both humorously and non-humorously indicated as the source of type 2 diabetes. The participants further noted that because a large portion of Native Americans were and remain lactose intolerant, the emphasis on dairy products became a source of additional contention. Inclusion of so much dairy in the commodity boxes brought discomfort to many Native Americans and so was looked on by many as another attempt to harm Native American communities. One participant noted that she always wondered what type of food the cheese really was because "it did not melt, and if it would not melt how were the people were supposed to digest it?" This comment was received by many participants with a bit of humorous agreement. Another participant stated that most of the contents of the commodity box "were not edible by humans and so was fed to the livestock". Still another talked about how everything was powdered and people thought "it could not be good to eat" and so it was left uneaten except as a last resort. However, many of these participants indicated that the real problem developed with the introduction of candies and soda. Whether it was at school or in the local stores, these products were discussed as major contributors to health problems including diabetes. Dr. Locust made reference to a study she conducted on some of the reservations in Arizona that associated the rise of type 2 diabetes with the rise in dental cavities. Her findings indicated that the closer the people lived to the stores, the more they suffered from both diabetes and dental cavities. The farther from the store, especially the children, the less likely they were to have either.

The conversations then turned from food sources to water rights. These comments came primarily from those in the American West. However, others, especially from the Northern areas, mentioned not the depletion of water, but the contamination of water as a significant contributor to unwellness. For those in western America, there was a great deal of discussion around the loss of water. In many cases, they talked of water being diverted to other primarily "white" farms or to power "energy plants" that did not serve, or provided limited services to, Native American communities. Regardless of the specifics, the loss of water meant not only thirst, but also the loss of healthy crops. Alternatives to drinking water included milk and soda, neither of which worked well in these communities. The alternative to traditional crops again became the use of commodity foods or the use of dry and canned goods from the local stores. An interesting discussion arose in terms of the loss of specific types of beans. According to some of the participants, Indigenous communities traditionally used food variety to promote wellness, both in gathering and in agriculture. For example, communities would grow a variety of beans, increasing both harvest potential and health benefits. The loss of water and land eliminated the agriculture diversity and so decreased the associated health benefits. This discussion was supported by research into tepary beans on Hopi land (Nabhan et al., 1985). According to the authors, the tepary bean was replaced by the pinto bean in the commodity boxes. The authors further note that the tepary bean has higher protein content while the pinto bean has higher carbohydrate content. The elimination of a single bean is insignificant if the people consume a variety of beans. However, when the diet becomes focused on a single bean source, the difference between higher protein and higher carbohydrates becomes significant. The discussion of the difference in beans became a popular topic in Tucson, with one participant stating, "[T]hat explains why my Grandmother kept telling us to eat this bean and not that bean." While the depletion of water in the American West prompted the previous discussion involving the loss of agriculture and healthy food variety, the participants from the Northern regions discussed water contamination. For these participants, the conversation focused on the pollution from factories and corporate farms. In these communities, the water remained, but the pollutants are perceived to have caused unwellness in Indigenous communities, a topic that will be discussed in the following section.

Regardless of what specific events led to the destruction of traditional ways of being, the destruction itself resulted in the fracturing of the Indigenous self. Individuals and communities were forced to seek survival in food and ways of life that caused a loss of balance and replaced wellness with unwellness.

PARADISE LOST: CONTINUED IMBALANCE

The fracturing of the four-dimensional self is not simply something that occurred in the past, it continues today. The already fractured pieces continue to splinter into ever-smaller pieces. Separations have increased between individuals and communities as assimilation has pulled Indigenous people into Western cultures with urbanization, media, and education. Within Indigenous communities, determination of legitimate descent has become an ever-increasing topic of conversation. Often these conversations contain elements of modern politics, government, and economics, which may oppose tradition. Historic and continuing tribal/national disruptions and separations reinforce the unbalanced self. Some participants stated that the struggle for legitimacy has overshadowed discussions of balance and wellness. One participant noted that the time spent "proving one's ancestry" focused the efforts of the individual on herself instead of allowing her to focus on the needs of those around her. When this issue was put before other participants, most agreed that it was important to make sure individuals were not making claims that could not be supported or that they were not acting contrary to Indigenous modes of ethics. However, they also tended to agree that individuals "show their true nature by their attitudes and behaviors." According to one participant,

> We traditionally allowed all people to come to the fire and then we watched. Those with negative inclinations or who were not living in the tribal way would show themselves. It was their behavior that made them part of the community. Sure it was important to know the family and introductions usually start not with names, but with places you were from. But good people can come from bad families and bad people from good families. You have to watch how they act towards others.

As this project is not a discussion of legitimacy or heritage, determinations involving these discussions will be left to those of wiser disposition. However, understanding that the issue exists illustrates yet another barrier to the dimension of self needed to promote balance and wellness. The alienation of individuals from the dimension of community further inhibits the promotion of the balanced self.

Along with issues of who qualifies for participation in community, the participants discussed additional factors that continue to increase the diabetes epidemic. The first factor discussed involved schools. While the majority of Indigenous students no longer attend boarding schools, which participants indicated contributed to the change in habits of both diet and activity, the current school systems, both on and off the reservations, also offer challenges in the attempts to curb or manage diabetes. To begin, sedentary lifestyles are reinforced by confining students to desks throughout most of the school day. One participant stated that "[W]e actually punish children for being active, creative and exuberant in schools. We encourage them to sit quietly for long periods of time and tell them to be quiet at all times. It is no wonder that so many have the idea that movement and exercise is bad or at least is not a natural part of life." There was little enthusiasm for the current physical education programs among the participants. The competitive nature involved in physical education classes, and school sports programs, can be counter to some Indigenous ways of being, which focus on cooperation rather than competition, causing conflict in the child and an aversion to the activity. Additionally, for those not athletically gifted or who enter school already overweight, the activities can be both daunting and socially awkward. Recently, there have been attempts to revitalize health education in schools by giving positive imagery of active lifestyles, yet the students still spend the majority of time sitting quietly and working at their desks. Participants seemed skeptical about the effectiveness of these programs.

The same skepticism arose in the discussion of school lunch programs. While efforts have been made to popularize fruits and vegetables, participants claimed that the lunches remained heavy in carbohydrates and contained sweets such as cakes and cookies. It was not the existence of these food varieties that bothered the participants, but rather the fact that many students ate only the sweets and carbohydrates and left the rest. One participant pointed out that the national standards for nutrition, adhered to in schools, were flawed from the start. He pointed out that the food pyramid, and now the food plate, has been taught and used in such a way as to indicate that the food types and proportions were the "ideal" for all people. The universality of this system belies the complex relation of individual to food, and in some cases ethnic biology to food. His contention was that such "one-size-fits-all" programs do not take into consideration biological or heritage issues such as lactose intolerance or diabetes. Participants discussed the possibility that a person's heritage could play a part in how well she digests certain types of foods. Setting aside the issue of heritage, individual body elements play a part in food requirements for wellness. Food intake, according to one participant, "should be considered with the same scrutiny as medicine intake, individual and heritage specific." Several participants indicated that they concurred with the analogy involving medicine, and that all food and drink should be seen as medicinal and as such understood to participate in spirit. "Since food both creates and assists in the maintenance of body wellness, great care should be used in its production and ingestion." For this reason, participants indicated that nutrition education should focus on finding a balance with the foods consumed that is appropriate for each individual's specific body needs. For those with a predisposition to diabetes, attention should be given as to how much and which types of grains and breads should be consumed, just as the dairy requirements and recommendations should be re-examined for those with lactose intolerance.

One participant offered an interesting perspective as to the historic nature of Native American foods, which were primarily alkaline rather than acidic as is more popular now. This distinction prompted a good deal of discussion as several participants stated that they had never thought of food in those categories. The individual who brought forth these ideas pointed out that not only did food in the raw state differ in alkaline and acidic categories, but also that in some cases cooking the foods would change their nature. His example of tomatoes, which are alkaline when raw but acidic when cooked, may explain why people with certain stomach challenges can eat raw but not cooked tomatoes without suffering negative results. Traditional alkaline diets would be consistent with dietary requirements to help avoid unwellnesses such as type 2 diabetes.

Several of the participants indicated that a movement back to a more alkaline diet warrants further investigation and some participants wondered if a change in traditional diet, such as a move to a more acidic diet, could be connected with "cravings" for certain types of foods. Most agreed that the "cravings" were probably based on familiarity, but some discussion involved ideas that certain types of foods could create or increase the desire for more of the same types of foods. For example, one participant said she was told by her doctor that carbohydrates promote cravings for more of the same or for sweets because of the way they are digested. Several mentioned that the more sweets they ate the more they wanted, but that if they stayed away from sweets the "craving" diminished. Their concern was for children who may have difficulty controlling these cravings or understanding the need to replace immediate gratification of taste with the long-term gratification of health.

Certainly the conversations, in most cases, evolved from basic concerns about schools and nutrition education to concerns about junk and fast foods. Not surprising, every participant mentioned the overabundance of these foods in the Indigenous diets. What may be surprising was the discussion as to why these foods are so prominent in some Native American diets. The participants indicated that while a multitude of factors play into the Indigenous consumption of junk and fast foods, poverty was a significant factor. Poverty was the most commonly discussed indicator of junk and fast food usage. The following are some of the comments made.

When the store is miles away and you have no car, you go when you can get there. When you're at the store you buy cheap food that lasts a long time. If you don't have a car, chances are you don't have a freezer or maybe not even a fridge. So, there isn't any storing food that goes bad. You may not have electricity to cook or it may not always be on because you can't pay the bill or just because you live in the middle of nowhere. Things that last a long time, packaged food that store, junk food that lasts these are what you buy. I will tell you pop tarts last a long time.

If the store is way out in the rural areas, it may not have much in it. So you buy what you can there and make it work.

For some that work all day, the prepared food is easier. There is no time to make big meals or to cook for long times. So you use what is fast. Then after working all day, you can do what you need to for your family.

The dollar menus are actually cheaper than buying healthier foods. Fruits and vegetables are expensive, especially for a large family. It is a cheap lunch if you are working, but it is also a way to get a lot of filling foods for a lot of people.

The preservatives and sweeteners in processed food, especially in junk food isn't good for anyone. The chemicals ingested must impact the body. So instead of good, healthy and natural foods, we are feeding ourselves and our children chemicals we can't pronounce and have no clue as to what they are. It is no wonder we are as unhealthy as we are.

According to some of the participants, the poverty that is so prevalent in Indigenous families also leads to choices of food over medication. Insulin may be seen as a luxury that simply cannot be afforded. For individuals who are caring for multiple generations or broader family groupings, the need for quantity over quality and the need to eliminate medicines in lieu of food are all too common. A second factor discussed was the role of the media in the promotion of fast and junk foods. The way these foods appear in the media promotes "cravings" for the foods and the people shown appear slim, vital, and healthy. The participants were in agreement as to the negative role of advertisement and product placement in the media. This factor may not be surprising, but it certainly should not be underestimated when it comes to influence on food choices, especially among children. When poverty issues are attached to these types of advertisements, the potential for negative impact increases. One participant pointed out that junk and fast food, especially from cheap menus, can be used to satisfy a number of people for little money. In addition to the affordability of junk and fast foods, there was concern about the misinterpretation of those outside of impoverished areas as to what foods are bought and why. "Healthy foods cost money and feed few" was a comment by one participant. Another participant explained the usage of cigarettes and diet drink among those in poverty. This individual stated that she had met several people in poverty, not just Indigenous individuals, who used these as cheap substitutions for food. Both tobacco and caffeine were mentioned as effective hunger suppressants. The use of these products allowed individuals to spend less on their own food in order to spend more on the food for their children. The individual who reported these practices expressed an additional concern about the advertisement of health drinks for both adults and children as possible substitutes for proper diets. All of these practices create problems for those prone to or already experiencing type 2 diabetes.

Mention was also made about the use of alcohol. The reasons given for alcohol consumption varied among the participants. The discussion ranged from the inability to process alcohol/sugar to the devastation of poverty and the lack of hope in Indigenous populations. The following are some of the statements collected from the participants.

> My dad told us that when they took the water, they gave the people alcohol to pacify them. This kept the people quiet while it killed them.

> In the 30s and 40s Phoenix got big and they drained half the water. They gave us alcohol to distract us.

> The people did have some fermented drinks, but they were for specific cere-monies or medicines. When the white man introduced alcohol as an everyday drink, the people lost their way. It has destroyed people and communities.

> Because the Indian people can't convert the alcohol in the pancreas, it goes straight to the brain destroying brain cells faster. They aren't alcoholics, but binge drinkers. They can stop for long times, but when they start, the desire for more becomes too much.

> Our youth have been destroyed by poverty and lack of hope. They turn to alcohol and drugs to find the feelings they hear about in the old days, the passion, the joy, the purpose. They have lost what was real to us long ago and there is nothing to take its place. So, they fill the hole with what is false. These things lie in offering hope and courage, but they aren't real. But then it is too late, the young people are caught.

There was one specific food discussed among participants that is important because of its evolution from simply food to a symbol of tradition. Frybread is not only a much loved food among Native Americans, but it has also become a symbol of Native American heritage. Participants agreed on their love of frybread covered in sugar, honey, made with pumpkin or as the base of a taco. Not one participant mentioned an aversion to frybread and several of them admitted to a near addicted status. However, participants also noted the negative impact of frybread on the individual diet. For those with type 2 diabetes the frequent partaking of frybread has a negative health impact. One participant stated that frybread has become a symbol of "Native Pride" similar to "American as apple pie;": "Native as frybread."

In a related, but slightly different vein, one participant brought up the effects of type 2 diabetes on mood. He said he had been to a seminar where a speaker began talking about how diabetes patients, especially older patients, would get into a negative mood cycle. As he understood the explanation, it is common to experience negative impacts on mood when one's blood sugar is compromised. In these moods, the individuals often range from irritable to combative and uncooperative. The individual may then, out of upset or depression, refuse to take insulin or refuse to eat properly. Furthermore, the individual experiencing these events may not realize she is being short-tempered or uncooperative. She may experience a depression that makes seeking balance through healthy choices too difficult or "not worth the effort." Individuals in these moods may turn to poor food choices such as junk and fast foods or alcohol out of indifference to self. The community dimension of self is essential to combat these experiences and situations.

One unexpected element in these discussions on imbalance as a contributor to diabetic unwellness came about after research indicated a possible link between persistent organic pollutants and diabetes. Research articles linking diabetes to DDT, dioxins, mercury, lead, and other industrial chemicals prompted the questioning of the participants on this matter. While the participants in the American South and West were unfamiliar with official research linking these chemicals to type 2 diabetes, Northern participants had knowledge of the connection. Much of this research is about Indigenous populations and points to the increasing links between these pollutants and type 2 diabetes (Longnecker & Michalek, 2000; Codru et al., 2007; Kouznetsova et al., 2007; Rahman & Axelson, 1995; Lee et al., 2010, 2007, 2011; Philibert et al., 2009; Carpenter, 2008). Some authors discussed the possibility that certain pollutants and chemicals, rather than obesity, could be primary triggers to type 2 diabetes. Regardless of whether or not these elements trigger type 2 diabetes, the general relationship between pollutants and diabetes requires further study. If a high correlation is found, the teachings as to how to avoid type 2 diabetes will have to be expanded from diet and exercise to the avoidance of these elements. The following are some of the responses to the possible connection between persistent organic pollutants and type 2 diabetes.

I hadn't considered the role of persistent organic pollutants in diabetes, but it makes sense. These chemicals must certainly impact the body and it isn't surprising that they would attack the areas of the body responsible for blood glucose maintenance.

It certainly seems that places that had high levels of diabetes on the reservation were also areas that had been heavily crop dusted in the past or were mined. All these chemicals we know ran into the water supply and they don't go away quickly. We are still seeing people around the old mining areas coming in with contamination issues and many of them are diabetic.

I am glad to hear that other triggers or exacerbating factors for diabetes are being considered. It is important to promote exercise and proper eating, but it is important to understand that there are outside factors as well. Too often individuals are blamed for their own condition, when we know that there are other factors including environmental and social. In looking at the role of POPs, people may stop blaming the victim or stop seeing those who are overweight as weak or as failing in some way. It has become all too common to dismiss the sociological, environmental and historic causes that impact a person. These shouldn't be an excuse, but they may be reasons for the situation. Certainly, the individual must take steps to help himself, but it takes a community, and a healthy community at that, to succeed.

The mining in Apache shut down in the 1940s but the chemicals used ran down into the water. People are still suffering from that water.

It is rather sickly ironic that POPs may contribute to, trigger or exacerbate type 2 diabetes especially in the case of dioxin. Dioxin builds up and stays in meats, fish, eggs and dairy. But diabetes diets are supposed to be heavy in protein. So, diabetics are often encouraged to eat those things rich in dioxin.

We have known about the link between pollution and sickness for a long time. Nobody listens when we talk and instead they just blame it on our weight or our poor eating habits. But when we know pregnant women shouldn't eat the fish, we know these pollutants are killing us.

As can be seen from this section, the persistent effects of colonization continue to contribute to imbalances in the self as seen in the diabetes epidemic in Indigenous populations. Loss of traditional societies, activities, and foods promote unwellness and inhibits the regaining of wellness. The previous factors involving nutrition education, media emphasis on improper foods and lifestyles, and the additional factors of descent, poverty, and pollution, create an environment where the fracturing of self becomes increasingly hard to avoid or to repair.

PARADISE REVISITED: ATTEMPTS TO BALANCE

While the "paradise" of the past may not be regained, it stands now in the memories of Indigenous populations as an ideal rather than an obtainable reality which may be revisited. None of the participants expressed a possibility of regaining the Indigenous existence prior to contact; and a couple indicated that such an existence would not be desirable even if it could be achieved. One participant stated that "Native American culture was never stagnant. Improvements and progress were part of life, but these were done with an understanding of harmony with all things." This final section is dedicated to the concerns and attempts, in Indigenous populations, to curb the diabetes epidemic. None of the participants expressed a belief that type 2 diabetes could be eliminated, but all expressed a belief that it could be controlled and severely reduced with, as one participant put it, "knowledge, choices and accessibility."

One participant wrote about his experience recently on a trip to the hospital. He went to visit three friends, all of whom had diabetes, and all of whom either already had or were awaiting amputations. His comment focused on how they were all his own age and all suffering in the same way. In response, another participant noted that she had been in the hospital recently, and that three of the four diabetic patients she was working with were now in comas.

Other participants stated that they themselves had diabetes or had relatives with diabetes. In fact, there was not one individual in these discussions that was not personally affected by type 2 diabetes. The need to combat this epidemic has prompted a movement to revitalize communities in an attempt to reassemble the shattered pieces of the self. Communities are coming together to support individuals with diabetes and are creating programs to encourage wellness in all age groups. Indeed, one of the more positive factors has been the encouragement of inter-generational activities. One participant pointed out the increase in the number of booths at powwows and Native American events dedicated to increasing knowledge about diabetes and other chronic illnesses. These booths offer information by Native Americans to Native Americans in the form of pamphlets, support, and community. Communities and governmental agencies are also beginning to form coalitions to address concerns such as diabetes in Native American populations. Additionally, recent legislation re-funded Native American health initiatives (Affordable Care Act, 2010). The potential for positive impact and improvement exists. However, the participants in these discussions were clear that the manner in which these programs are implemented is critical to success.

The participants were largely in agreement that while exercise and diet are significant, they often fail if they are not implemented within an inclusive Indigenous understanding of existence. The participants talked about embracing traditions and ceremonies, bringing back thought patterns and actions that embraced the concepts of the four dimensions of self. Participants were concerned about the alienation of individuals from themselves and from their heritages. Reconnecting with societies and traditional beliefs was a recurring theme. The discussions of reconnecting the mind, body, spirit, and community were couched in words of hope. The resurrection of hope seemed to be the focus of many participants' efforts in promoting wellness. The following are some of the statements made by participants.

> I spend most of my day giving hope and positive energy. At the end of the day, I am exhausted from these efforts.

> It is a constant surprise to me just how much hope is missing and how giving even a little hope can create wondrous events.

> Sometimes I am so sad at the negativity these people feel. They seem to live in such darkness. And then I remember that I'm supposed to be one of the Hope Warriors and I have to find the positive in the world to pass on.

One participant talked about the need to focus on balance and positive energy, "while difficult at first, it becomes a habit after a while." The problem she noted with chronic illnesses such as diabetes is that there is no "fixing it." "There is no cure for type 2 diabetes, there is only coming to balance with it and understanding that it is part of you. Fighting with it or ignoring it, won't make it better. Coming to balance with it is the only way to find peace." Another participant stated that "[W]hen I stopped fighting and accepted that

I had diabetes, it became almost a companion. I wouldn't say we were best of friends; but more like my poor eyesight it is something that needs attention, but doesn't control my life."

Under the auspices of Indian Health Services, Yvette Roubideaux has established initiatives and promoted programs that address diabetes in Native American populations (Roubideaux, 2012). The emphasis of these initiatives is on tribally directed, but federally supported, programs that address a holistic approach to diabetes. These efforts tie the individual and community together in an attempt to stop the epidemic. Tribally specific projects are being reported with increasing frequency, such as the Kickapoo "... Fight against Diabetes" described in *This Week In Indian Country Today* (2012) and the Zuni Diabetes Project (Leonard et al., 1986). The National Diabetes Education Program has developed programs and materials including *We Have the Power to Prevent Diabetes* (2008) and *The American Indian and Alaska Native Community Partnership Guide Supplement* (2012). These programs offer support to those attempting to reestablish traditional concepts of balance and wellness.

In addition to these efforts, research into traditional Indigenous foods and issues Indigenous of health is becoming more prevalent. *Gathering the Desert* (Nabhan, 1985) offers insight into traditional desert foods. *Decolonizing our Diets by Recovering Our Ancestors' Gardens* (Mihesuah, 2003) discusses the recovery of ancient diets as a means to promoting healthier lifestyles. The idea that at least some traditional foods and ways of being can be promoted increases the hope among Indigenous populations for the restoration of wellness by balancing the four dimensions of self.

While the "the four dimensions of self" is not a traditionally stated construct, this terminology has been used in this chapter to facilitate an understanding of the interaction of individual and community as a means of combating the diabetes epidemic. Promoting balance in the interaction of body, mind, spirit, and community may result in new and effective approaches to the treatment of chronic illnesses. The information offered here is not intended to encourage anyone to try to take on Indigenous ways of being, but to suggest that Western treatments of chronic illnesses, such as diabetes, could benefit from an understanding of Indigenous knowledge of self and balance. The use of participant dialogue was supplied to support and explain historic and current situations, as well as to communicate the projected hope for the future. The goal of the project has been to emphasize that within Indigenous populations, spirit and community are necessary components in cosmology and are imperative to understanding the concept of wellness.

REFERENCES

American Diabetes Association. (2012). *Native American programs.* Retrieved from www.diabetes.org/in-my-community/programs/native-american-programs/
Basso, K.H. (2000). *Wisdom sits in places: Landscape and language among the western Apache.*Albuquerque, NM: University of New Mexico Press.

Cajete, G. (2000). *Native science: Natural laws of interdependence.* Santa Fe, NM: Clear Light Publishers.

Cajete, G. (2004). *Look to the mountain: An ecology of Indigenous education.* Asheville, NC:Kivaki Press.

Carpenter, D.O. (2008). Environmental contaminants as risk factors for developing diabetes. *Reviews on Environmental Health, 23*(1), 59–74.

Centers for Disease Control. (2011). *Trends in Diabetes prevalence among American Indian and Alaska Native children, adolescents, and young adults—1990–1998: Fact sheet.* Retrieved from http://www.cdc.gov/diabetes/pubs/factsheets/aian.htm

Codru, N., Schymura, M.J., Negoita, S., Rej, R. & Carpenter, D. (2007). Diabetes in relation to serum levels of polychlorinated biphenyls and chlorinated pesticides in adult Native Americans. *Environmental Health Perspectives, 115*(10), 1442–1447.

Department of Health and Human Services. (2012). *Diabetes in American Indians and Alaska Natives facts at-a-glance.* Retrieved from http://www.ihs.gov/medicalprograms/diabetes.

Kouznetsova, M., Huang, X., Ma, J., Lessner, L. & Carpenter, D.O. (2007). Increased rate of hospitalization for diabetes and residential proximity to hazardous waste facilities. *Environmental Health Perspectives, 115*(1), 75–79.

Lee, D.H., Lee, I.K., Steffes, M. & Jacobs, D.R. (2007). Extended analyses of the association between serum concentrations of persistent organic pollutants and diabetes. *Diabetes Care, 30*(6), 1596–1598.

Lee, D.H., Steffes, M.W., Sjodin, A., Jones, R.S., Needham, L.L. & Jacobs, D.R. (2010). Low dose of some persistent organic pollutants predicts type 2 Diabetes: A nested case- control study. *Environmental Health Perspectives, 118*(9), 1235–1242.

Lee, D.H., Steffes, M.W., Sjodin, A., Jones, R.S., Needham, L.L. & Jacobs, D.R. (2011). Low dose organochlorine pesticides and polychlorinated biphenyls predicts obesity, dyslipidemia, and insulin resistance among people free of diabetes. *Public Library of Science Journal, 6*(1), 1–9.

Leonard, B., Leonard, C. & Wilson, R. (1986). Zuni diabetes project. *Public Health Report, 101*(3), 282–288.

Longnecker, M.P. & Michalch, J.E. (2000). Serum dioxin level in relation to diabetes mellitus among air force veterans with background levels of exposure. *Epidemiology, 11*(1), 44–48.

Lovern, L.L. & Locust, C. (2013). *Native American communities on health and disability: A borderland discussion.* New York, NY: Palgrave Macmillan.

Mankiller, W. & Wallis, M. (1993). *Mankiller: A chief and her people.* New York, NY: St. Martin's Press.

Marcus, H.R. & Kitayama, S. (1991). Culture and the self: Implications for cognition, emotion and motivation. *Psychology Review, 98*(2), 224–253.

Mihesuah, D.A. (2003). Decolonizing our diets by recovering our ancestors' gardens. *The American Indian Quarterly, 27*(3), 807–839.

Nabhan, G.P. (1985). *Gathering the desert.* Tucson, AZ: University of Arizona Press.

Nabhan, G.P., Weber, C.W. & Berry, J.W. (1985). Variation in composition of Hopi Indian beans. *Ecology of Food and Nutrition, 16*, 135–152.

National Diabetes Education Program. (2008). *We have the power to prevent diabetes.* National Institutes of Health Publication No. 085525. NDEP–73. Retrieved from www.YourDiabetesinfo.org

National Diabetes Education Program. (2012). *American Indian and Alaska Native community partnership guide: Supplement and activities plans.* Retrieved from http://ndep.nih.gov

Patient Protection and Affordable Care Act (2010). Pub. L. No. 111–148, §2702, 124 Stat. *119*, 318–319.

Philibert, A., Schwartz, H. & Mergler, D. (2009). An exploratory study of diabetes in a first nation community with respect to serum concentrations of p,p'-DDE and PCBs and fish consumption. *International Journal of Environmental Research and Public Health*, 6, 3179–3189.

Rahman, M. & Axelson, O. (1995). Diabetes mellitus and arsenic exposure: a second look at case-control data from a Swedish copper smelter. *Occupational and Environmental Medicine*, 52(11), 773–774.

Roubideaux, Y. (2012). *Special diabetes program for Indians update*. Indian Health Service: Washington, DC. Retrieved from: www.ihs.gov/medicalPrograms/Diabetes/index.cfm?mc

Smith-Morris, C. (2006). *Diabetes among the Pima*. Tucson, AZ: The University of Arizona Press.

Thompson, V.C. (1997). Independent and interdependent views of self: Implications for culturally sensitive vocational rehabilitation services. *The Journal of Rehabilitation*, 63(4), 16–20.

United Nations. (2009). *State of the world's Indigenous people*. United Nations Publication ISBN 92–1–30283–7. Retrieved from www.un.org/esa/socdev/unpfii/documents/SOWIP_web.pdf

United Nations. (January 14, 2010). *State of the world's Indigenous peoples*. Retrieved from www.un.org/esa/socdev/unpfii/documents/SOWIP_Press_package.pdf

Wendell, S. (2008). Toward a feminist theory of disability. In A. Bailey & C. Cuomo (Eds.), *The feminist philosophy reader* . Boston, MA: McGraw-Hill, 243–254.

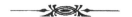

CHAPTER 11

IFÁ DIVINATION: A METHOD OF DIAGNOSING AND TREATING CHRONIC ILLNESSES/*ÀMÓDI* AMONG YORUBA PEOPLE

Akinmayowa Akin-Otiko

The possibility of illness is a human reality that we face daily and has created in every culture methods of responding to illnesses. This reality moves from the realm of ordinary reality when an illness does not follow the expected course or lasts longer than anticipated. In the Western biomedical paradigm, such a course may be labeled chronic. But for the Yoruba, such a course is not labeled chronic; it is rather labeled as having a supernatural cause. It is at this point that a Yoruba traditional healer turns to *Ifá* divination. This conceptualization is not unique. Many cultures incorporate the idea that suffering during an illness may be the result of some spiritual imbalance just as the relief from suffering may come from the same spiritual source.

Traditional Yoruba are usually reluctant to begin any undertaking without first consulting *Ifá*. Idowu (1996) noted that before a betrothal, marriage contract, birth of a child, after the birth of a child, at every successive stage in a person's life, before a king is appointed, before a journey is made, in times of crisis, in times of sickness, at any time and at all times, *Ifá* is consulted for guidance and assurance (p. 78).

For the Yoruba, reality is rooted in both the physical and the spiritual worlds. Yoruba traditional healers may relate to the physical/natural world of reality without the need for supernatural intervention. But there is the belief and practice of employing *Ifá* divination/spiritual help when there is the feeling of need for spiritual intervention and this can be for any aspect of life including health.

Ifá divination is "a geomantic type of divination, a system that has 256 *Odù* (verses or chapters) which a *babaláwo* is to learn by heart" (Simpson, 1994, p. 73). A *babaláwo* is both the "father of secret" (Bascom, 1969, p. 81) and *onísègùn* (healer) that is trusted. *Babaláwo* are diviners and healers who are the custodians of *Ifá* corpus, they are regarded as "the chief medical consultants in crisis time" (Osunwole, 1989, p. 225). Abimbola (1976) referred to *babaláwo* as the "guardians, counselors, philosophers and physicians of their various communities" (p. 18).

One can only become a *babaláwo* after years of rigorous training. In most cases they begin their training between the ages of 7 and 12. The length of time spent in training depends on the ability of the trainee, and usually lasts between 10 and 12 years. The trainee is expected to learn how to use the paraphernalia of the divination system (the *ikin* and *òpèlè*). Once familiar with these, he begins to learn and to commit the verses of the 256 *Odù* to memory, with particular attention paid to the 16 principal *Odù*. There are no fixed numbers of ese-*odù* (verses of each of the *Ifá* literary corpus) that the trainee must learn before he qualifies for initiation (Abimbola, 1976, p. 19). Some hold that six verses of each of the 256 *Odùare* required, while some others hold that one must learn 16 verses of each of the 256 *Odù*. It is only after the trainee has learned and understood how to use the divination tools for diagnosis and prescription that he is initiated as a *babaláwo*. Initiation is usually not the end of training, as *babaláwo* are expected to always learn from one another. It is usually said that *Babaláwo tó kó'fá kó'fá tó ní òun ò kó'fá mó, ti inúu rè ni yíò run* (if a *babaláwo* stops learning how to divine, the knowledge he already has will diminish); and *Onísègùn tó kó oògùn mó oògùn, tó ní òun ò kó oògùn mó, ti inúu rè ni yíò run* (if a healer stops learning the use of medicine, the knowledge he already has will diminish).

Each of these 256 *Odù* has its own divination signature and *ese* (the verse of the *Ifá* literary corpus). It is believed that each of the 256 *odù* has hundreds of verses traditionally associated with it. The signatures are determined through the use of either *òpèlè* (divination chain that has eight cowries attached to it) or *ikin* (group of 16 palm-nuts). Once a signature is determined, the content of the verses explains to the diviner the nature of and the treatment for the illness being diagnosed; because the *Ifá* literary corpus is "an ancient well-preserved oral literature, which is the basis of a highly systematized and effective traditional healing system used by the Yoruba" (Parrinder, 1976, p. 124).

Ifá divination is employed to diagnose and treat cases that are perceived to be chronic illnesses (*àmódi*) because it is the avenue used to access a body of religious directives with a basic purpose of determining "the correct sacrifice necessary to secure a favourable resolution of the problem confronting the client" (Bascom, 1969, p. 60). This is why "*Ifá* may be regarded as the most important *Òrìsà* [divinity] of the Yoruba people" (Farrow, 1926, p. 3). For the Yoruba, "*Ifá* is believed to have been sent by *Olódùmarè*, the Almighty God, to use his profound wisdom to put the earth in order" (Abimbola,

1976, p. 9). *Ifá* is called *Akéré-f'inú-sogbón* (the small person with a mind full of wisdom), *Akóni-lóràn-bí-iyèkan-eni* (he who gives one wise advice like one's relative), and *"Obirikiti a-pa-ojo-iku-da'* (the great one, who alters the date of death)" (Ajayi, 1996, p. 1).

In the following excerpt, the role of *Òrúnmìlà* (the divinity that is directly linked with *Ifá* divination, and sometimes used as a synonym for *Ifá* divination) in human life is likened to that of the calabash-mender (someone who repairs broken human situations). This is because he daily protects humans from danger, and could therefore be said to mend human life as one mends calabash.

> When a cross-bow loses its string,
> It dances all over the ground.
> *Ifá* divination was performed for *Òrún-mìlà*
> *Ifá* was going to mend the life of the king
> of *Ifè*
> As one who mends a broken calabash.
> (Abimbola, 1976, p. 154)

More than the general purposes for which *Ifá* divination is used, Parrinder (1976) observed that *Ifá* divination plays a huge role in Yoruba traditional healing, especially in the diagnosis and treatment of chronic illnesses. With *Ifá* divination, the *babaláwo* is able to unveil the cause of the illness and make necessary prescriptions. This points to *Ifá* divination as a "vital method of communication between the *babaláwo* and the patient during health consultations, making this aspect of illness management focus on a holistic cure and ritualistic competence" (O. Jegede, 2010, p. 41).

Ifá divination is prominent in Yoruba traditional healing practice as a method of diagnosis because some supernatural factors such as bewitchment, sorcery, curses, aggrieved spirits of ancestors, and the breaching of cultural taboos can cause illnesses. According to Sawandi (2010), Yoruba healers believe that human beings are vulnerable to both physical and spiritual illnesses, which may be caused by oppressive forces known as *ajogun*, "belligerent enemies and powers that work against man" (Abimbola, 1976, p. 152). Illnesses caused by these forces usually defy biomedical solutions in such a way that it becomes paramount to look at the cultural environment of the patient to see if there is an imbalance resulting from a disregard of social, cultural, or traditional norms, in order to treat them.

During *Ifá* divination, "the *babaláwo* possesses a higher level of perception and is in full control of his senses. During [divination] he attains a high level of spirituality which enhances his ability to draw on deeper information from the world of spirits" (Jegede, 2010, p. 43). With *Ifá* divination, the *babaláwo* takes the patient to his or her own origin or to the origin of the condition in order to trace what may be responsible for the symptoms or illness found in the patient.

The *babaláwo* believes that as soon as the cause of an *àmódi* is known, the relevant treatment becomes achievable. This characteristic makes it difficult for Yoruba people to accept that there is anything like "*àrùn tí ò sé é wò*" (incurable illness). Illnesses are perceived to be incurable only when they are located solely within the realm of material and sensual reality.

How Does *Ifá* Divination Represent Chronic Illness?

From the understanding of the content of the *Ifá* literary corpus, *babaláwo* are known to make distinctions between *àìsàn ara* (physical illness) and *àmódi* (chronic illness). *Àìsàn ara* is known to have explainable natural causes in which symptoms are understood within existing categories, making diagnosis possible with the use of ordinary diagnostic tools.

For example, Buckley (1997) acknowledged that in Yoruba traditional medicine there are categories of diseases caused by *kòkòrò* or *aràn* (bacteria or parasites) in which there are links between the symptoms and the cause or agent. This categorization allows for normative prescriptive treatment because the symptoms are logical consequences of an understood cause. *Ifá* divination is not employed in the diagnosis and treatment of *àìsàn ara* because *àìsàn ara* in its diverse forms is not regarded as chronic illness. But in the case of *àmódi*, symptoms do not have specific links to particular physical cause, thereby making diagnosis difficult.

Ifá divination gains relevance in the diagnosis and treatment of *àmódi* because it addresses the inexplicable or supernatural causes of illness. *Olódùmarè* is believed to have endowed *Òrúnmìlà* with the power to use words and herbs to heal regular illnesses; and with *Ifá* divination to determine the causes of chronic illnesses; and to prescribe effective therapies and methods of application in their treatment.

Yoruba traditional healing practice adopts some "techniques used . . . which seem to contradict both scientific knowledge and common sense" (Buckley, 1997, p. 17). Jegede (2006) stressed the link between Yoruba traditional healing and religion. For him, "religion and medicine are connected and are ever crossing each other. Thus, African therapeutics is medico-religious. It includes the use of divination, rituals, and sacrifices as well as incantations, from aetiology diagnosis to the management and treatment of diseases" (p. 64).

Therefore, traditional healing practices are an indispensable "part of the rich cultural tradition of a Yoruba town," an indication that even though these practices "in many respects should be regarded as distinct from the mainstream of traditional Yoruba religion, like many other parts of Yoruba culture distinct though, it is, it is inextricably intertwined with it" (Buckley, 1997, p. 1).

Ifá divination emphasizes causes of illness within the context of the supernatural or unexplainable. Simpson (1994) found that traditional Yoruba medicine incorporates practices that address natural causes of diseases as well as supernatural causes. Yoruba traditional healing practice divides causes of illness into the categories of the natural (or explainable) and supernatural (or unexplainable). It is believed that supernatural illnesses may have culturally known but not always explainable causes. This distinction is linked to the contention between Western medicine and Yoruba traditional medicine as to what constitutes illness: "Too much emphasis of modern medicine on germ theory of disease has made it lose sight of other factors as recognized by traditional medicine" (Jegede, 2010, p. 56). Supernatural causes of illness do not fit into the logic and sequence of Western science and practice.

This concept of unexplainable causes of disease has generated much debate among practitioners and scholars of Western medicine andanthropology. This concept embraces the validity of supernatural causes of illness such as magical practices, sorcery, witchcraft, curses, aggrieved spirits of ancestors, and the breaching of cultural taboos.

Witches are believed to have *ajogun* (belligerent enemies and powers that work against man) at their disposal to impose afflictions on human beings who have no protection or who have offended them. Witches are believed to be capable of "making a woman temporally infertile or permanently barren, they can prolong pregnancy, cause miscarriage, make delivery difficult, induce frightening dreams and sleeplessness and drain people's blood supernaturally" (Jegede, 2010, p. 28). In these cases, the supernatural is understood to be largely the cause of *àmódi*.

There are two major categories of unexplained illness: (1) those caused by supernatural forces resulting from the influences of spirits or human agents and (2) those caused by spiritual penalties resulting from sinning, breaking taboos, or caused by the choices the individual's *orí* (one's personality soul) made from heaven. These causal elements are supernatural, but this has not prevented them from being recognized and accepted by Yoruba traditional healers as causing *àmódi*.

The early symptoms of this class of illnesses may first take the form of *àìsàn ara* (naturally caused illnesses), which later becomes unresponsive to treatments employed by the patient, his/her family member, or primary health care provider (*onísègùn*). *Àmódi* can be manifested by physical and psychological/mental symptoms, which may obscure the true unexplainable cause (supernatural).

What Makes an Illness *Àmódi*?

In Yoruba traditional healing practice, an illness is regarded as *àmódi* when the use of ordinary diagnostic methods and treatments are ineffective. For example, the bodily/physical symptoms manifested by the patient may not match the suspected cause, or test results for the suspected agent may be negative. In Western medicine, such an illness might be attributed to a psychological or emotional problem. *Àmódi* has been described in *Ifá* literary corpus, *Ogbè atè* (*Ofò ire*) as

> The day you were coming from heaven to earth
> Three of you turned to three cross roads,
> Three broad and spread rocks,
> Each of you separated and entered *Ilé-Ifè*,
> *Òrúnmìlà* bore children in *Ilé-Ifè*.
> But the others did not bear children.
> After a while
> They conspire to disturb the children of *Òrúnmìlà*
> *Òrúnmìlà's* children were afflicted with different diseases,
> They had the look of a paralysed person,
> *Òrúnmìlà* invited *Àtàpán tèrukù mole*,
> His own divination student.
> *Òrúnmìlà* asked that *Àtàpán tèrukù mole* should divine for him.
> He offered sacrifice, but it was not accepted.
> He invited *Apansáká yoró, Sìgìdì meji omo Olòtò*,
> Who is also *Òrúnmìlà's* divination student.
> He also descended from heaven,
> He too tried to heal *Òrúnmìlà's* children,
> But did not succeed.
> Then *Òrúnmìlà*, headed for heaven,
> To meet with *Olódùmarè*,
> *Òrúnmìlà* told *Olódùmarè* that,
> His companions that went with him to earth,
> Have been troubling his children on earth.
> His children have been having different serious sicknesses,
> They had the look of a paralysed person.
> He reported that he invited his divination students,
> They tried, but the children were not healed.
> This has made me come to you, *Òrúnmìlà*.
> *Olódùmarè* instructed that *Òrúnmìlà* should prepare:
> A yard of white cloth, one tortoise, one snail,
> *Eso* leaf, male and female *edan*,
> *Olódùmarè* then instructed *Òrúnmìlà* to prepare one thousand two hundred.
> He was instructed *Òrúnmìlà* to gather all these items together,
> And burn them together on his return to the earth.
> But he was to leave the money and the white cloth in heaven,
> For the diviners in heaven to continue to use in interceding for him,
> So that blessing will be his on earth.
> *Òrúnmìlà* went to *èjìgbòmekùn* market,
> He bought all that was prescribed,
> He left the yard of white cloth and the money in heaven,
> And returned to earth with the other items,
> He burnt them as instructed by *Olódùmarè*,
> He mixed the ashes with pap and drank,
> He also gave some to his children to drink.

Not too long, Òrúnmìlà's children started to eat,
And started to drink, they recovered from the disease,
They recovered from their chronic illnesses.
Òrúnmìlà resolved to use masquerade leaf to prevent all chronic illnesses,
That are manifest in his children,
Such that they will live long on earth.
A tortoise still crawls in its old age, same with the snail,
Don't stain my white garment, I am wearing white,
That witches cannot destroy the lives of my children,
I have offered a thousand two hundred, drain all evil from my body, from my children's body.
Use Ogbè atè, to drain all the evil of somatoform disorder away,
From my body, from my children.[1]

From the narrative above, one finds the children of Òrúnmìlà suffering from àmódi that proved difficult to treat until Òrúnmìlà performed the ebo (prescribed sacrifice) as directed by Olódùmarè. This narrative sets the context for the diagnosis and treatment of àmódi in Yoruba traditional healing practices; and shows that for the Yoruba, chronic illness/àmódi is curable, based on the distinction between, àrùn tí ò sé é wò (incurable disease) and àrùn tí ò gbó òògùn (a disease that cannot be cured with medicine). For the Yoruba people, this distinction is possible because medicine is not the only means by which human illnesses can be cured: "The concept of incurability of a particular disease does not exist in African traditional religion and medicine" (Jegede, 2009, p. 23)

The Yoruba believe that every illness in existence today had existed and been treated at some point in history. The babaláwo diagnoses the present disease by consulting with the Ifá literary corpus through the use of Ifá divination to discover the cause of the disease and the treatment that was used in the past. For the babaláwo, the existence of àrùn tí ò gbó òògùn (disease that cannot be cured with medicine) requires cures that are beyond medicine, thus making the use of Ifá divination for the diagnosis and cure of àmódi necessary.

Mbiti (1969) noted that "diseases attributed to both naturalistic and supernatural causes can be treated by traditional healers who exist in each African village" (p. 160). In this case, a traditional healer will be

a person who is recognized by the community in which he lives as competent to provide health care by using vegetable, animal and mineral substances and certain other methods based on the social, cultural and religious background as well as on the knowledge, attitudes, and beliefs that are prevalent in the community regarding physical, mental and social well-being and the causation of disease and disability.

(Ampofo & Johnson-Romauld, 1987, p. 39)

Acknowledging supernatural causes of illness provides a basis for the acceptance of àrùn tí kò gbó òògùn (disease that cannot be cured with medicine).

For the Yoruba, there is an understanding that invisible realities (or supernatural realities) are possible causes of illnesses, especially when an illness is not explainable within the established illness and health-care paradigm.

How Does *Ifá* Divination Respond to Chronic Illness/*Àmódì*?

Once an illness is diagnosed to be *àmódi*, the *babaláwo* moves treatment to the realm of *Ifá* divination. At this level both palliative and curative measures are sought. The patient is helped to understand the source of the illness as well as the requirements for recovery. At the point of diagnosis, the patient is expected to begin to experience some level of psychological relief prior to the commencement of his/her treatment. Jegede (2010) noted that "before the introduction of Western medical science, [for the Yoruba] traditional medicine was used in the diagnosis, treatment and management of bio/psycho/social disorders and illnesses" (p. 2). When an illness defies every natural means and methods of diagnosis, the *babaláwo* moves on to the use of *Ifá* divination as a diagnostic tool, because historically, "herbal preparations, rituals and incantations, as reflected in the *Ifá* verses (*Odù*), provided effective therapy" (Jegede, 2010, p. 2).

To overcome the difficulty in diagnosing *àmódi*, the *babaláwo* follows three stages in *Ifá* divination. The first stage begins with the client confiding in *Ifá* by speaking to either the *ikin* or *òpèlè*. By doing this, "it is believed that the client has communicated his wishes through the divination instruments to *Ifá* himself who will then provide an answer, through the appropriate *odù*" (Abimbola, 1975, p. 22). After this, the *babaláwo*,without having heard what the client said to *Ifá*, picks up the divination tool, then casts the *òpèlè* or the *ikin*. He begins to chant the *ese* of the *odù* that appears.

During the second stage, the *babaláwo* addresses particular questions. He asks whether the conditions signal *ire* (good) or *ibi* (evil). Once *ire* or *ibi* is known, the *babaláwo* asks *Ifá* the nature of the *ire* or *ibi*: Is it natural or is it caused by *àwon iyà mi* (witches) or any other force? These questions shape the direction of the investigation. After the questioning, the patient is invited to tell the *babaláwo* about the relevant parts of the *ese Ifá* that apply to his/her situation. This narrative will help the *babaláwo* to analyze the *ese Ifá* that was previously chanted. Both the *babaláwo* and the patient then agree on the treatment for the *àmódi*. The third stage is the process of *ótán tàbí ókù?* (is this all or is there still more?), when the *òpèlè* is used to ask *Ifá* if the prescription is sufficient. If it is not sufficient, the same process will be used to ask *Ifá* what else is to be added. Once *Ifá* indicates that the prescription is sufficient, the *babaláwo* and the patient are assured of appropriate treatment.

Treatment of Chronic Illness/*Àmódi*

Treating *àmódi* has always been a practice of the *babaláwo*, even though they would prefer to prevent *àmódi* rather than treat it. It is said that "*bí òní se rí, òla kìí rí bè, níí mú kí babaláwo dá Ifá oroorún, wón wá ní kìí sé oroorún mó, bí kò se ní ojojúmó,*" (divination is done weekly because each day has its problem, but now in our days, divination is done daily, not weekly anymore). For the *babaláwo,* divination may function to protect humans from the attacks of *ajogun* and to prevent things that would have resulted from *àì ko béèrè* (lack of divination).

The concepts of preventive and curative care are situated in the day-to-day cultural practice of the Yoruba: "The average Yoruba man would try by every means to avoid any violation of taboos so that he could maintain a good relationship with the supernatural beings" (Jegede, 2002, p. 325). Some of these practices include:

1. *Èbè/ìyónú àjé/àwon àgbà* (appeasement of supernatural pow- ers/witches): *Èbè* is used "for protection against witchcraft poisoning and making sure that all medicine retain their potency" (Osunwole, 1989, p. 228). *Èbè* is also a form of appeal to *Olódùmarè,* a chosen divinity or a force, for the purpose of blocking possible sources of chronic *àmódi.* It is a plea to prevent the afflictions that may come upon a client or members of his/her family.

2. *Só ara fún èèwò* (avoidance of taboos): Taboos for the Yoruba peo- ple are known as "*a kìí se é*" (things that are not done). It is believed that divinities can see things done in secret and so punish whoever breaks "*a kìí se é*"; explaining why the occurrence of *àmódi* or misfortunes that are not understood, inspire a belief that some wrong ("*a kìí se é*") has been committed.

3. *Ìwà-pèlé* (good character/gentleness) and *Ìmò ìwàn ara eni* (not going beyond one's bounds): Yoruba people believe that *Ìwà-pèlé* protects one from the attack of *àwon ìyà mi* (the witches). *Ìwà-pèlé* is regarded as "sufficient armour against any untoward happening in life" (Idowu, 1996, p. 162). It guides the actions of individuals and helps to avoid incurring the wrath of *àwon ìyà mi* or any of the *òrìsà.* *Ìwà-pèlé* symbolizes virtues like *Ìwà-ìrèlè* (humility), *ìsò òtító* (telling the truth), *Ìmò ìwàn ara eni* (not going beyond one's bounds), and *Ìkó ara eni ní ìjánu* (being cautious).

4. *Ètùtù/ebo* (sacrifice): For the *babaláwo,* *Ètùtù/ebo* is required for per- sonal safety. Sacrifices are expected to be offered to *òrìsà* (divinities) and *òkú-òrun* (ancestors) to protect individuals from danger. Jegede (2002) noted that to prevent the interference of evil machination, "certain sacrifices (*ètùtù*) must be offered as may be directed by the oracle (*Ifá*) through a diviner (*babaláwo*)" (p. 324). A popular saying among the *babaláwo* is that *ikú ò kí je oúnje eni, kí ó tún pa'ni* (death does not eat a person's sacrifice/food and still kill the person): this saying expresses the power of *ètùtù.*

5. *Egbò-igi ìyónú/èbè àwon àgbà,* (use of herbs that protect against the attack of witches). There are different known herbs that protect people from the attacks of *àwon àgbà* (witches). For example, the Yoruba believe that *Èpo Òbò* (the bark of *Spondianthis prussii* tree) has some antidotes against the

attacks of witches. It is said that *Àjé kìí rorò kó je eérú, Àjé kìí rorò kó je Òbò*
(no matter how powerful a witch is, it dares not consume ashes or *Òbò*). The
name of a similar herb, "*Àjé kò bàlé*" (*Crotton Zambesicus*), literally means
witches do not perch on it. Another is "*má fi owó kan omoò mi*" (*Solanum
dasphyllum,* which literally means, *do not touch my child*). These barks and
herbs are taboos for "*àwon àgbà*".

6. *Esè nbálè/Ìkosè-wáyé* (divination at birth to find out what a child will
become). Among the *babaláwo*, "on the third day after a child's birth, the
oracle is consulted. This rite is called *Ìkosè-wáyé* or *Esè ntáyé* (the first step
into the world)" (Idowu, 1996, p. 192). The rite is meant to find out what
the child will become and what destiny he/she has chosen. If there are things
to be corrected, the rite is meant to inform the corrective process. The rite
also reveals the child's taboo so that it can be avoided. *Ìkosè-wáyé* or *Esè ntáyé*
is a way of avoiding sickness or conditions that may affect the future of the
child.

When these preventive methods are ineffective or unobserved and *àmódi* is
not prevented, the *babaláwo* does not lose hope, because he still believes
that effective treatment is possible by prescribing the content of the identified *Odù*. The signature determined through the use of either *òpèlè* or *ikin*
identifies the *odù* that will diagnose and prescribe treatment for the *àmódi*.
In Yoruba traditional healing practice, it is believed that *àmódi* do not occur
without identifiable causes.

Sofowora (2008) observed that *Ifá* divination is used to diagnose the
origin and nature of illnesses and to proffer solutions by prescribing relevant *àkóse Ifá* (medicines as contained in the chosen *Ifá* literary corpus) and
ebo/ètùtù (rituals) (p. 43). This process is possible because "the *babaláwo*
(*Ifá* priest) knows the type of diseases and their cure through *Ifá* divination"
(Jegede, 2010, p. 42).

The prescribed treatment may consist of herbal remedy, which usually contains healing attributes as well as symbolic spiritual significance. This was
evident in Buckley's (1997) observation that "incantations may be used in
medicines which are directed against 'supernatural' agencies or to counteract
sorcery" (p. 140). The treatment of *àmódi* has three components that can be
described as three siblings in traditional Yoruba healing practice: e*bo lègbón*
(sacrifice, the oldest), *oògùn l'àbúrò* (medicine, younger), and *ogbón/ojú- inú
l'omo iyèkan won lénje lénje* (wisdom/experience, their sibling).

1. *Ebo* (sacrifice): From the tradition and teachings of the *Ifá* literary corpus, it is known and believed that *Ifá kìí bale kí o má yan ebo* (once there is
divination, there must be a prescribed sacrifice). Whether the *odù* (*Ifá* literary corpus) indicates good or bad (whether the patient's condition will have
a favorable resolution or not), the patient is expected to offer some kind
of sacrifice: "It is the belief of the Yoruba that if the prediction of *Ifá* is
good, a sacrifice will help to further make it come to pass, and that, if the

prediction is evil, a sacrifice will help the client to dispel the evil" (Abimbola, 1976, p. 35).

Ebo in particular is why a *babaláwo* is not called "*adá un se*" (one who acts alone). He is known as *olórìsà* (one who relates with the divinities). *Ebo* facilitates communication with the divine by being "sent" on an errand to look for favor from *Olódùmarè*. The material constituents of *ebo* may be grouped into two: regular items and items for specific occasions. Regular items, *obì, epo, èko* (kola-nut, palm-oil, and solid pap), are always present, while other specified items may include goat, dog, pigeon, fowl, red-oil, beans, eggs, pieces of white cloth, or other items to keep the soul at rest.

Ebo is offered to a chosen deity for two reasons: first, as the quota or contribution of the patient to his/her process of healing; second, to acknowledge and appease the divinity that *Ifá* has chosen as *aládìmú* (witness to the affliction). In other words, *ebo* is a means of asking for help from the divinity identified in the *Odù*. With *ebo*, it is believed that whatever is sought will be received.

A prescribed *ebo* may be *àkórú*, meaning that all the stages and sacrifices mentioned in the *ese-odù* (verses of the *Ifá* literary corpus) must be performed; or it may be *ògángán*, meaning that a specific sacrifice in the narrative of the *ese-odù* will suffice for the treatment of *àmódi*. With *ebo*, *Ifá* directs the patient to appease the *òrìsà* who has been identified as the *aládìmú;* because the chosen *òrìsà* would have witnessed the affliction of the patient, and therefore knows what to offer in order to appease the forces responsible for the *àmódi*. Once the *òrìsà* is chosen, *Ifá* prescribes what to offer to the chosen *òrìsà*.

When *ebo* is being prepared, the *babaláwo* begins to narrate the story of the patient, and calls the patient by name and the patient's mother by name (e.g. X the child of Y); then narrates the purpose for the invocation of *òrìsà* (to grant release and ease the suffering of the patient); and appeals to the *òrìsà* to accept the items that have been brought as *ebo,* stressing past occasions in which the *òrìsà* accepted the same *ebo*.

Once the *òrìsà* has been invoked and the *ebo* prepared, the *babaláwo* takes the *ebo* to the identified venue so that the other agents[2] of sacrifice can partake in the offering and plea for the release and healing of the patient.

Èsù (the deity that interfaces between good and evil) is seen as the mediator for humans. He mediates between either the *òrìsà* and *àwon ìyà mi* or between heaven and earth. He is responsible for taking *ebo* from the place it is offered to the designated force or *òrìsà*. *Èsù* will only refuse *ebo* when the *ebo* is not good enough or if either the *òrìsà* or *àwon ìyà mi* refuses to accept the *ebo*.

For the *babaláwo*, ebo is very effective: *àdúrà l'ebo, kò sí ohun kan tí a rúbo sí tí kìí dèrò* (sacrifice is prayer; there is nothing that is not resolved after a required sacrifice is properly offered).[3] *Ebo* cleanses out the *owó ayé* (influence of the witches) before the administration of herbs or medicine. It is believed that without *ebo*, prescribed herbs or medications will not be as effective as it ought to be in treating a patient's illness.

2. *Oògùn* (medicine) is the second sibling in the treatment family of *àmódi*, and follows *ebo*. Every *babaláwo* is considered a physician. He can prescribe ordinary medication without divination. But in the case of *àmódi*, ordinary medicine is not the only *oògùn* that the *babaláwo* uses. In this case, *oògùn* includes *àkóse Ifá*. *Àkóse Ifá* is the prescription contained in *Odù-Ifá* (*Ifá* literary corpus), which may be supported with the *babaláwo's* general knowledge of ordinary *oògùn*. *Àkóse Ifá* may include herbs, animal parts or anything else that was used in the cases recorded in *Odù-Ifá*.

Àkóse Ifá (medicinal ingredients prescribed by *Ifá*) is only known to *babaláwo* since they are the custodians of the *Ifá* literary corpus. This knowledge makes the *babaláwo* better equipped than the *adáhun se* to treat *àmódi*.

3. *Ogbón/ojú-inú* (wisdom/experience) is the third sibling in the family of treatment for *àmódi*. Every *babaláwo* recalls his *ogbón/ojú-inú* to help in the present context, in addition to the *ebo* and the content of the prescription from the *Ifá* literary corpus. Because the patient must be treated both physically and spiritually, the *babaláwo* draws inspiration from his wealth of experience; he employs what he has found to be good and complementary to the found prescription from the *Ifá* literary corpus. *Ogbón/ojú-inú* recalls what helped in earlier situations but is not present in the particular *odù* that prescribed the treatment that is currently being followed.

Once the three siblings of treatment are incorporated, and visible progress is observed in the patient, the *babaláwo* carries out an evaluation to establish whether healing has taken place. He uses the same divination tools that he used for diagnosis but they are now employed to determine whether *ó tán tàbí ó kù?* (is this all or are there more things to be done?). This process confirms either that the healing is complete or that there are still more things required for healing to occur. Once healing is achieved, the patient is declared healed and the patient appreciates *Ifá*.

CONCLUSION

The concept of *àmódi* in the understanding of the Yoruba portrays the existence of the natural and supernatural causes of illness. *Àmódi* may be prevented through certain day-to-day cultural practices; or may be treated through the use of *Ifá* divination. McClelland (1982) noted that each *Odù* "form a body of medicine with two aspects, the curative and the preventive" (p. 104).

This understanding is germane to providing holistic care for chronic illnesses among the Yoruba: "The greatest advantage of African traditional medicine is its holistic approach to medical problems and misfortunes whereby both organic and psychological attributes of disease or illness are considered together" (Sindiga, 1995, p. 21).

Like every aspect of life in the Yoruba worldview, health may be affected by the supernatural. "Disease and misfortune are regarded as having socio-religious foundations. Consequently, the treatment process must go beyond addressing the symptomatology of disease to discovering its deep-seated causes and subsequent ways of preventing it from recurring" (Mbiti, 1969, p. 170).

The only time a *babaláwo* will not treat a patient with *àmódi* is when he is instructed by *àwon ìyà mi* (the witches) to not proceed with treatment. This happens only in the cases of *àkótán* (when a patient is completely taken by the witches), which implies that the patient's body parts have been shared among the witches and cannot be returned.

In such instances the *babaláwo* believes that *èsù* and *àwon ìyà mi* have refused the *ebo* that was offered to them. Once this happens, the procedure for treating the illness in question is taken beyond the reach of the *babaláwo*, then only *Olódùmarè* (almighty God) can intervene on behalf of the patient. If any *babaláwo* continues to treat such a patient, he (*babaláwo*) will be punished, either by being killed or by having the disease transferred to him. It is at this point that the patient may become disappointed and lose hope in being treated by *Ifá* divination.

The inexplicable but culturally understood causes of illness create the need for contextual understanding and interpretation of health conditions in order to achieve the best possible outcomes. There is no longer a single method for interpreting and relating to illness. There are now many complex biomedical treatments and technologies, as well as the need for the integration of cultural perception and understanding of health and illness. These diverse approaches to treatment account for why it is "not uncommon to see patients in hospitals permitting themselves to be treated by modern medicine during the day and having recourse to the recipes of traditional medicine at night" (Ampofo & Johnson-Romauld, 1987, p. 51). This, in no small way, has promoted the holistic approach to healing and more precisely it has reduced that barrier for the treatment of *àmódi* among the Yoruba.

Given the reality of multiple approaches to treating *àmódi*, there is need for dialogue between the practitioners of Western and Yoruba traditional medicine, with the hope of improving on both methods, thereby creating the possibility of having the two paradigms complement each other in a holistic way for the good of patients.

NOTES

1. Translation was done by the author.
2. Once *ebo* is offered, it is expected that agents like the air, rats, birds, dogs, lizards, even man (especially mad people and beggars) will assist in taking the *ebo* to the *òrìsà* by partaking of it. Once this happens, they join to plead for the patient's release. This process is believed to have been witnessed by the agents that took part, the earth and heaven (the chosen deity and *Olódùmarè*).
3. Interview with Wande, Abimbola at his residence in Oyo town, on February 23, 2011.

References

Abimbola, W. (1975). *Sixteen great poems of Ifá*. Paris: UNESCO.
Abimbola, W. (1976). *Ifá: An exposition of Ifá literary corpus*. Ibadan: Oxford University Press.
Ajayi, B. (1996). Ifá divination process. *Research in Yoruba Language and Literature*, 8, 1–15.
Ampofo, O. & Johnson-Romauld, J. D. (1987). *Traditional medicine and its role in the development of health services in Africa*. Background paper for "The Technical discussions of the 25th, 26th and 27th sessions of the Regional Committee for Africa". Brazzaville: WHO.
Bascom, W. (1969). *Ifá divination: Communication between gods and men in West Africa*. Indiana: Indiana University Press.
Buckley, A. D. (1997). *Yoruba medicine*. New York: Clarendon Press.
Farrow, S. S. (1926). *Faith Francies and Fetich, Yoruba paganism*. London: Society for Promoting Christian Knowledge.
Idowu, B. E. (1996). *Olódùmarè: God in Yoruba belief*. Ibadan: Longman.
Jegede, A. S. (2002). The Yoruba cultural construction of health and illness. *Nordic Journal of African Studies, 11*(3), 322–335.
Jegede, A. S. (2010). *African culture and health*. Ibadan: Book Wright Publishers.
Jegede, O. (2006). From disease etiology to disease treatment: An exploration into religion and the Yoruba therapeutics. *Orita, 60*(20), 60–68.
Jegede, O. (2009). Traditional religion and HIV/AIDS in Nigeria. *Orita, 42*(2), 18–33.
Jegede, O. (2010). *Incantations and herbal cures in Ifá divination: Emerging issues in indigenous knowledge*. Ibadan: African Association for the Study of Religion.
Mbiti, J. S. (1969). *African religion and philosophy*. Ibadan: Heinemann Books.
McClelland, E. (1982). *The cult of Ifá among the Yoruba: Folk practice and the art*. London: Ethnographic Ltd.
Ogbè-Atè. (n.d.). *Ifá* Literary Corpus. Unpublished oral tradition of the Yoruba people.
Osunwole, S. A. (1989). Healing in Yoruba traditional belief system (PhD thesis). Institute of African Studies, University of Ibadan.
Parrinder, E. G. (1976). *African traditional religion*. London: Sheldon Press.
Sawandi, T. (2010). Yoruba medicine: The art of divine herbology. Retrieved from http://www.planetherbs.com/theory/yorubic-medicine-the-art-of-divine-herbology.html.
Simpson, G. E. (1994). *Yoruba religion and medicine in Ibadan*. Ibadan: Ibadan University Press.
Sindiga, I. (1995). African ethnomedicine and other medical systems. In I. Sindiga, C. Nyaigotti & M. P. Kanunah (Eds.). *Traditional medicine in Africa*. Nairobi: English Press Ltd.
Sofowora, A. (2008). *Medicinal plants and traditional medicine in Africa*. Ibadan: Spectrum Books Limited.

CHAPTER 12

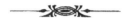

INANNA'S WAY: A PERSONAL JOURNEY INTO THE UNDERWORLD

Ruth Krall

Earth I am
Fire I am
Water, Air, and Spirit I am[1]
The morning and the evening star are mine
Lions sit at peace with me in secluded courtyards
Dolphins pull my chariot in the sacred pools
Thunder and lightning speak my will
I am Inanna! I am the moon's daughter! I am the Queen of Heaven![2]

INTRODUCTION: MY ILLNESS NARRATIVE

In a personal encounter with endometrial cancer, I needed to learn how to recover a secure sense of myself as a whole person. In my search for a pathway back to sense of personal wellness, I turned to the mythology of ancient Sumer. In particular, I turned to the myth known as the *Descent of the Goddess* (Wolkstein & Kramer, 1983). In this myth, Sumer's important deity, the Goddess Inanna journeys into the underworld of death and suffering.

In 1995 I survived two surgeries that followed a biopsy report of endometrial cancer. The first surgery removed the malignancy. After fully waking from anesthesia, the surgeon told me that no malignant cells were found outside the uterus. He thought I had an excellent chance of living for a long time. I set myself to the business of recovering from the dual assault of surgery and anesthesia. I began walking every day. I rested. I ate healthy foods. I accepted immediately the opinion that I would live. Joy at being alive flowed into me and through me like a strong springtime river. Joy invaded my spirit. Joy sustained me in the first days after surgery. I would live.

The surgical wound, however, did not heal well. It herniated and I had to return to surgery. Following the repair of the herniated wound, I again moved back into restorative actions: walking, sleeping, visiting with friends, and eating healthy foods.

Almost a month after the hernia repair, the wound opened once more. This time I had an open wound, the result of an abdominal seroma. The surgeon told me that the body's open post-surgical wound would now need to heal itself. In short, I would need to live with and care for an open body wound while the body itself directed my healing. I would not be re-sewn. No physician would preside over my healing. Instead, I would need to wait for the body to heal itself. The body would need to preside over its own healing if I were to return to full health. I was devastated and I was terrified.

For more than a year I lived with an open abdominal wound that steadily and slowly healed. But its scarring was deep and permanent. Each day during those months the body's wounds called me insistently to care for my inner spirit's wounds.

In the years before my malignancy was diagnosed, I had lived in grief. In each of the preceding six years, someone of great importance to my life had died or an important relationship had failed. I had tried to do my grief work with each death or loss, but when a college classmate and close friend died at age 50 from breast cancer, I was bereft. I was overwhelmed by staggering, wordless grief. I simply held it inside and carried it as my own share of the world's grief. I had no language skills capable of speaking to anyone at this desolate inner space.

My own diagnosis followed my friend's death by five weeks. I was initially quite sure that I was going to follow her into the land of death. But each time I heard that thought in my head, I simultaneously found a strong desire to live. I did something that was uncharacteristic of my personality. I reached out to all of my friends and colleagues and said, *ask your own gods that I might live*. I explored the realms of conventional and alternative possibilities. I began a series of therapeutic touch sessions. In one of these sessions, I entered a state of altered consciousness and found a vortex of energy entering my body though the body's center of balance.

Before these surgeries, I held to a strong belief in the power of the life force to bring about physical and emotional healing. Now, however, faced with the body's open wound I crossed into a world of anxiety, fear, and anger. I was terrified by the need to touch and take care of this wound several times a day.

One night, shortly after the seroma dumped my body fluids on the concrete floor of my basement, I was alone in my home. I heard my own voice screaming, *I hate you body, for doing this to me*. I was so shocked by my words that I retreated into an immediate, total, and withdrawn emotional silence. I immediately understood that this was not an attitude that would foster mind–body–spirit healing. Reflecting upon this moment of enraged shouting, I made the decision to change this imagery and emotional experience into an attitude of seeking to cooperate with the body-self rather than assault it with my rage.

In the midst of all of this emotional upheaval, my body steadily and slowly moved toward healing. The scarring was deep and permanent. Each day during that year, the body's wounds called me to recognize deeper and earlier wounds of the spirit and psyche. With a clinical therapist's help, I confronted ancient personal out-of-body experiences, a near-death experience, childhood trauma, and instances of dissociated terror. With therapeutic help, I touched ancient wounds that had left disturbed energy fields in their wake.

With the help of my primary health care practitioner, I created a complex team of healers. Each of them reassured me that my strong belief in the power of the life force to heal was essential. Each of them acknowledged my terror while not indulging it. Each of them helped me to decode into a recognizable language that which previously had been wordless and totally chaotic. With slow steps I entered another form of psychic space, a layer of consciousness I had not previously encountered or explored.

Spontaneous healing imagery began to erupt. For several months I imaged the cellular structure of my abdomen being recreated. Every time I cared for my body's wound, I sang an adaptation of a little children's song: *inch by inch, row by row, gonna help my body grow*. As I sang I imagined healthy cells at work clearing out debris and replacing scar tissue with living cells. I imagined a cellular bricklayer choosing cells and placing them in just the right spaces, leaving no pockets of air or fluid for bacteria to enter and infect the wound. All three images are the body-minds attempts to cooperate with my request for healing imagery to emerge. None is rational. None could have been planned logically. This is the beauty of guided imagery work.

One day as I sang, I became aware that a large fish was swimming in the open wound of my abdomen. Asking what it was, it said its name was sturgeon. In the inner, non-rational world of spontaneous imagery, a large sturgeon appeared to help me keep my body wound clean. I knew almost nothing about these great fish. When I talked to my primary care physician, she said something like, *Oh, Ruth, that's wonderful. They are some of the most ancient living organisms that we know. In imagery work, this fish will help you keep your wound clean and healing.*

As I continued to work with my body and my psyche, I encountered wells of grief and exploding zones of panic. In doing energy work, energy cysts moved and shifted and then drained. I simply tried to stay present to whatever emotional response emerged as I dealt with a body that seemed to have turned on me. When I hit zones of terror and overwhelming sadness, I tried to find the inner lesson. I found the sturgeon's cleansing presence in the field of my inner world to be reassuring. As I deliberately and carefully worked with my inner sturgeon, bricklayer, and gardener, I also realized that most people would think I'd lost my rational mind.

Sensing my deep inner loss of balance and some unspeakable anguish, each healer encouraged me to seek help in the creative forces that were less dependent upon logical, analytical thought. When poetry began to emerge, each healer was willing to read it and to talk with me about it.

Sensing in me a primitive mix of confusing emotions (rage, despair, and unremitting anxiety), each healer encouraged me to find the way into my terrors and to believe that I was strong enough to make it through the land of the living dead back into the land of the fully living.

At one point in the process I heard one of my clinicians say, "When you can accept all of this body and psyche chaos as your teacher and be grateful to it, then life's own healing can begin to flow into your life, no matter what the specific outcome in your body." This resonated within me so profoundly that I knew it to be truth. In my post-surgical encounters with physical wounds and weakness, I was guided to acknowledge and to seek healing for inner emotional and spiritual chaos as well.

In the middle of my recovery year, in a moment of synchronicity, I traveled to a professional meeting in philosophy and medicine at Pacific Medical Center in San Francisco and heard Jungian analyst Jean Shinoda Bolen read from her book, *Close to the Bone*. She described the Sumerian myth of Inanna's journey as one that could be helpful to guide individuals in their illness journeys. In the middle of her lecture she described a friend's encounter with cancer. For her woman friend the mythic Inanna and her recorded journey into the underworld was a journey that brought understanding and comfort. That evening Bolen recommended the myth's teachings to the assembled physicians, nurses, and other healers.

In *Close to the Bone: Life Threatening Illness and the Search for Meaning*, Bolen (1996) elaborates upon her intuitions about the importance of Inanna's journey as a way to conceptualize the chronic realities of illness, which compromises the body–spirit–psyche integrity of the person who is ill.

> Metaphorically and actually, illness and hospitalization strip us of what covered and protected us in many ways... the journey is similar to Inanna's. There are still gates we go through which strip us of persona and defense; we become exposed and bare-souled. The stripping away makes it possible for us to reach depths within ourselves that we might otherwise not reach, where whatever we consigned there or abandoned or forgot of ourselves suffers the pain of not being remembered or of not being integrated into our conscious personality or allowed expression. (pp. 31–32)

The day after hearing Bolen lecture, I hunted down a library copy of Wolkstein's and Kramer's (1983) compilation of Sumer's mythic stories about Inanna. I began to research the goddess and her narrative. As a theologian and former seminary student, I already knew about Inanna. However, until the evening of Bolen's speech, Inanna was simply one of the bronze-age deities who populated the world of antiquity. I immediately found Inanna's story to be compelling. I sought to allow the ancient myth to enter dialogue with my own actual narrative of struggle and search. In particular, I began with therapeutic help to look at the questions raised by my post-surgical encounters with a disrupted and disorderly psyche and body. I began to search for deep acceptance and deep joy as the womb of my healing.

As you read my retelling of this ancient story of Inanna's journey into the underworld of death, have compassion for yourself. Open your own spirit and heart to know and understand your personal and unique journeys through life's continuous cycles of loss, grief, and transformation. Inanna's passage from life into the bleak underworld of death teaches us about giving ourselves over to life's important work with us.

INANNA: ANCIENT SUMER'S GODDESS

Who was Inanna and what was her journey? What we know about her has been brought into our contemporary era as scholars have located and translated Bronze Age Sumer's clay cuneiform tablets which have been recovered from today's landmass of Iraq. Thousands of years ago, her priests, priestesses and scribes carved stories about Inanna and her place within Sumer's cosmology. They left them behind as Sumer's power waned and Inanna's temples were abandoned.

The mythic Inanna was a goddess. In her own era she was the most powerful deity in the Sumerian pantheon. Her story, according to Pritchard (1961), sheds light on Sumero-Akkadian-Babylonian religious beliefs. Worship of her was born in prehistory and her lineage is unclear. As with many succeeding goddesses, she appears to have appropriated powers and symbols of lesser deities into her own.

Sumer was as influential in its time and place as was Ancient Greece to another era. Sumer's influence followed the trade routes and it is believed by some historians that evidence of Inanna's influence and importance can be found as far west as England and as far east as India and China. As century followed century, her names as a dominating goddess changed just as political powers changed and empires changed. Because of her many names and her many iconic representations as, for example, the Queen of Heaven, today's scholars trace her to Aphrodite/Venus in the later Greco-Roman centuries. In addition, many of her iconic and representative symbols have become associated with Christianity's Virgin Mary (Baring & Cashford, 1991).

Her worship centers occurred within two different ethnic groups. In the south, in Sumer, the goddess was called Inanna. Stories about her from this place were centered on temples in Sumer's major cities. To the north, the Semitic people known as the Akkadians called their leading goddess Ishtar. Many of Inanna's attributes and iconic symbols were taken over by Ishtar. The particular myth that I have chosen to use is known as the Sumerian Descent of Inanna. In the Sumerian story, Inanna hears voices that command her to journey to the underworld ruled by her sister Ereshkigal. As she makes her decent, she must cross through seven gates. At each gate she must give up an object that signifies her rule and her power in the upper world.

A similar yet slightly nuanced myth appears later in history as *the Akkadian Descent of Ishtar*. The two descent stories represent somewhat different perspectives on Inanna's personality. In the Akkadian story she is bolder in her behaviors at the underworld's gate. In this version she pounds on the door to the underworld and demands entrance.

In my retelling of the Inanna myth, I have chosen to stay within the constraints of the earlier Sumerian version while remaining aware of the later Akkadian one.

In *The Descent of Inanna,* the clay tablets describe the journey of Inanna from her home in the heavens where she rules as daughter of the moon and queen of the date palm oasis. In the narrative she decides to journey into the underworld domain that is ruled by her older sister Ereshikigal. Her reasons for making this journey are unknown to us.

In Sumer's stories about Ereshikigal, we learn that she lived in a lapis lazuli palace in the middle of a great underworld cave where the shades lived in darkness and were covered with dust. The relationship of the two sisters is not explained in great detail. Pritchard (1961) raises the question of whether Ereshkigal was Inanna's enemy as well as her sister. Other Jungian-influenced authors such as Reis (1991) and Perera (1981) raise the question of whether or not Inanna and Ereshkigal form one complete archetype. In such a view, Ereshkigal represents the resentful, denied, buried, despised, silenced, sacrificed, or forgotten aspects of the self.

The clay tablets tell us that when she heard the voices of the underworld, Inanna immediately dressed in the regal garments of her rule as goddess of the sky and earth. In the extant text that we have, however, it appears as if she had a premonition that not all would go well during her journey. Before she began her journey, she advised her loyal servant Ninshubar to watch for her return. Warning Ninshubar that she might not be able to leave the underworld in order to return to earth by a certain time, she requested Ninshubar to contact the gods to ask them to search for her and rescue her.

Leaving Ninshubar behind, she traveled toward the underworld. Arriving at the entrance to Ereshkigal's realm, she had to pass seven gates or thresholds and meet the demands of seven gate guardians. At each gate she was forced by that gate's guardian to give away a garment, a piece of jewelry, or some other valued sign of her rule as queen of the upper worlds.

Arriving at the seventh gate, she was stripped of all remaining garments, jewelry, and signs of her rule. She was forced to crawl naked into Ereshkigal's presence. Here Ereshkigal was joined by the Anunnaki, the seven dreaded judges of Sumer's underworld.

Her elder sister was not happy to see Inanna and fixed on her the eyes of death. Turned into a corpse, Inanna hung on the peg of death like a slab of decaying meat. For three days and three nights (the nights of the dark moon) she hung there.

When Inanna did not return on time, her servant Ninshubar asked various Sumerian gods for help. Each God refused to change the rules of the realm of death except Enki, the god of wisdom. To help Inanna return to life, Enki created small genderless creatures that crept into the underworld. Their only mission was to rescue Inanna. As instructed by Enki, they sprinkled on her the food and waters of life. Following this sprinkling, Inanna returned to full life.

Faced with her now reborn and living sister, Ereshkigal agreed that Inanna might return to the upper world of earth and sky. However, she insisted that the rules of her realm of death must be followed. A substitute needed to be brought back to the realm of death.

As she traveled home, Inanna encountered her mourning servants and refused to condemn these faithful servants to take her place. Encountering her mourning children, she likewise refused to condemn them to take her place.

However, as she came to her seat of rule she found her lover-consort Dumuzi sitting in the place of rule. He was sitting in a chair carved out of the world tree. Discovering that he had not mourned her absence at all, Inanna immediately gave Dumuzi to Ereshkigal's demons so that they could carry him back to the underworld in her place. She then resumed her rule.

In this Sumerian myth of death and resurrection, the goddess Inanna completed the cycle of life to which the underworld's voices called her. She traveled into the world of death. As she reemerged from the land of death into the land of earth and sky, she returned to her role as goddess of the moon and the date palm oasis. By her return earth's fertility was once more assured and the cycle of the seasons was once again shaped into life's ongoing order and repetition. The moon returned to the sky and her star (Venus) showed itself.

What then is Inanna's own story? What do the recovered finds of archeologists tell us about her life and times? What must it have been like for a goddess to give up all of her divine powers to the power of death? What must it have felt like to lose sight of her star in the sky? What must it have meant to her to leave the stability of her chair of rule that was carved from the world tree? What did it mean to her to leave the comfort of the date palm oasis for a rugged journey into the underworld? What did she experience as she kept losing more and more of her garments, her jewelry, and her symbols of rule? What fears did she have? What doubts? When we read the original sacred myths and poetry of Sumer, we find that Inanna's story teaches us about the inevitability of suffering. We find that it also teaches us about the amazing powers of faithful love to transform suffering into resurrection and renewed life.

THE SONG OF LIFE SINGS US: PERSONAL REFLECTIONS ON SUFFERING AND HEALING

Inanna's Way bears testimony to the life force that flows in and through each one of us and that will continue to flow when our bodies return to the dust from which we were created. Life has borne us out of the womb of past generations and continues to give birth to itself in succeeding generations. For this moment we are simply a manifested vessel of consciousness into which Life has poured flesh, breath, and spirit. For this period of time we know as our individual life, we are simply a water skin of life's consciousness. Life moves in and through us as she wills. Life brings us to breath, and for as long as we live, Life breathes us.

We participate with Life by living but we cannot control Life as she moves among us, breathing each one of us into life as we know it and bringing us to consciousness. When our own individual life ceases to be breathed, Life will continue to bring consciousness into all subsequent manifestations of her ongoing being and becoming.

Every individual life knows times of death, destruction, suffering, and loss as well as times of resurrection and reanimation of the life force. No human individual can escape the underworld's shadowy wisdom for life.

Inanna's passage from the underworld back into life provides us with an important foreknowing. Even when we are most trapped in awareness of our own suffering, we need to know that our continuing life contains the present moment of transcendence. Transformation is always possible.

Because we love life; because we love others; because we love ourselves: each of us must bushwhack and cut open our own trails through the wilderness of suffering. The moment when the wilderness of our suffering closes in around us is the moment when we know we are lost. In the moment that we realize we have lost our way, we concomitantly find ourselves standing in strange doorways that both beckon to us and repel us. Having entered the pathway into the dark night of the soul, we discover altars in places where we least anticipate shrines and burial vaults where we most desire to worship Life.

SLUICE GATES

> In seeking a way across the raging river;
> In seeking a way to escape these drenching rains;
> In seeking a way into gentle shelters with firelit hearths;
> In seeking a way to cover my ragged nakedness with soft, dry fleece;
> I merge with the wind and rain.
> I slip through to the altar of the river's gods.

Upon entering into life-changing boundary situations, we begin, if we are wise, to prepare for an arduous journey. In the moment when we hear the voices of our own underworld calling us, we know that they call us by our many names. Intuitively we realize that we are trapped into a journey we would avoid if at all possible. However, upon hearing these underworld voices calling us, we know immediately that there is no way to avoid them. There is no way to avoid making the journey into the dark night of our suffering.

LARGE EARTHQUAKES

> I have crossed through a gate I did not see.
> I have passed under a portal I did not know existed.
> Innocence has been mauled

Simplicity has been assaulted
Contentment has been attacked
Vulnerability has been abused
There are secret corridors here
There are chaotic labyrinths here
Harmony has been corroded
Trust has been disrupted
Joy has been buried alive
Abundance has been plundered
I have passed through a doorway I did not recognize
I have passed over a threshold I did not perceive

Sensing that hard times lie ahead for us, we mobilize our resources so that others may watch over us. No one, it is true, can walk through the overgrown wilderness thickets of our own personal suffering for us. No one can even walk with us through our personal gates of loss and grief. But, knowing that we are lovingly attended to and watched over, we find hope that we may be able to find an honorable way to travel into the depths of our ancient grief and our current suffering, and in those depths, find healing.

Tossed against the doorway of illness and its concomitant physical and emotional suffering, we intuit that our journey will change us, and our perception of the world, forever. Times of life-threatening illness; times when we lose our powers in the world; times of strong grief; times of great fear; times of struggle with the unnamed and unknowable: these are all times of hearing the call of the world of death. Each of these experiences can provide the impetus for us to explore our own underworld of the shadows and the shades. Each of these can take us into nether worlds whose meaning to us is so deep that we have no words adequate for the task of making our way.

As we struggle with the inner chaos of voicelessness, wordlessness, and fear, we realize the nearly total loss of our powers of control in the world. As we struggle with the absence of adequate maps, oracles, portents, and prophecies, we discover that it is imperative to befriend our ongoing existential experiences of pain, anxiety, terror, rage, and despair. We discover, as we journey, that we must face and acknowledge the inner experience that so devastates us and lays waste to our usual powers in the world. In our sense of being lost, we realize we must make peace with the experience of being lost.

OBSCURE BORDER

Yesterday I crossed borders
But knew not how I passed from one land into the second.
There were no border guards
With guns at the ready to prevent my passing.
There were no petty functionaries
With stamps and inks to mark my papers
Or to deny my travel rights.
There were no gates to seal the boundaries

To foreigners and aliens—all those who do not belong.
There were no trained dogs with bared teeth
To stop me from straying.
Yesterday I crossed borders
But knew not how I passed from one land into the second.

Somewhere in the wilderness (or the bleak arid desert) of our own partic-ular journey into the soul's dark night, we begin to reflect on our life and our current troubles. In these actual moments of memory, turmoil, panic, and despair, we attempt to hold onto sustaining memories of centeredness, security, and joy.

We begin, then, to create meaning out of this present moment of suf-fering. In our intense self-examination, something deep stirs within us and we remember what it was like to feel well and whole. We stretch toward that remembered wholeness with intense desire. No longer totally separated from our own self; no longer totally alienated from the life force that contin-ues to live in us; no longer sensing our absolute separation from others: we slowly open ourselves to whatever it will be that finds us and heals us. In that moment of surrender and opening, a well of healing waters shows itself to us and we begin to drink.

Tasting the remembered artesian waters of life, we recognize that our jour-ney has already changed us and is continuing to change us. We recognize that we are a metamorphosis in process. With this recognition, we begin the slow acknowledgment to ourselves and others that we can never return to who we were in the moment just before our journey into life's underworld began.

LARGE WATERFALL

To get to this spot
I walked into uncertain canyons
And rock crevices so narrow
I knew I could not find my way back
The way I came.
To get to this point
I walked across dunes so high and windswept
I thought I might drown,
Unseen and un-mourned,
Under barren, shifting rivers of sand
To get to this place
I slid down mountainsides so ragged
I thought I might fall straight down
Into isolated and undisclosed ravines.
I could not think about them without trembling.

A wild grief erupts because we are no longer who we were. A rough-handed terror claims us because we do not yet know who we are now. Dread invades and shadows our brooding because we cannot know the outcome of our journey until it is completed. We feel the psychic tug of our wounds and scars. Simultaneously, however, we feel the strong tug of the life force calling us forward.

There is no way to successfully abort the journey and return to wholeness. The only way to find a full, abundant, and living life is to continue. The only way to return to the upper world of the living is to yield to the transforming processes of the underworld—those processes of dying and resurrection that continuously move in and through us.

THE SOUL'S BIRTHPLACE

> I am unrecognizable to myself
> Standing here
> In harsh winds and rain
> With clothing that does not conceal,
> Skin that does not protect.

The path out of the wilderness of suffering begins with this time of inner reflection. The way begins with our own deep inner processes of searching for the meaning of suffering in our particular life. In this time of reflection and deep searching we eventually learn to trust our personal experience. We eventually learn to honor suffering's wisdom for our lives. Gradually we come to accept the presence of suffering as our most reliable guide through the wildness of the dark night into which life has tossed us.

WALLS AND GATES OF STONE

> The descent is slow.
> Each step is just one stone away from a broken body—
> From a body that is unable to rise again.
> The horizon is hidden:
> The path covered with long shadows.
> In the distance I see palm trees
> And a huge pool of turquoise water.
> With outstretched arms, I begin to run.
> The mirage fills my nose with the scent of hibiscus and flowering plumeria.
> It comforts my feet.
> It soothes my wind-scarred eyes.
> It bathes my skin in rapture.
> I rush forward to swim in its waters.
> Entrance, however, is denied.
> Posted guardians of the gate deny me access.

In learning to be present to the experience of suffering as our teacher and guide, we begin to experience a deeper joy that travels with us in spite of access, in spite of cure. We are not only suffering and dying. We are being reborn into life. We begin to recognize that each moment in which Life breathes us into being, we are embodied life. Life not only suffers in us and with us. Life also rejoices in us and in itself. Even in the midst of the chaos of not knowing whether we will live or die; in the midst of not knowing whether we will succeed or fail miserably in our search for life: Life herself pours the waters of healing all around us. In the moments of our journey when healing flows into us and through us; in the moments when the waters of life connect with us: we enter into moments of truthful resurrection.

> Reflections from the World of the Shadow Trees Naked and suffering
> I hang between the worlds
> And hope life is stronger than death.
> Alone and bleeding
> I struggle between the worlds
> And wait for the waters that contain death.
> Isolated and weeping
> I search between the worlds
> And discover the soul's labyrinth understands death.
> Abandoned and despairing
> I dance between the worlds
> And trust the heartbeat's rhythms to transform death.
> Silent and speechless
> I hear the music between the worlds
> And begin to sing my resurrection.

Immersed in the healing waters of life, we find a song singing us. It is the song of Life and as long as we breathe it is always present within us. Hearing the song of Life singing deeply within our consciousness, we begin to sing our own song back to her. We sing and Life sings back. Life sings and we sing back. In the mutual song, we encounter embodied joy.

If we are to emerge from these deep, gray, wordless underworlds of our encounters with life's difficult will for us, we must bow before the gates of death and pray that the vital song of the life force has not forgotten us. The sorrows and losses that we take into the land beyond words must become our teachers if we are to live equitably with their terrifying presence. In the moment of acceptance of our situation exactly as it is (no more and no less), our sorrows and our losses become our transforming powers.

THE WORLD'S OFFERINGS

> It is said that suffering makes us wise
> And becomes our truest teacher.
> It is said that suffering is a result of sin
> And by repenting we can stop its ravaging of our spirits.
> It is said that suffering is due to our attachments
> And all we need to do is to let them go.
> It is said that suffering is inevitable

And by accepting our fate we can live honorably.
It is said that suffering is karmic
And by this life we redeem our past lives.
It is said that suffering is what makes us most human
And that we can offer it our thanks.
It is said that suffering is caused by our weakness
And by choosing to be strong we can grow beyond it.
It is said that suffering is our rite of purification for rebirth
And by embracing it we are transformed.
It is said that suffering connects us most deeply with others
And by drinking from the well of suffering we learn, at last, compassion.

Brought into suffering by our life and its journeys, we eventually reach a place of multiple impasses. Any path that we can see in front of us appears to us as a wrong path. We are stuck. We cannot go back the way we came. We cannot see the path ahead of us. We resent the apparent "unfairness" of life. We call upon denial to manage our suffering. We call upon anger to mobilize our failing resources. To no avail!

Nevertheless, even in the middle of our suffering, Life continues to call to us. We sense that we must move forward and that by our choices we will create our future. We encounter fears so ancient they have no reasonable names. In the silence of our suffering, we intuit an even deeper silence of healing. We open inner doors of the spirit—doors we previously had no knowing of—and we find new spaces in which to create and live our ongoing lives.

Encountering in our own personal experience (as if for the first time in human life) these ancient and archetypal stories, our naïve innocence is shattered. Our deepest intuitions tell us that once called by unknown voices to make such a journey, we cannot refuse. Thrown into suffering by the gods, the fates, or by life itself, we sense with a deep foreknowing that our life trajectory has been permanently changed.

BIRTHING WOMAN

A woman who decides, however she decides,
To give birth to a new self
Nevertheless shrieks loud grief for her old dead self
But *silently* so no one may hear her.
The loss of easy habits and conventional gestures;
The absence of midwives boiling water;
A deep inner ambivalence about such a pregnancy:
All of these, and more, snake-like
Create a shedding of identity.
A familiar, beloved and comfortable skin must be left behind.
Coming to a moment just before the moment of her birthing
She squats in the time of the dark moon
And ponders what she has done.

In that fertile darkness of brooding silence and waiting
She enters the night sky to divine the signs.
With awe and reverence she weaves herSelf
A bright red ribbon to wear around her left wrist.
She crochets an indigo silk sleeping cap
To protect her from hostile winds and
Embroiders a cashmere dreaming blanket to shelter her fears,
To comfort her times of aloneness.

We know with a deep wordless knowing that to have any hope of being reborn into wellness and wholeness, we must move into and through our pain. We must learn how to embrace it as our teacher. The journey into such a mythic dying to our previous self paradoxically becomes a journey into deep healing. Begun in suffering, this journey becomes nothing less than a passage into spiritual transformation of the individual.

GIVING BIRTH

She has risked creation
She has become a she-goddess pregnant with a new universe
She is going to give birth to herSelf.
Her labor has just begun.

This is the wisdom of Inanna's journey into the underworld to meet her older sister Ereshkigal. This is the wisdom of our own stories of moving into our own underworld stories. The cycle of life is a continuously moving circle of living and dying; of dying and living. Accepting this, we begin a journey of deep, inner transformation. In this journey, suffering gives way to acceptance and joy. As long as we live, Life is with us. Understanding this, we come to understand that Life moves always within us to bring us renewed life. As we accept the realities of our life exactly as they are, we begin to understand that all life is sacred. Life's sorrows, suffering, grief, pain, rage, terror, and despair are sacred in their ordinary presence within our lives. As we reach deep within ourselves to find the resources to survive suffering, we discover that it is not only in the good and happy times of our lives that we discover Life's amazing steadfastness to us.

During the crisis of physical illness, I encountered *The Descent of the Goddess Inanna*. In my attempts to make sense of a body that I felt had betrayed me by not healing easily from a surgical wound, I found that Inanna's descent mirrored my own confusion about how to return to remembered wellness and wholeness. In my fears and terrors about future blindness due to macular degeneration I was lost in a forest and all around me were shadow trees. The path to healing appeared blocked no matter which direction I faced.

Needing to reconcile, in some manner, my own life's history with my hopes for the future, I needed to acknowledge what was dead or lost. I needed to encounter that which was still dying. To be born again,

I responded with passionate identification to Inanna's own troubled and troubling journey. As a clinician and healer, I now needed to seek healing. I began the unwanted but necessary process of laying bare the suffering inside.

LIVING WATERS

Come close:
Let your waters heal me.
Sing to me and I will sing back to you
Embrace me in your love.
Help me surrender to life's beauty.
Come closer:
Let your waters heal me.
Sing to me and I will sing back to you.
Carry me skywards while I reach towards the sun.
Help me surrender to life's dance.
Come closer still:
Let your waters heal me.
Sing to me and I will sing back to you.

In the story of Inanna's descent into the underworld of death and its shades, we find the story of Inanna's transformation. As she returns to life, earth's rich fecundity returns with her. Returning to life through the gates of death and loss, an ancient story of transformation and resurrection appears. As we make cyclical journeys into life's more dense realities of suffering, we find Life is there with us as well. To hear our own song, indeed to hear Life's song, within us in the midst of suffering, we must become quiet and still within our spirit. When we reach a certain inner stillness, suffering begins to yield to acceptance. Acceptance allows us to ask of our suffering what it will teach us. In that moment, the healing waters of life flow unrestricted through us and around us. We find that we are not alone. Life is with us. Recognizing her presence we are overcome by joy.

Now, 15 years after my malignancy surgeries and their aftermaths, I have found my way back into life. Now continuing to live with an uncertain visual future, I have begun living in the present moment. Each day I am aware of the wonderful gift of seeing in this day, of living in this day. Each day I celebrate the breath of Life.

A SONG FOR THE SKY

On this day my breath is strong and pure:
I breathe and know I am breathing.
On this day my ears are attentive:
I listen and know I am hearing.
On this day my eyes are open:

I look and know I am seeing.
On this day my pace is measured and steady:
I walk and know I am walking.

A SONG FOR THE OCEANS

On this day my heart is at ease:
I open it and know it is opening.
On this day my mind is peaceful:
I still it and know it is quiet.
On this day my spirit is free:
I unfetter it and know it is celebrating.
On this day my body is awake:
I touch it and know that it knows me.

A SONG FOR THE FOREST

On this day my voice is playful
I tease the gods and hear their ripples of laughter.
On this day my hands are graced
I play the flute and hear its sweet cadences.
On this day my legs are strong
I climb steadily and recognize the path.
On this day my life is content
I look within and find joy.

What I find each morning is such gratitude to the life force for sustaining me through my struggles to re-member and to reorder my life and journey. I find such abiding joy in the present moment of my life where earth's beauties surround me.

I do not believe that Life's goal for us is to celebrate and worship our wounds. Rather, the necessity of our life is to integrate all of our experiences into a foundation for future life. The life we lived before and the life we now live will reveal their secrets to us if we will be quiet enough to listen.

One of our unique life tasks is to learn how to assimilate all aspects of our unique life journey as a teaching. We must learn how to search for Life's lessons in a cyclical process that creates the inner matrix for transformation and resurrections.

The inner balance of destruction and creation; of death and resurrection; of lost stories and epiphanies; of losing and finding: this is a fragile balance that shifts and moves and dances with us. Gradually we learn to trust this inner balance. That which is most alive within us reaches toward and embraces life in all of its complexities. Our inward destructive and creative forces begin to work with each other in a new synthesis, in a new set of harmonies.

Slowly, day by day, I continue to assimilate awareness about acceptance and gratitude. Rereading the poetry years later, I can recognize moments of transforming metaphors. I can find the moments when a subtle shift from clutching pain and grief began. I find moments when a genuine celebration of being alive began to pulse in my veins like wild improvisational dancing. I found myself releasing fear, terror, rage, and despair. One of the most important metaphors from my therapeutic process was a teaching about celebrating breath itself—about allowing myself to be breathed by Life and to find this current, present-moment breath to be sufficient.

What has surprised me the most is the spontaneously recurring comment from a wide variety of friends and colleagues: *these days you seem so much more at peace with yourself.* When I pause with them, I understand that they rightly perceive some vast changes in my inner world. I am growing in patience. I am growing in gratitude. I am growing in acceptance of that which is (as opposed to being depressed at that which is no more or greedy for what is no longer possible).

There has been trauma in my life. I am much less victimized by its history in my life than I was in 1995—when my surgically altered body spoke a simple message to me: *Pay Attention! This time in your life is very important. Don't miss the opportunity to learn, grown, and change.*

By creating the manuscript and poetry of *Inanna's Way*, I began to tell the story of my wounds and of my strong desire to regain a full and joyous life. My particular story as a particular woman blends into Inanna's archetypal story of violence, illness, loss, suffering, dys-ease, and death. In beginning to share the story and poetry outside of my immediate friendship group, I found that these themes became visible to other men and women as they too dealt with various forms of personal suffering.

During the past several years (while the *Inanna's Way* story and poetry rested on my home office shelves) I kept asking myself and I kept asking colleagues and friends, *Is this simply a personal story for close friends and family to understand?* In an elongated process of questioning my own motives for releasing the story into a different sphere than the private one, I decided that if Inanna's story or my own story could be useful to other women and men who have lost their own sense of a trusted and beloved body, then it was important to leave behind my intense personal sense of privacy in order that others who needed her story could hear the story of the Goddess Inanna for themselves.

INANNA II

Good morning, Sun
Good morning, Earth
Good morning, Cool Mists
Good morning, Soft Breezes
I am Inanna.
I am daughter of the moon and queen of heaven;
Protector of the date palm oasis and full granaries;
My star in the heavens shines in the morning and in the evening.

I have returned from my sister Ereshikigal's cave.
I have come back into life.
I have returned to you.
In my hands once more are the powers granted me by the gods.

NOTES

1. This is a spiral dance chant I learned from Matthew Fox at a Body and Soul Conference in Seattle, WA, sometime during the 1990s.
2. The poetry in this chapter is my own and involves a retelling of Inanna's story.

REFERENCES

Baring, A. & Cashford, J. (1991). *The myth of the goddess: Evolution of an image.* London, UK: Arkana/Penguin.

Bolen, J. S. (1996). *Close to the bone: Life-threatening illness and the search for meaning.* New York, NY: Scribners.

Perera, S. (1981). *Descent to the goddess: A way of initiation for women.* Toronto, Canada: Inner City Books.

Pritchard. J. B. (Ed.). (1961). *Ancient near eastern tests relating to the Old Testament* (3rd ed. with Supplement). Princeton, NJ: Princeton University Press.

Reis, P. (1991). *Through the goddess: A woman's way of healing.* New York, NY: Scribners.

Wolkstein, D. & Kramer, S. N. (1983). *Inanna: Queen of heaven and earth: Her stories and hymns.* New York, NY: Harper and Row.

CHAPTER 13

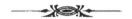

In Spite of: Reflecting on My Son's Pain and Suffering

Noel Boyle

> *The courage to be is rooted in the God who appears when God has disappeared in the anxiety of doubt.*
>
> —Paul Tillich

I hope to explain how Christian theologian Paul Tillich has helped me think about the pain and suffering endured by my severely disabled son named Ciaran (keer-in). Conversely, by reflecting on Ciaran's life, I hope to illuminate the concrete and lived meaning of Paul Tillich's abstract theological and philosophical claims. I hope the end result is a general framework that might help anyone dealing with chronic pain and illness.

CIARAN I: " . . . IN THE ANXIETY OF DOUBT"

On May 27, 2000, when he was six months old, Ciaran had his first seizure. It lasted 35 minutes. The emergency room physician said it was a febrile (fever caused) seizure, relatively common in young children. Ciaran was sent home. My wife Jessica protested, firmly stating her belief that something serious was wrong, and that we would be back.

Two days later, we were back. Ciaran's second seizure, unlike the first, was not a typical rhythmically convulsing event. It was what we later learned to call an atonic seizure, a type of seizure characterized by loss of muscle control and tone—a sort of semi-conscious wet noodle state. We arrived at the emergency room and the seizure was stopped with intravenous (IV) medications.

It had lasted 45 minutes. Ciaran was admitted to the hospital for a battery of tests. The next day, May 30, he was suffering from some sort of infection or reaction; he spent the entire day screaming inconsolably as the result of some unknown agony. Test results indicated nothing. A neurologist was consulted and Ciaran was prescribed an anti-seizure medication. He was released the next day.

Life-threatening seizures began to occur every four or five days. During this time, nearly all of his seizures were over 30 minutes long and associated with varying degrees of respiratory failure, ranging from events in which he would lose some color in his lips to events in which he would stop breathing altogether. In June of 2000 a pattern developed in which he would have a seizure, be rushed to the emergency room, be given IV medication to stop the seizure (after the emergency medication that we had at home failed), be admitted for overnight observation and testing, and have only a couple of days of respite before another terrifying seizure would restart the cycle.

On one such occasion, we rushed him to the emergency room, seizing and blue, nearly 15 minutes into a seizure. Knowing that his veins were extremely difficult to access, the nurses began working immediately to start an IV. At first, there was one working on his left arm. She tried and failed a couple of times. Another nurse started working independently on the right arm. She also failed a couple of times. Ten minutes later, 30 minutes into the seizure, there was still no IV access. Ciaran was convulsing; the respiratory therapist was manually pumping air into his lungs using a bag and mask. Two more nurses joined in the IV attempt, one on each leg. The doctor was standing at the head of the bed; she was trying to start an IV in his scalp (regularly done in such small children). I stopped counting at 30 failed attempts to start an IV; 30 times, they inserted a needle and accomplished nothing. Thirty-five minutes into the seizure, the doctor attempted placement of an intraosseous line (IO), using an object that looked to us like a meat thermometer. She poured iodine over his little left leg and climbed onto the table. Using her body weight, she drove the wide four inch needle directly into his shin bone. As she explained to us later, there is a soft area in the shinbones of very young children. Despite being unconscious and still seizing, Ciaran cried out in response to the pain. They connected the medication tubing to the IO line. But before the medication could be delivered, the line stopped working. Leaving the IO needle sticking out of his shin, she called for another one. The second time it worked; IO access was established, and the seizure was stopped. As I looked at my son in the emergency room unresponsive, recovering from a seizure, with two four-inch needles sticking out of his tiny shins, I realized that less than an hour earlier, he was playing on the living room floor at home. Four days previously, he had been released from the hospital after a similar, slightly less horrific incident. It would be only about five days before he went through something similar again.

During a mid-July 2000 appointment at the Mayo Clinic, we became acquainted with video EEG monitoring, a tool used for advanced diagnosis of seizure disorders and an indispensable tool for surgical evaluation. The goal of the test is to determine, as precisely as possible, the location of the brain tissue generating the seizures. The EEG technician literally glued about 20 wires to Ciaran's head. As Ciaran could not be made to understand what was happening, he had to be wrapped tightly in a sheet with his arms folded in, a technique with a deceptively benign name: papoosing. After the wires were glued to his scalp, his head was wrapped in gauze so that he could not pull at the wires. The wires themselves were bundled and routed through the back of his gauze-wrapped head, looking like a long pony tail of brightly and variously colored strands. Then he was placed in front of a video so a seizure could be captured.

Unfortunately, Ciaran seizure began shortly before they were to hook him up to the EEG machine. We knew the pattern; the emergency medications that they administered in order to stop the seizure would ensure a few nearly seizure-free days. And so it was. For seven beautiful days, Ciaran played in his crib and the immediate area that was (mostly) in range of the video camera. In the end, the Mayo physicians could tell us only that he had a seizure disorder of unknown cause, nature, origin, and trajectory.

Over the next two years, Ciaran's seizure disorder grew in complexity and intensity. By the spring of 2002, he was having nearly every type of seizure recognized by neuroscience. Generalized tonic-clonic seizures racked his whole body. Tonic seizures contracted every muscle in his body, making it difficult even to force air into his lungs. With secondarily generalizing seizures, Ciaran howled in abject terror, knowing he was about to lose conscious contact with the world. During partial seizures, in which only some defined part of the body convulsed, he threw himself at the nearest loved one and clutched with agonizing force. Gelastic seizures caused him to laugh uncontrollably and maniacally. During myoclonic seizures, one or more of his limbs jolted a single time and he briefly lost consciousness; clusters of such seizures made life seem to him like a movie in which short pieces have been spliced out. During those two years, we saw no developmental progress whatsoever, most particularly in terms of speech and language.

On April 27, 2002, Ciaran was scheduled for brain surgery at Children's Hospital of Michigan in Detroit. As Ciaran lay between Jessica and me on the night before the first of two scheduled phases of the surgery, we counted nearly 150 myoclonic seizures during a single hour. He was on enough depressant medication to sedate a horse and still going through the cycle of increasing clusters of little seizures, up to hundreds a day, that persisted until the clusters ran together into a life-threatening episode of *status epilepticus* (non-stop seizure), followed by a day or two of respite before the clusters started again.

The purpose of the first surgery was to set up a very fine resolution video EEG. The surgeon removed the skull plate on the left side of Ciaran's head. He placed tiny electrodes, laid in rows and columns on several pieces of silicon, directly on the surface of Ciaran's brain. He then replaced the skull plate, leaving wires protruding through little holes in the back of Ciaran's scalp. Afterward, the wires were connected to a computer, EEG recording was begun, and a camera was trained on Ciaran's bed. Then the swelling began. Both eyes became blackened and swollen shut. The skin on his face, stretched by the swelling, was shiny, hard, and seemed as brittle as fine china. For three days, he lay like that and seized while they mapped the hundred or so locations on his brain that were most directly responsible for his seizures.

On the fourth day, he went back into the operating room and had two sections of the left half of his brain removed. Specifically, most of the frontal lobe and the posterior half of the temporal lobe were resected. The parts of his brain responsible for conscious control of movement were left intact. The doctors were very clear that the remaining portions of the left hemisphere were also involved in some of his seizures (as was the right hemisphere). Their hope and expectation was that, with the most epileptogenic brain tissue resected, the remaining tissue would "settle down" and the impact of his seizure disorder would be greatly mitigated.

The other possibility that they mentioned is what happened, instead. The remaining left brain became markedly more epileptic, as though the parts of his brain that they removed were previously suppressing the epileptic discharges from unresected portions. In particular, the part of his brain responsible for conscious control of movement (the primary motor strip) became more epileptogenic. A new pattern emerged, its gruesome regularity recorded on the dry erase board in his hospital room. It began with a rhythmic twitch in his big right toe. Over a period of six to eight hours, the twitch would involve the other toes, then also the ankle, then the leg, the right arm, and the right side of his face. Once his face started twitching, the seizure would generalize and his whole body would convulse as he faced another life threatening event of respiratory suppression and *status epilepticus*. The staff on the neurology unit would intervene, giving him up to 2.5 mg of Ativan (a breathtaking amount). The closest the staff could come to stopping the seizure was getting back to the point where only the big right toe was twitching. And it would start over, repeating every six to eight hours.

Ciaran spent eight days going through that cycle over and over again while they ran more tests, looked at more scans, and held more conferences. At one point, the neurologists decided new EEG information was necessary (after all, they were now dealing with an anatomically different brain). Just a few days after his first two surgeries, they were gluing electrodes directly on the fresh surgical wound. He screamed until he vomited and passed out.

The decision was made to remove the entire remaining left hemisphere, a procedure called a hemispherectomy. Surgery was scheduled for May 8, 2002. As I carried him toward surgery, I knew that, by removing the primary motor strip we were creating a permanent physical disability where none currently existed. I was hopeful, however, given the doctors' assurances that this final surgery would likely be the end of his seizures. The primary neurologist even predicted that Ciaran would learn to talk within a few months. As we rounded a hallway corner and faced the entrance to the surgical prep area for the third time in two weeks, Ciaran recognized the place. He lost it. He screamed, squirmed, hit me repeatedly in the face, and grabbed the door frame in a vain attempt to avoid going over the threshold.

We had been told that, when Ciaran woke up from surgery, he would have no control over the right side of his body; it would be very bad at first but would improve in time. When Ciaran awoke, he could not sit up because he could not control the trunk muscles in the right half of his body. He could not hold up his head, as he could not control the muscles on the right side of his neck. When attempting to drink, water oozed out the right side of his mouth. When trying to eat, he would choke as he was unable to sense that food on the right side of his mouth was inadequately chewed. The third night after surgery, as he was beginning to recover from the immediate surgical experience, we were awoken by the sound of him using his healthy left arm to savagely and repeatedly smash his unresponsive right arm against the metal rails of his hospital crib. Later that day, he had a 15-minute seizure.

That was 10 years ago. Though generally medically stable, he still has a major seizure every few days and he has little seizures every day. He has not progressed developmentally since shortly after his first seizure. He has a 10-month-old mind in a 12-year-old body. He is entirely without language. We call him "Gigantibaby." He is affectionate and often stoic. He still likes to do the things that he liked to do when he was six months old: wander around looking for mischief, throw things, bang objects against the wall or on the ground. He hits people sometimes, but he intends no malice; we call it percussive affection. He spends a great deal of time snuggling. Though there have been years at a time when we literally did not see him smile, today he seems more pleased with life than at any time since the first seizure.

After discharge from Detroit Children's Hospital in June of 2002, he spent about six weeks at Mary Free Bed Rehabilitation Hospital in Grand Rapids. By the time he was discharged from there, he was taking a few steps unassisted. Within a few months, he was walking effectively, though with a profoundly unbalanced gait. A year later, in the spring of 2003, Ciaran developed hydrocephalus (fluid in the skull) as a delayed complication from the hemispherectomy. He spent about 70 nights in the hospital, mostly in intensive care. He learned to walk for a third time in the months that followed.

Just last year, in 2011, Ciaran had surgery to correct and prevent the worsening of a slowly unfolding hip displacement caused by a decade of walking with a terribly lopsided gait. Surgeons sawed through the right femur, just below the hip, and rotated the bone about 40 degrees before putting the leg back together with a metal plate. To keep the foot properly in line, they did essentially the reverse procedure to the tibia. A week after the surgery, still bedridden from the operation, the plate came dislodged from the bone; the bone fractured at a lengthwise angle and the screws that were supposed to be holding the bone together were puncturing the soft tissue of his thigh. Though the cause was unknown, doctors speculated that a seizure might have had the force to pull the newly positioned muscle so hard against the bone that something had to give. During emergency surgery, the plate and screws were removed and a nail, running inside the bone marrow along the entire length of the right femur, was inserted. As I write in August of 2012, that surgery was done about 10 months ago. Though he can take some independent steps, he has made sadly little progress in learning to walk for a fourth time.

Early in his childhood, walking around aimlessly in search of mischief was one of Ciaran's favorite things to do. Eating was another. As I mentioned, initially after the hemispherectomy, Ciaran could not swallow water because it would just spill from the right side of his mouth. With time and effort, he returned to a diet of solid food. But hospitalization with hydrocephalus was a setback to his eating; he left the hospital with a feeding tube but still receiving most of his nutrition by mouth. Soon after that discharge, he nearly choked on a hot dog. A few weeks later, a piece of carrot lodged just below his windpipe was removed in the emergency room. He has refused to eat by mouth since.

In 2009, Ciaran was playing when we noticed that he was being quite protective of his left arm. As that is the only arm he can use, and physical contact is his preferred means of interacting with the world, his behavior was more than unusual. At my wife's insistence, we took him to the emergency room. The physician initially said the arm was certainly not broken. After all, Ciaran was not crying. When the physician examined and rotated the arm, Ciaran merely winced. X-rays confirmed that his ulna was fractured. His arm was in a cast for six weeks. He never did cry about it. I suppose that he just didn't bother.

Thus far, I have dwelt on Ciaran's physical/ bodily suffering and the immediate emotional ramifications. But there is another, easily overlooked manner in which Ciaran suffers: he is *isolated*. Ciaran never learned to speak and it is not entirely clear why; left hemispherectomy patients are typically able to use language normally or nearly normally. He lacks the motor dexterity and cognitive capacity to learn sign language. Presented a multitude of times with communication boards, he simply throws them. Ciaran cannot express any of his feelings, beliefs, or wishes except in very rudimentary ways. When put in his car seat, he has no way of knowing whether he faces a 10-hour car ride to see Grandma, a 5-minute ride to the grocery story, or a 20-minute ride to the hospital for another operation. In recent weeks, he has taken to occasional soft weeping. We don't know whether it is an allergic reaction causing red and watery eyes, a new kind of a seizure, a sadness over something he cannot do, a longing for a particular toy that he cannot find, or an overwhelming feeling of anxiety and despair. My wife and I often say that we wish we could spend just 10 minutes inside his head, to experience the world as he experiences it, to live from his point of view. But it is impossible to know how Ciaran experiences the world. He cannot tell me what it is like for him; he cannot create poetic or descriptive introspective language. My own life is too unlike his for me to imagine what it would be like for me to be him; seemingly arbitrary and endless suffering is simply too foreign to me. I have dreamed that I had half of my brain cut out, but I have no idea whether the experiences in my dream at all resembles what it is like to be Ciaran. I spend more time with him than I do with any other person; yet I know less of his point of view and his feelings than those of my most casual acquaintances.

Obviously, I have focused on the hard parts of Ciaran's life, the parts that are theologically troubling, interesting, and potentially fruitful. Before doing some theology, I wanted to establish clearly and unequivocally that Ciaran suffers.

DIGRESSION: DISPENSING WITH SIMPLISTIC THEOLOGY

I reject theologies that somehow deny or diminish Ciaran's suffering. Such theologies are powerless and false. Sadly, such theologies are common; I frequently encounter well-intending people and loving family members offering me simplistic comfort in response to Ciaran's story. People have tried to reassure me that Ciaran's seizure disorder was planned by a loving God, that God comforts Ciaran during seizures, or that Ciaran's suffering is somehow illusory.

The most direct form of such theology denies Ciaran's suffering wholesale. Just as Jesus died for our sins, Jesus intervenes in Ciaran's life to suffer for him; Ciaran literally does not suffer at all because Jesus suffers in his stead. The only motivation I see for holding such a view is a profound desire to believe that Ciaran does not suffer despite all the evidence to the contrary. Wanting something to be true is no reason to believe that it is (a lesson too commonly forgotten or overlooked). Deciding what you want to believe and then constructing a theology to support your beliefs is to make your own wishes, instead of truth, the ultimate standard of your theology. That is ultimately a form of narcissism.

Though such direct denials of Ciaran's suffering are rare, indirect denials are common and equally pernicious. I often hear that Ciaran's suffering is part of a wise and loving plan being implemented with meticulous care by an omnipotent God. While not denying the fact of Ciaran's suffering, this theology holds that Ciaran's suffering is both good and meaningful, as it is a necessary part of something infinitely good. Embracing this theology involves submitting to the will of a being whose plans I cannot understand but, on faith, must accept. It offers comfort in the threefold contention that suffering has a purpose, that the purpose is worthwhile, and that I should never expect to understand the purpose. These represent, of course, standard and noble theological themes of mystery, faith, and submission to the divine.

However, these themes are misapplied here and this too is a theology I simply cannot accept. First, this theology strains logic. A God who figures out which little children must suffer for the sake of His larger plans seems neither good nor loving, no matter how much God loves those who suffer. Such a God is a master manipulator. Under no other circumstances would we find it reasonable to expect someone, especially a child, to suffer on the basis of a promise that "I, the one doing this, am wise enough to know it is good for this child to suffer. Just trust me, as you lack the wisdom and foresight to know—as I do—that the suffering I impose upon this child is actually good and purposeful." Such reassurances should be met here as they would be else-where: with something far stronger than suspicion. I am, of course, familiar with the long tradition of accounting for the presence of evil in a world that is, on the whole, good. However, the intellectual force of such apologetics dissolves in the face of a suffering child. If there is a loving God, He grieves for Ciaran's suffering and is powerless to stop it.

Second, such theology seems motivated only by an attempt to deny the manifest. In 2006, we learned that the underlying cause of Ciaran's condition is a random mutation of his SCN1A gene that occurred during conception. Ciaran has a rare condition called Dravet syndrome. Of course, it is coherent to assert that God caused the genetic mutation. However, the only plausible motivation for such a view is dogmatic adherence to the claim that everything happens for a purpose. That is something that I wish I could believe, but see no reason to believe. An honest assessment of human life reveals random events behind much of what happens. An honest assessment of Ciaran's life recognizes that the genetic mutation did not have to happen, that Ciaran's life would likely have been very different—and very much better—if the mutation had not occurred. An honest theology must open space for true and deep grieving about his suffering, for the loss of the life he might have led; not offer implicit suggestions that Ciaran's suffering is to be met with some kind of mutant celebration of God's mysterious purpose.

In a comment that usually comes in close proximity to the claim that Ciaran's suffering is part of a loving God's plan, people often praise our strength and tell us that God knew what He was doing giving Ciaran to par-ents like Jessica and me. God, as is often said, never gives you more than you can handle. Though I know it well intended, I find such a comment offen-sive. First, I cannot handle being Ciaran's parent. I cannot handle watching him suffer. To say God has given me no more than I can handle is to negate before inspection any claim that I have been harmed or damaged by the demands of parenting Ciaran. At the very least, it is to imply that such harm would reflect my inability to live up to a God-given potential. It lays upon me an expectation that I will handle Ciaran's suffering with grace and joy, or be blameworthy and blasphemous. Second, if it is categorically true that God never gives people more than they can handle, then God has not given Ciaran more than Ciaran can handle. That is plainly false. Ciaran's seizures have attacked his mind, undermining his cognitive and reflective capacities. In trying to handle "what God has given him" Ciaran is in an absolute bind. The very part of him that handles or fails to handle things is precisely that part which is damaged. To say that Ciaran has not been given more than he can handle is to deny the destructive nature of his seizure disorder. Nei-ther Ciaran nor we have handled his suffering. We have simply preserved of ourselves what we could, and braced ourselves for the future.

When I encounter these theological approaches, I try to remember that the people I am talking with are more interested in offering comfort and support than in theological analysis. And I realize that no one knows what to say. Though I would like to be comforted and supported, it is far more important to me that Ciaran's suffering be acknowledged. I long for a theological response to Ciaran's suffering, but above comfort, I long for truth.

The first section of this essay established Ciaran's suffering as a fact. Given the reflections of this section I now go further. Any responsible theological response to Ciaran begins from an even harsher truth: Ciaran suffers meaninglessly. In my own spiritual journey, I have found such an intellectually responsible theological response by reflecting on the work of Paul Tillich.

Tillich I: " . . . when God has disappeared . . . "

Paul Tillich was a mid-twentieth-century German Protestant theologian and philosopher who moved to the United States when the Nazis came to power in 1933. His work brought the insights of existentialist philosophers such as Jean-Paul Sartre to Christian theology. The end result of this work was a re-appropriation and renewed understanding of many of the central concepts and doctrines of Christian thought.

Laying an extraordinarily abstract, but necessary, foundation for his theological insights into how we might confront suffering, Tillich writes that being is prior to nonbeing; being is a more fundamental concept than nonbeing. Though no single account of the meaning of "being" in Tillich's work could be exhaustive, etymology suggests something like, "that which exists" or, as he puts it, "the ground of everything that is" (1952, p. 34). However exact is the definition of "being," "non-being" is simply its negation. "Nonbeing" has no meaning outside the meaning of "being".

Contrary to Tillich, one might think that being and nonbeing are non-overlapping categories in that whatever comprises being (whatever exists) does not comprise nonbeing and that whatever comprises nonbeing (whatever doesn't exist) does not comprise being. Tillich thinks this line of reasoning mistaken in its implication that without being there is only nonbeing. Instead, Tillich points out, without being, nonbeing cannot "be." Without being there is—to speak loosely—nothing for nonbeing to negate. In different language, without something, there is not even nothing. As Tillich puts it, "nonbeing belongs to being, it cannot be separated from it" (1952, p. 179). Being "embraces" nonbeing; being has nonbeing "within" it (1952, p. 34). Though abstract, and expressible only in metaphor and paradox, the basic point I hope is clear enough: nonbeing depends on being.

Given this dependency, "no actual negation can be without an implicit affirmation" (1952, p. 176). For example, the sentence, "there is no hope" is a negation that makes sense only within an implied affirmation of hope. There must, in some sense, be a persistence of hope in order to feel any significance in a denial of hope. More generally, to negate something is precisely that: to negate *something*. The presence of this *something* in the nega-tion demonstrates that negation and negativity are experienced only on the grounds of a persistent, if only implied, affirmation and positivity. For every negation or negative experience, one can ask what affirmation or positive experience persists in that it is being negated.

In this way, nonbeing "opens up" being, offers a "window" into being (1952, p. 178). The contemplation or experience of nonbeing, by setting us already within the contemplation or experience of being, creates a point of access to being. In the experience of nonbeing there is always the possibility that one can move through nonbeing toward an experience of the being that lies behind it. Being is so overwhelming that we finite creatures cannot approach or contemplate it directly; nonbeing is our finite point of access. We need a ground upon which to gaze at being, itself. By way of analogy, the sun is too bright for our eyes to see; but very dark lenses, in themselves excluding light, can allow us to see the sun.

Moving toward application, Tillich's definition of "anxiety" is "the state in which a being is aware of its possible nonbeing" (1952, p. 35). In what he calls "shorter form," "anxiety is the existential awareness of nonbeing." Put maybe too loosely, there is nonbeing enclosed within human being. When we experience the nonbeing that is contained within our being, the resulting feeling is anxiety.

Tillich describes three directions from which nonbeing threatens all human beings, and three corresponding anxieties: death, condemnation, and meaninglessness. Anxiety about death is "the most basic, universal, and inescapable" (1952, p. 42). All humans die; to live a human life is to know, and be uneasy about the fact that, one will someday no longer be alive. In other words, anxiety about death threatens our being directly in that it threatens our basic self-affirmation (the simple declaration that "I am"). Our very ability to say "I am" (an expression of being) is threat-ened in the recognition that it will one day be true that "I am not" (an expression of nonbeing). The second anxiety, the anxiety of condemnation and guilt, threatens a particular form of self-affirmation, specifically moral self-affirmation ("I am good"). To live a human life is to be faced with morally ambiguous situations in which we are anxious that we have behaved immorally. Facing such situations, I myself ultimately am not only the accused but also the accuser, the jury that decides that case, and the judge who deter-mines the rules of evidence. Any moral authority over me gains its power precisely in that I have endowed it with authority. Thus, in feeling the anxiety of condemnation, we are anxious that "I am good" (an expression of being) ought to be replaced with "I am not good" (an expression of nonbeing). The third anxiety, the anxiety of meaninglessness, threatens human beings' spiritual self-affirmation ("I matter"). To live a human life, especially in our times, is to feel the loss, or possible loss, of an ultimate source of meaning, the loss of a "spiritual center" (1952, p. 47). The institutions and doctrines that have traditionally provided an ultimate source of meaning waver, and our current culture is unable and unwilling to replace them. In feeling the anxiety of meaninglessness, we are anxious that "my life has meaning" (being) might be replaced with "my life has no meaning" (nonbeing). To sum up, human existence or human being asserts itself by saying, "I exist in a good and meaningful way." That human existence, that human *being*, contains within it, the threat of nonbeing that we feel as anxiety about death, condemnation, and meaninglessness.

Tillich describes these anxieties as "existential" in that they are part of our existence; we cannot live without experiencing them. Therefore, no genuinely satisfying theology can grow in the wake of their denial. Yet, much mainstream religion attempts to avoid these existential anxieties by denying that nonbeing necessarily threatens us from these directions. Such theology places comfort above truth; the attempted evasion of nonbeing comes at the cost of embracing falsehood. Worse, such avoidance fails. After all, these anxieties are existential; they are bound up in our existence and cannot ultimately be evaded. Theologies built upon denying the threefold threat of nonbeing (death, condemnation, meaninglessness) are not believable. Even the people who advance such theologies know, in their lived experiences, that they are not true. Clearly indicating that Tillich is a bold and radical Christian theologian, much of what is considered central Christian doctrine amounts to denying the threefold anxiety.

People try to escape the anxiety of death by asserting the soul is immortal. Instead of seeing the doctrine of the immortality of the soul as indispensable to Christian faith, Tillich sees it as a misguided and futile attempt to escape the fact that we are all aware of existentially. "For existentially everybody is aware of the complete loss of self which biological extinction implies" (1952, p. 42). In short, Tillich maintains that everyone knows—not intellectually but in their lived experience—that the soul is not immortal. People try to escape the anxiety of condemnation with dogmatic adherence to a rigid moral code. Instead of advocating a strict religious morality, Tillich sees such rigid moralities as springing from the misguided and futile attempt to eliminate the moral ambiguity that is inherent in human existence. The attempt is futile because people still feel the anxiety of advancing a morality that has no more objective basis than anyone else's. People try to escape the anxiety of meaninglessness by holding that everything is part of a pre-conceived divine plan. Instead of seeing the hand of God in all that occurs, Tillich claims that such beliefs arise from the misguided and futile attempt to find objective and pre-ordained purpose and meaning in life. The attempt is futile because, whatever intellectual machinations they advance, in the recesses of their souls people experience the inherent meaningless of life.

In asserting these existential anxieties, Tillich offers an analysis essentially the same as atheistic existentialists such as Jean-Paul Sartre. The fundamental human affect is anxiety; we are thrown into the world without guide or purpose and forced to choose what we will do and be. The atheistic existentialists, however, are content to proclaim the death of God, point out the intrinsic meaninglessness of the world, and leave it at that. Building on his account of the relationship between being and nonbeing, Tillich seeks the implicit affirmation lurking behind the explicit negations offered by an honest confrontation with anxiety. The move is inherently paradoxical. It is as if Tillich says, "given that God is dead, let us go in search of the living God."

TILLICH II: " . . . THE GOD WHO APPEARS . . . "

If we embrace our anxieties, instead of running away from them, we can ask whether there is courage to be, in spite of the anxiety. Tillich's intellectual hero is Martin Luther, the sixteenth-century leader of the Protestant Reformation against the abusive Christian hegemony of the Roman Catholic Church. A central concept for Luther, as for Tillich's response to the three-fold anxiety, is *trotz* ("in spite of"): Do not deny mortality, but ask what of a person's essence persists *in spite of* the fact of death. Do not deny moral unacceptability, but ask what acceptance persists *in spite of* condemnation. Do not deny the intrinsic meaninglessness of the world, but ask what meanings can be constructed *in spite of* it.

The best way to understand Tillich's theology is to begin with more familiar Lutheran reflections on guilt and condemnation. Much conventional theology of Luther's day amounted to denying one's unacceptability in the eyes of God. Wealthy patrons gave enormous sums to the church in order to gain some feeling of assurance that, in the eyes of God, it was as though their sins had never occurred. Luther found such purchased comfort to be implausible and misguided: no one can buy sinlessness from God and no human is worthy of God's presence. The question, as Luther saw it, was not how to become worthy of God's acceptance but to ask whether there can be acceptance by God *in spite of* our unacceptability. Luther offered an affirmative answer. The courage to morally self-affirm *in spite of* our guilt and worthiness of condemnation is found, to quote Tillich's account of the Lutheran approach, in "accepting acceptance in spite of being unacceptable" (1952, p. 166). Such acceptance is made possible by a personalized vision of God. By establishing and nurturing a direct and personal relationship with God, one is able to experience His infinite forgiveness. By embracing the leading anxiety of the age Luther developed a theology that spoke to the spiritual needs of the day while reinterpreting the very nature of God.

According to Tillich, however, the specific content of Lutheran theology no longer seems believable or speaks to current spiritual needs. Just as Martin Luther's theology embraced the anxiety of condemnation that dominated his age, Tillich's approach embraces the anxiety of meaninglessness that dominates our age. Though it leads to theological conclusions that Luther would not have accepted, Tillich calls on us to confront this newly emergent direction of the threat of nonbeing and to embrace it. Thus, just as Luther taught to accept acceptance in spite of being unacceptable, Tillich seeks to forge a theology that finds meaning in the acceptance that our lives are inherently meaningless.

Like Luther, Tillich's beginning leads ultimately to a re-conception of God. Referring to the "God of theism," Tillich describes the traditional

Protestant conception: "the personalistic image of God, the word as the tool of creation and revelation ...the idea of a divine purpose, the infinite distance between creator and creature" (1952, p. 183). Referencing Nietzsche's declaration that God is dead, Tillich says that the contemporary anxieties of doubt and meaninglessness can only be taken on if the God of theism is transcended. In one sense, this is an atheistic move on Tillich's part: the traditional conception of God is no longer believable or spiritually effective (which is what Nietzsche meant when declaring God dead). However, recognizing that every explicit negation implies an affirmation, Tillich is in a position to ask about the positive conception of God implied by the death of the God of theism.

As Tillich sees it, embracing the anxiety and meaninglessness makes it possible to see that the traditional conception of God is a symbol. The loss of power in this traditional symbol allows us to ask, more clearly than ever before, about the literally true conception of God that has existed all along behind the symbol of God as person, conscious will, and creator. When the symbol is swept aside, the symbolized comes into view. So, in a deeper sense, it is entirely mistaken to say that Tillich's move is an atheistic one. The ultimate conclusion of Tillich's rejection of the traditional conception of God is the emergence of a deeper and more genuine conception of God, a conception that was the true and living force behind the traditional conception all along. Tillich refers to this as "the God above God" (1952, p. 186) or, alternatively, the "God beyond God" (1952, p. 188) or, alternatively again, "the God who transcends the God of the religions" (1952, p. 188). He says precious little about the precise nature of the God above God, except suggesting that He is not to be thought of as "a being beside others"; he critiques the traditional conception of God that "He is a being, not being-itself" (1952, p. 184). The God beyond God is being itself.

The implications of this reinterpretation of God's nature are dramatic. Recall that nonbeing, contained within being, opens a window into being; and that the existential anxieties of meaninglessness, death, and condemnation indicate a direction from which nonbeing threatens human beings. So, embracing existential anxieties opens a window into being, and thus into the true nature of God. As I described earlier, much contemporary theology seeks God by avoiding existential anxieties by using a belief in the immortality of the soul, adhering to rigid morality, and asserting that everything is planned by an all knowing and loving God. If Tillich is right, such avoidance is precisely counterproductive: it blocks access to that which is sought. The true point of access to God, the way to grasp the true nature of the divine, is to embrace existential anxieties, making it possible to encounter the living God standing behind dying symbols. As Tillich put it in the famous last sentence of his book, *The Courage to Be*, "*the courage to be is rooted in the God who appears when God has disappeared in the anxiety of doubt*" (1952, p. 190, emphasis in original).

Tillich thus offers a strategy for encountering difficulty in life: Embrace hard truths, refuse simple comforts, and look for the theological and spiritual opportunities that thereby become available. Having acknowledged the fact of Ciaran's suffering, and having refused the easy comforts of simplistic theology, it is time to ask whether spiritual redemptions thereby arise.

CIARAN II: "THE COURAGE TO BE IS ROOTED IN ..."

Ciaran suffers for no reason. Valuing truth above comfort, and believing that no genuine spiritual insight comes by avoiding anxiety, I will deny neither Ciaran's suffering and isolation, nor the meaninglessness of it. I will not embrace a theology that offers comfort at the expense of truth. Instead, I take my lead from Paul Tillich. I ask whether joy exists *in spite of* suffering. I ask whether relationships flourish *in spite of* isolation. I ask whether meaning emerges *in spite of* the pointlessness of his agony. In short, I ask whether Ciaran's life, honestly confronted as it is lived by him, is a life worth living.

Authentic affirmative answers to these questions do not and cannot come easily. Easy answers to hard questions are almost always false. Nevertheless, I find that genuine affirmative answers do come.

There is joy *in spite of* Ciaran's suffering. It would be easy to point out that Ciaran experiences some amount of pleasure. There are things he does because he finds them fun, and there are outward displays of that pleasure. He likes to play with his toys, tapping them on various surfaces; he likes to throw things; he likes to move around and explore his environment. Occasionally, though rarely, he will squeal in delight during these activities. However, his pleasures do not outweigh his pains. If, as some philosophers have maintained, what matters in life is the balance of pain and pleasure, his pleasures are far from adequate for justifying his pain. But none of this is to the point.

To understand what importantly persists in spite of Ciaran's suffering, it is necessary to distinguish joy from pleasure. Pleasure is fleeting, bodily, and rather easy to attain. It is the feeling of "having fun"; pain is its opposite. In fact, as opposites, pain and pleasure are closely conjoined. Pain interrupts the pleasure of an experience. And many pleasurable experiences, such as drinking alcohol, lead directly to pain when overindulged. It is also characteristic of pleasure (and pain) that it produces nothing; when the pleasure ends nothing persists, except perhaps a strengthened desire for pleasure. Not coincidentally, pleasure, though not inherently immoral, does not imply virtue or goodness.

Contrary to pleasure, joy is more difficult both to grasp and to experience. Joy might be defined as basking in the glory of being. Perhaps a better definition is that joy is the lived experience of loving the world. Unlike the fleeting nature of pleasure, the experience of joy helps to sustain itself in the soul. Unlike the unproductivity of pleasure, joyful experiences have enduring significance. We may look fondly back on our moments of great pleasure, but we only vaguely remember the feeling of them. Recollections of our most joyful moments, however, transport us back to the feeling, the value, and the majesty of the moment. As joy inherently involves meaningful and valuable engagement with the world, joy is inherently good and virtuous. Though it can be hard to feel joy during painful experiences, joy is compatible with suffering. In fact, when both joy and pain are present, the presence of joy diminishes the existential importance of pain in a way that pleasure cannot. In itself, the persistent and profound suffering that marks Ciaran's life is intolerable to the human spirit. A little bit of interspersed pleasure does nothing to change that. But joy does. Where there is joy in spite of suffering, suffering can be tolerated because it is, at least, suffering endured in a magnificent world.

Ciaran is joyful. He has not been made timid or withdrawn by his suffering. His curiosity about his environment is unquenchable. He relentlessly seeks new corners of the world to explore. Though I cannot get inside his head, every outward sign indicates that he has a deep and persistent love of the world. One day, when Ciaran was about a year and a half, we rushed him to the emergency room seizing, not breathing. To prevent severe brain damage from a lack of oxygen, a breathing tube was inserted into his trachea and he was placed on a ventilator. After the seizure stopped, he was transferred to the pediatric intensive care unit (PICU), standard practice for a patient on a ventilator. An hour and a half later he had removed the breathing tube himself and was breathing on his own. Soon, he was sitting up and showing signs of being hungry. Just an hour more and he was rocking so hard in a high chair that the chair was moving toward the medical equipment that he wished to investigate. When his food came, he gleefully smeared macaroni and cheese on the glass doors of the PICU and was promptly discharged. As far as I know, he is still the only patient admitted to the PICU on a ventilator and discharged home on the same day. Though that is just one story, it is typical of the hunger that Ciaran has for life. *In spite of* his suffering, Ciaran loves being in this world and finds it endlessly fascinating. And that is enough.

There is relationship *in spite of* Ciaran's isolation. It would be easy to point out that there are people who love Ciaran and that he returns their affection. It is worthwhile, but easy, to point out that I have never known anyone who gives himself over so totally to being held. Sometimes, as I hold him, he relaxes so completely that he seems to have been poured into my arms. As wonderful as that is, it is not really to the point.

All people, especially those in despair, long to be held. Richness in human living involves more than receiving affection; one must also reach actively into the lives of others, opening a reciprocal connection and a mutual exchange. Ciaran has precious few such relationships, but they are all the more precious for being so few. Though he sees my mother only a few times a year, when they are together Ciaran gravitates to her and she becomes the center of his attention. His teacher, Beth, was able to learn things from Ciaran that allowed her to better serve her class of severely disabled students. She created an environment that led to freer and more natural interactions between the children. Ciaran, in turn, enjoys going to school and always delights in seeing

Beth. In writing, I cannot prove that these are genuinely reciprocal relationships; but if you could see Ciaran's eyes when he is with these people, you would understand why I believe that they are.

Perhaps Ciaran's capacity for reciprocal relation is most directly shown by the different ways he responds to two different, and both wonderful, home care nurses. His former nurse, Dana, was energetic and Ciaran responded to her presence with energy. His current nurse, Candace, is more reserved and Ciaran responds to her with a gentler quietude. Ciaran responds differently to these two loved ones because they are different themselves; such variation is most naturally described as reciprocation and sincere interaction. Naturally, my wife and I have the most special relationships with him. He smiles when he sees us after an absence; he likes, for whatever reason, to sit on our heads when we try to sleep in later than he does. He is more affectionate when we are openly sad; he is more energetic when we are openly excited. He does not understand the causes of our emotions, but he is able to understand their nature well enough to respond appropriately. My own relationship with him is one that I understand less than any other relationship that I have. I know only that there is something going on in Ciaran's mind, that he seeks out connection with me, and that our relationship is important to him not only logistically but also emotionally. But I also know that it is a relationship without pretense, hidden motivations, or empty politeness. Ciaran's relationships are unusual, perhaps irrevocably mysterious to those involved in them. They are also caregiver, not peer, based. But they are important, both to Ciaran and to those with whom he relates. *In spite of* the isolation caused by the uniqueness of his life and his lack of language, Ciaran loves and is loved in reciprocal interaction. And that is enough.

Though it may seem paradoxical, there is meaning from Ciaran's suffering *in spite of* the meaninglessness of Ciaran's suffering. As a result, Ciaran's life is worth living, though that worth is found only in the works and actions of others. Usually, the worth of a life is a function of the works and actions of that life. Has the person served the needs of others? Has the person expanded human culture with artistic, scientific, or philosophical accomplishments? Has the person achieved virtuosity in some inherently worthwhile activity like running, carpentry, or brewing beer? Has the person manifested self-control, embodying virtues such as courage, moderation, and justice? Is the person a true and ennobling friend? A life generally has value, meaning and worth because affirmative answers can be given to some or many of the preceding questions. Though I suppose it unpopular to point out these days, mere life is not of value; actions and accomplishments make life valuable. Those who attain excellence have what the ancient Greeks called *eudaimonia*, misleadingly translated as "happiness" and meaning something much more like "the objectively best human life." The Greeks knew, though we have largely forgotten, that merely to live is not worthwhile; to live *eudaimonistically* is worthwhile.

For Ciaran, *eudaimonia* is unattainable. Ciaran has not, cannot, serve others or learn to brew exceptionally good beer. He is absolutely not a model of self-control. Yet, because of Ciaran and through Ciaran, many others do move toward *eudaimonia*. Ciaran's younger brother, Teagin, is the most certain example. Jessica and I have always told Teagin that caring for Ciaran will never be his responsibility; Teagin's life need not be shaped by Ciaran's care in the way that ours has been. Nevertheless, Teagin plausibly imagines a future in which Jessica and I are physically unable to meet Ciaran's needs. When that day comes, Teagin believes that Ciaran will need him. Teagin intends to be ready. That is heavy stuff for a 10-year old to contemplate, but it is just one way in which Teagin is more compassionate and mature for being Ciaran's brother.

More generally, though Ciaran does not serve the needs of others, he has needs that others serve. A similar structure applies for some of the other questions relevant to the worth of a life. Ciaran has produced no science, but science has been produced through and for him. Ciaran is not courageous, as he lacks the foresight and reflective skills to see danger approach and willingly and wisely face it. But Ciaran has inspired courage in others through the tenacity with which he faces life. Ciaran is not truly anyone's friend, as he lacks the cognitive and linguistic skills to genuinely share activity and to build collaborative purpose; besides, friendship is, by definition, a relation between peers and Ciaran is generally uninterested in his peers. But many friends have genuinely shared the activities of Ciaran's care and collaboratively sought to build purpose for Ciaran. *In spite of* the fact that Ciaran is not a bearer of *eudaimonia*, he is a conduit of *eudaimonia*. And that, too, is enough.

Conclusion

I love Ciaran. It breaks my heart to watch him endure so much pain. I am sincerely grateful to the loving family and friends who have tried to offer me comfort. Without diminishing my gratitude, I admit that I have generally not found comfort in what they have said. We are all lost in the experience of suffering, but we should not seek easy answers. Ciaran offers only a strikingly extreme example of the nonbeing that threatens us all as human beings. Understanding the sufferings that inevitably mark human life is a far more difficult theological task than people want to accept, one in which adherence to doctrine is less important than authentic acknowledgement of the lived suffering of human life. Tillich's framework is a profound tool for all who wish to share in his courage to acknowledge the deep causes of suffering found in each human life. But it doesn't offer the comfort of emotional reconciliation. Nor should we seek emotional reconciliation with suffering; I will never find it acceptable that Ciaran suffers so deeply. Tillich's theology provides the comfort that comes from realizing that my grief over what Ciaran has suffered and lost, and your grief over what has been suffered and lost in your life, is the beginning of truly seeing the meaning and value in what remains. Using Tillich's framework, we can build the courage to truly grieve and, yet, to know that we are blessed to live lives rich enough with love and meaning that there might be something to grieve about. Being Ciaran's father is a joy.

By genuinely confronting his suffering, I have refused the comforts of simplistic theology. In refusing, I have come closer, far closer, to "the God who appears when God has disappeared in the anxiety of doubt."

REFERENCE

Tillich, P. (1952). *The courage to be*. New Haven, CT: Yale UP.

CHAPTER 14

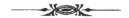

SPIRITUALITY, CHRONIC ILLNESS, AND HEALING: CONCLUDING REMARKS AND ONGOING INQUIRY

Michael J. Stoltzfus and Rebecca Green

A collection of chapters like this one is difficult to tie up in a neat little bundle that answers a question, recommends a solution, solves a problem, or presents a specific piece of evidence for application to practice. Many of us in the practice disciplines are left dissatisfied if we feel like we have not made some sort of positive measurable progress along a linear path of inquiry. But those of us from the less quantitative disciplines are sometimes over-satisfied with ambiguity, assuming that there is no such thing as quantifiable progress. For people who live with chronic illness in the real world, the reality usually lies somewhere in the middle. People who live with chronic illness every day have to address all of it, the objective measures of disease they face in blood glucose, c-reactive protein, tumor necrosis factor, white blood cells, CT scans, and liver enzymes; the subjective experiences of pain, fatigue, loss, love, fear, and grief; and those real parts of life that include both … bank account balances, insurance coverage, parenthood, marriage, and employment. Those of us who dwell on scholarly, academic, and practical disciplines owe it to those people and to ourselves to not only meet in the middle ground but also move more freely in general among worlds, or rather, within the greater world where we dwell together. It is perhaps this idea of meeting in the middle, or dwelling together in the world or *blending*, that is the greatest overarching theme of this collection, the theme that we feel is most important. Despite the fact that the contributors come from many divergent backgrounds, disciplines, religions, cultures, and methods, all have in common a desire to understand what it means to live with chronic illness; and despite the diversity of approach, there are common themes threaded throughout the accounts; and a new, enhanced understanding that can be operationalized into specific recommendations for future inquiry.

For the chronically ill, disease is often an intrinsic element of being alive, a permanent feature of living where people must learn to integrate their illness constructively into their sense of personal, social, medical, vocational, and spiritual self-identity. The nature of such a challenge requires a personal and relational response that may be quite different from the acute care model of disease where isolated individuals seek diagnosis, treatment, and cure. A helpful distinction, utilized by contributors throughout this volume, can be drawn between disease talk and illness talk. Disease talk, which is what one hears from many health-care professionals, tends to reduce the body and mind to a physiology that is measured and organized. Illness, by contrast, is the experience of living with the disease. Facing an ongoing illness that highlights the fragility of the human experience can provide a connection to the exploration of spirituality and healing. Indeed, spirituality and healing are about how people face the paradox of illness and wellness, tragedy and triumph, despair and hope, pain and joy, religion and culture that are always shifting and changing. The perpetual inner and relational adaptation to this dynamic paradox is described in this book by a variety of spiritual terms like awareness, grace, balance, or mindfulness and is addressed by a multitude of spiritual healing practices like chanting, meditation, prayer, yoga, and a host of distinctive embodied rituals.

Multiple authors from diverse contexts and perspectives have suggested how chronically ill people may begin to approach their experience as newly authentic when they stop assuming that fixing their diseased body is necessary to accepting it or even loving it. Encounters with ongoing illness not only evoke the deepest and most complex of emotions including fear, anxiety, humiliation, and alienation, but also open the door to new awareness and healing. As people move from experiencing themselves as passive victims of disease or viewing disease as an enemy to be eradicated to experiencing themselves as active creators of meaning and purpose, they may entertain new thoughts, feelings, and relational dynamics. We hope we have provided a vision in which health care providers can facilitate this meaning-making through new ways of viewing themselves, their patients, and even illness.

Chronic illness, spirituality and healing involve an ongoing journey where there is no final arrival, no instrumental purpose to be pursued, attained, and completed. Central questions involved in the spiritual healing journey include: How do people, families and communities live well, learn from, and discover meaning in the midst of living with the uncertainty and vulnerability associated with chronic illness experience? What does physical, mental, spiritual, and relational healing mean when cure is unlikely? Healing goes far beyond individual physical cure or psycho-physical health. A chronic condition requires perpetual balance actively constructed by the person moment to moment, day to day. This kind of balance or healing involves a transformation of the whole person in all of their social, cultural, spiritual, personal, economic, and medical contexts. Healing cannot be reduced to or associated exclusively with only one of these contexts. Rather, balance is created in the midst of the very multidimensional complexity of personal and social dilemmas. Healing places an emphasis on becoming whole in mind, body, spirit and relational dynamics with a deliberate focus on integration and acceptance within the limitations of any given disease or circumstance.

Throughout the book there is recognition and discussion of the unique meanings spirituality, chronic illness, and healing have for each person and the inability of biomedical or religious models to capture these shifting horizons of meaning into an abstract or objective category. This dynamic not only presents ongoing problems for people living with chronic illnesses but also offers creative opportunities for insight and awareness. For example, individuals with chronic illness have first-hand exposure to the limitations and sometimes narrow views of conventional medicine, conventional religion, and conventional cultural responses to disease; many are looking for alternative ways to gain understanding about their illness and incorporate spiritual insight, practice, and self-understanding to help achieve healing. Healing, then, is a dynamic process, not a fixed state that can be achieved and maintained. Spirituality, too, is not a static event associated with objective meaning, but rather an active process associated with emergent meaning. As such, blending spirituality, chronic illness, and healing engenders an emphasis on ongoing creative transformation as people, families, communities, and health-care providers and institutions respond to evolving circumstances.

Viewing dynamic situations and relational dynamics as opportunities for learning rather than as barriers are presented as important components to healing in many of the spiritual traditions and practices presented in this book. Dwelling on the present moment and acceptance of things as they are rather than how we would like them to be may be seen as important complements to the more instrumental purposes of biomedical treatment which tend to focus on desired outcomes. Multiple authors stress the importance of diverse ritual-making activities due to the unique ability of rituals to bring the mind and body together in full attention to the present moment through the embodied integration of thought and action. In addition, diverse ritual expressions like chanting, meditation, prayer, yoga, sutra-copying, or visualized healing imagery often are rooted in the process of embodied spiritual practice rather that striving for some future goal. Likewise, reflective practice can facilitate a personal transformation of the health-care provider, so that he or she is able to imagine better ways of responding to patients with chronic illness and not reducing clinical encounters to lab results or some other measurable objective outcome.

Multiple contributors from diverse disciplinary and cultural contexts stressed the importance of cultivating a non-dualistic experience of reality where health and illness are not viewed as adversarial but experienced as relational components of a broader whole, which requires ongoing balance, resiliency, and response. Balance and resiliency tend to be detached from a desire for certain results due to the complex nature of spirituality in the context of chronic illness. Indeed, it is critical for people with chronic illness to not allow their spiritual resilience and ongoing quest for balance to be limited by a desire for specific health outcomes as this might lead to loss of hope when disease symptoms persist.

Viewing illness, vulnerability, and lament as normal parts of individual and collective life and as opportunities for spiritual cultivation and healing are vitally important in the context of chronic illness experience. People with chronic illnesses can teach other people, health-care providers, and religious traditions how to integrate pain and uncertainty into an expanded view of spirituality and healing; an understanding not rooted in isolated control or future cure. The existential condition of vulnerability, pain, and fear often prompts resignation or alienation, yet it also presents opportunities for resolve and transformation. Health-care providers and systems must create new ways in which they can facilitate such resolve and transformation; rather than resignation or alienation both in themselves and among patients with chronic illness.

A powerful temptation, long recognized by diverse spiritual traditions and addressed by multiple contributors in this volume, is to only find life meaningful when one is pain free, safe, healthy, self-sufficient, or "normal." The temptation is fed by the illusion that it is possible to somehow free oneself from disease and pain, and is reinforced by the way our society views health as good or ideal and illness and bad or abnormal. The perpetual uncertainty affiliated with chronic illness experience may help people to overcome this temptation by recognizing the limits of measuring healing in terms of self-sufficiency or specific health outcomes and the abundance of discovering healing in terms of relational dependency and care. This type of healing is centered on the realization that tomorrow may or may not bring new medical treatment but that healing is available nonetheless through concrete acts of loving-kindness available in the present moment.

Spiritual traditions as a whole tend to embrace frailty and vulnerability as inevitable elements of the human condition while viewing suffering and healing as arising, in part, from the conditioned ideas or emotions that individuals attach to particular experiences of pain or disease. For example, when the chronically ill become attached to the idea of individual cure, these individuals may find such attachment increases their sense of suffering while doing little to increase their sense of healing. For people thus attached, the biomedical focus on cure that they encounter in clinical settings may further alienate them from potential spiritual healing.

There is a practical necessity for health-care professionals to habitually consider what is "normal" and to think of pain and disease as deviation of normal. Health-care providers utilize a body of expert knowledge to know exactly what clinical signs and symptoms are significant heralds of disease, and what lab values indicate an aberrant response in what they perceive should be a normal body. Interventions are aimed at returning the body to as close to the norm as possible. Success is determined by how close to normal the patient comes. This way of viewing patients and illness is a prime example of how expert knowledge creates a clinical cage in which professionals exist. Health-care providers sometimes become so limited by their field's narrow categories that they may have trouble conceptualizing ways in which "not normal" might even be acceptable, much less preferable to "normal." Unfortunately, all too often health-care providers ensnare patients with chronic illness in this cage with them, and rather than empowering patients for healing and possibility, clinical encounters tend to foster patients defining themselves in terms of abnormality or not meeting optimal outcomes. Providers need to begin to think of ways in which they can not only free patients from disease processes, but also free themselves and the patients from narrow understandings and approaches to health, well-being, and healing.

The inexplicable but culturally understood causes of illness create the need for contextual understanding and interpretation of health conditions in order to achieve the best possible outcomes. There is no longer a single method for interpreting and relating to illness. There are now many complex biomedical treatments and technologies, as well as the need for the integration of cultural perception and understanding of health and illness. The many diverse religious traditions, cultural contexts, illness narratives, disciplinary perspectives, spiritual practices, and experiences of healing presented in this book help to broaden the conversation, and, in doing so, loosen the conventional categories and expand perspectives of care and approaches to healing.

Spiritual awareness and practice seek to discover a means of maintaining grace, balance, or mindfulness in the midst of joy and pain, suffering and healing, as human life is sure to involve the full gamut of these experiences. In this context, the human community as a whole might be viewed as a chronically ill community where spirituality and healing are present in the midst of vulnerability, dependency, and the relational comfort and care that may result. In this context, providers and the health-care establishment are as much in need of ongoing healing as are sick people and populations.

The common themes threaded throughout the contributors' essays and narratives resulted in an enhanced understanding of chronic illness from those themes reflected in the original call, and also provide a blueprint and specific direction for future inquiry. As a result of this work, we have identified and recommend further inquiry into the following themes.

• The critical nature of human relationship as a facilitative medium of holistic well-being for those who live with chronic illness. Specifically, we recommend scholarly inquiry into the relationship between provider and patient as healing medium itself, or as treatment itself, not just as an avenue for treatment or therapy. Additionally, the exploration of the therapeutic mutuality of the provider/patient relationship should be explored: For example, how does the patient help the provider become a better practitioner? How can the patient be empowered to become a healer of self and others?

- *Blending* (rather than *augmenting*) biomedical care with care practices from other spiritual, religious, and cultural traditions and disciplinary perspectives. Repeatedly we recognized in the contributions the theme that those who experience chronic illness incorporate biomedical care as just one element of a multidimensional life experience of illness. Those of us who practice in a specific disciplinary area and care for these patients must become adept at helping them incorporate elements of care into their lives, rather than the other way around. In order for this to occur, richer dialogue and more meaningful, intentional interactions must occur between and among disciplines; and in environments where patients go about their everyday lives.
- The role of individual reflective insight in understanding medical, spiritual, religious, and cultural rituals and practices associated with wellness and illness. People who have chronic illness and providers of their care must begin to look beyond the accepted societal understandings and definitions of wellness and illness in order to create new, positive meanings and experiences. If educational institutions institute this type of reflective thought and practice among students of the health professions, it can have an enormous impact on the lives of the patients they will care for in the future.
- Components of healthcare practices that focus on the holistic wellbeing of people with chronic illness by creating positive meaning out of suffering and loss. For example, we recommend investigating specific practice interventions, for both provider and patient, that are designed to promote patient well-being even when objective indicators of illness may be present and even worsening.

These are just a few themes and related recommendations that we, the editors, were able to glean from the rich and varied accounts provided by our contributors. But the real value of a work like this is in its ability to create a different vision for each reader; to spark unique lines of inquiry that we have not seen or considered; to provide solace or an answer in a personal story that speaks clearly to you in a way that it does not to me. Our assessment is that this is just the beginning of many visions, inquiries, and stories that will add to a greater and evolving understanding of what it means to live with chronic illness.

INDEX

Note: Locators with letter 'n' refer to notes

CPSIA information can be obtained at www.ICGtesting.com
Printed in the USA
LVOW05*2104260914

406142LV00003B/29/P